PREFACE

I grew up at Mount Saint Joseph's Orphan Asylum, which evolved into a delinquent girl's home in the early 1970's. I was cooped up there until I was a legal adult. I have had an interesting, convoluted life which has taken me around the block, and then some. I've collected oodles of sordid stories and experiences.

As the years staggered by, I found myself writing small rants and various articles for offbeat publications, nothing remotely sexually oriented at all. Then BOOM! it hit me like a stiff dick in the face, I had found my true passion; giving relationship/sex advice. I, being blunt and outspoken, listened to all my friends constantly ask for my help in matters of the heart and bedroom. When they did not listen to my boisterous advice, they always wished they had...thus the idea for a column.

Mz. Conduct's House of Sin gathered fast and loyal fans from all around the world via the internet and local stripper magazine. My columns have been called humorous, informative, and brutally honest with just a pinch of moxie. So, after all these years and all the inquiries when there would be a book, voila! This is dedicated to all of you.

This is also dedicated to my amazing son, the tried and true attorney at law, Ben. I want to be just like him when I grow up. And to the love of my life, Patrick, who has painstakingly worked on this with me, thank you for enduring all my scandalous stories.

Mz. Conduct's House of Sin

Good Advice from a Very Bad Girl

Now is the winter of dis–contents!

"The best time for planning a book is while you're doing the dishes." 9

"Life's a rash, and there's death and the itching's over." 13

"The only way I would take up jogging is so that I could hear heavy breathing again." 18

"We're all in this alone." 22

"Enemies are so stimulating" 25

"If I don't drive around the block, I'm pretty sure to make my mark. If I'm in bed each night by ten, I may get back my looks again. If I abstain from fun and such, I'll probably amount to much. But I shall stay the way I am because I do not give a damn." 28

"Sex is never an emergency." 31

"Imagination is intelligence with an erection." 34

"If the world were a logical place, men would ride side-saddle." 37

"Sex is an emotion in motion." 41

"Sometimes being a bitch is all a woman has to hold on to." 44

"From the moment I was six I felt sexy. And let me tell you it was hell, sheer hell waiting to do something about it." 48

"Too much awareness, without the accompanying experience, is a skeleton without the flesh of life." 52

"Imperious, choleric, irascible, extreme in everything, with a dissolute imagination the like of which has never been seen, atheistic to the point of fanaticism, there you have me in a nutshell, and kill me again or take me as I am, for I shall not change." 55

"Do you really think it is weakness that yields to temptation? I tell you that there are terrible temptations that it requires strength, strength and courage, to yield to." 58

"I've and got hampers and hampers of ironing and my diet pill is wearing off!" 61

"You better run me up to that hotel room, cuz baby, you got me hotter than Georgia asphalt." 64

"I shot my mouth off and you showed me what that hole was for!" 70

"The only people for me are the mad ones, the ones who are mad to talk, mad to live, mad to be saved, desirous of everything at the same time, the ones who never yawn or say a commonplace thing, but burn, burn, burn like fabulous yellow roman candles." 73

"How could I become a destitute woman when I have all these treasures locked in my heart?" 77

So this guy walks into a bar. He looks around and sees no one. He sits at the bar and orders a drink. All of a sudden he hears a voice say "You're sure a good looking guy!" He turns around, but still sees no one. Puzzled, he sips his drink and again a voice says "You are such a sexy man!" This time he asks the bartender what the deal is, he's hearing voices yet no one is in the place. The bartender points to the bowl of peanuts on the bar and says "It's the peanuts". The guys says "What the hell are you talking about?" and the bartender says "They're complementary". 81

"What is most beautiful in virile men is something feminine; what is most beautiful in feminine women is something masculine." 84

"Take what you can use and let the rest go by." 87

"The older I grow, the less important the comma becomes. Let the reader catch his own breath." 90

"Did you ever feel like the world was a tuxedo and you were a pair of brown shoes?" 94

"We were once so close to Heaven/Peter came out and gave us medals/Declaring us 'The Nicest of the Damned.'". 97

Mz. Conduct's House of Sin

Amy: "The hell with it. I shall become a bitter, twisted hag with nothing but rouge and one-liners to disguise the emptiness of my existence, and I shall drown the memory of numerous loveless affairs in a tsunami of vodka." Tulip: "I think gin's more traditional." 100

"It's the way you love me down. Every time we kiss you bring out the woman in me. Every time you holler out my name you set me free. I am a sex-o-matic venus freak when I'm with you." 104

"Cunt" is not slang, dialect, or any marginal form, but a true language word, and of the oldest stock. It is a derivative of the Oriental Great Goddess known as Cunti, or Kunda, the Yoni of the Universe 108

"Is sex dirty? Only if it's done right." 111

"Life is a banquet and most poor suckers are starving to death." 114

"Maybe some women aren't meant to be tamed. Maybe they need to run free, until they find someone just as wild to run with." 118

"My God, I haven't been fucked like that since grade school." 121

"Happiness lies neither in vice nor in virtue; but in the manner we appreciate the one and the other, and the choice we make pursuant to our individual organization." 124

"The truth can't hurt you/it's just like the dark/It scares you witless/but in time you see things clear and stark." 128

"I took a deep breath and listened to the old brag of my heart. I am, I am, I am." 132

"Cherish forever what makes you unique, cuz you're really a yawn if it goes." 135

"Time wounds all heels." 138

"All really great lovers are articulate, and verbal seduction is the surest road to actual seduction." 140

"Do you dream of impossible things?" asked the fairy. "Never" replied the girl, "for I am filled with wonderful dreams of all the things that are possible." 143

"What do I have to rebel against? I don't know, what da ya got?" 147

"You can turn off the charm. I'm immune." 150

"You cumming is sexy, me going is sexier." 153

"With a rebel yell, she cried more, more, more." 157

"Baby, sometimes you just take me right over that rainbow." 161

"I know everybody here wants you. I know everybody here thinks they need you. I'll be waiting right here just to show you how our love will blow it all away." 165

"There's nothing wrong with having bags under your eyes as long as you have shoes to match." 169

"There's nothing to writing, all you do is sit down at a typewriter and open a vein." 172

"Moral indignation is jealousy with a halo." 175

"If you're truly wild at heart then you'll fight for your dreams. Don't turn away from love...don't ever turn away from love." 178

"We are going to go to europe, and swill french wine, yell with the greeks, barter with the italians, and lick the sunrise of the east...we will conquer the world, one martini at a time." 182

"A positive attitude may not solve all your problems, but it will annoy enough people to make it worth the effort." 186

"When women go wrong, men go right after them." 189

"Of all sexual aberrations, perhaps the most peculiar is chastity." 192

"You can't start it like a car, can't stop it with a gun." 196

"It is not enough to conquer; one must know how to seduce." 200

Good Advice from a Very Bad Girl

"Happiness lies neither in vice nor in virtue; but in the manner we appreciate the one and the other, and the choice we make pursuant to our individual organization." 205

"Life is clay, honey, and I have a Deluxe Play-Doh set!" 208

"Okay, I gotta be honest with you. I only listen to you about half of the time and the other half I just nod and smile and wait for your pants to come off." 212

"It was so cold I almost got married." 216

"Good judgment comes from experience, and often experience comes from bad judgment." 220

"Everything has cracks, that's how the light comes in." 224

"Art has treated erotic themes at almost all periods, because eroticism lies at the root of all human life." 228

"I never write in the daytime. It's like running through the shopping mall with your clothes off. Everybody can see you. At night...that's when you pull the tricks...magic." 232

"Dancing is the perpendicular expression of a horizontal desire." 236

"What really makes us is beyond grasping, way beyond knowing. We give in to love because it gives us a sense of what is unknowable. Nothing else matters. Not in the end." 240

"Never let a domestic quarrel ruin a day's writing. If you can't start the next day fresh, get rid of your wife." 243

"If you love something, let it go. If it comes back, great. If not, it's probably having dinner with someone more attractive than you." 248

"The proper behavior all through the holiday season is to be drunk. This drunkenness culminates on New Year's Eve, when you get so drunk you kiss the person you're married to." 252

"You live but once, you might as well be amusing." 256

"Penetrating so many secrets, we cease to believe in the unknowable. But there it sits, nevertheless, calmly licking its chops." 260

"Love is a fire, but whether it is going to warm your hearth or burn down your house, you can never tell." ...264

"Razors pain you; Rivers are damp. Acids stain you; And drugs cause cramp. Guns aren't lawful; Nooses give. Gas smells awful; You might as well live." 270

"A liberated woman is one who has sex before marriage and a job after." 274

"Life is rated X. It is not rated R." 278

"I may be the outlaw, darlin', but you're the one stealing my heart." 282

"It's best not to be too moral—you cheat yourself out of too much life." 286

"Generally, by the time you are Real, most of your hair has been loved off, and your eyes drop out and you get loose in the joints and very shabby. But these things don't matter at all, because once you are Real you can't be ugly, except to people who don't understand." 291

"I've come here to be drugged, electrocuted and probed, not insulted!" 295

"They sharpen their knives on my mistakes." 299

Just as she was about to speak, there was a knock on the door. It was Sister Kimi, the dessert nun. "I thought you'd all like some sweets," said the adorable nun, pushing a tray filled with mouth-watering cookies and cakes. Cherry noticed she was wearing a habit that came to well above her shapely knees.......................303

"The prettiest dresses are worn to be taken off." 307

"The piano has been drinking, not me, not me." 311

"Speak in French when you can't put together English, keep your toes out when you walk, and always remember just who you are." 316

"Elegance has a bad effect on my constitution." 320

Mz. Conduct's House of Sin

"He who asks a question is a fool for five minutes; he who does not ask a question remains a fool forever." .324

The bitch is back! My fiftieth birthday seemed to unravel a stream of airborne events that picked me up, carried me as high as the largest pines, and then sent me corkscrewing, head over heels, ass backwards into this wedded bliss. Yes, that's right, Mz. Conduct is married! Here is the story of how Mr. Conduct came to be…..328

Hey, Don't Look at Me That Way!

"The best time for planning a book is while you're doing the dishes."
–Agatha Christie

Some men have redeemed themselves this week, and some have dug themselves a brand new proverbial grave. An improper example: me wearing anal beads for an entire eight-hour workday only to have the date broken that evening...ugh! The ebb and flow of things can be exhausting and a girl can get a royal headache, but a nice, soothing shave and soak with a stiff martini should do the trick. Holy hatbox full of sex toys! I realize I'm running low on razors and gin! This is not a good thing. How can one continue to be a smoldering seductress when this happens? Well, I pride myself on being resourceful and I will find a way. Speaking of resourcefulness, here is a little summer beauty tip, I've found that in the hot weather, when your hair needs an extra bit of stay-there-damnit, and your crotch is all moisty slick, a little bit of snatch sweat makes for a great aromatic hair mousse. Oh, get over it!

My dear bosom buddy, The Lil' Princess and I went to one of our favorite dives this week. (Yes, I love a dive bar with character and stories. I relate, okay?) We sauntered into the dark, smoky, Chinese Karaoke bar, my latest boy and ex-boyfriend in tow. It's the bar with the spider-web-patterned ceiling and the always drunken, quarreling gay boys. There's more than one in every city, you just have to know where to find one. So, after many cocktails, and my boys making fun loving fools of themselves, struggling with Nirvana and Peter Gabriel tunes, the pseudo divas got on stage. The Lil' Princess was naughty and picked the hideous and tedious Donny Osmond song, "Puppy Love." I wanted to sing, "Diamonds are a Girl's Best Friend," but was talked out of it by my ex. He explained how incredibly long it was and once I got up there, I'd be sorry...and so would everyone else. He did have a point, as I couldn't carry a note if it was in a handbag from Saks. I pouted for an appropriate amount of time and finally decided to share the stage with the Lil' Princess. There I was, the place packed now with a motley crew of an audience, all eyes on the royal smut

Mz. Conduct's House of Sin

queens. The ridiculous music began to play and the goofy lyrics rolled. We were laughing so hard we almost peed our panties, if we had had any on. Gawd, we were a mess, but honey, we looked great! When our voices strained for the notes and our eyes for the words, and all else failed, we decided to just make out with each other. Big sloppy girl smooches right there on stage, and that's how we gathered our applause for the evening. We've already made plans to slink back some night and seduce that cutie-pie Karaoke boy who ran the show. He had a bird's-eye view of our ample behinds and we could feel him breathing hard behind us, and lordy lordy, with sideburns to die for. Oh, what Mz. Conduct will do for those manicured, Elvis sideburns, uh huh.

Dear Mz. Conduct,

I started reading the columns you posted and after reading them I'm still so confused. It seems like most of those people don't have very good self-images like I do. Everyone says I am pretty, cute and that I look like Britney Spears! Anyway, I guess your advice was okay and everything, but you seem so—well, blunt! Take me, for example. People always ask me questions about why I'm so happy all the time? Why I never worry about anything. I just tell them not to worry, that things will always get better. I never tell them why I'm so happy. (You'll see why pretty soon!) Anyway, now I am so confused!

A week ago, when I was being 'nice' to my employer (because he said his wife wouldn't do what I always did), guess what? He fired me the next day? I couldn't understand why. The rest of the guys where I work told me not to take it personally, because they all said I was way better than any of the other girls when I made them feel good. I thought that's what all the girls did? Why do you think he fired me? He said he heard me in the rest room stall with a couple of the guys and he wouldn't put up with that kind of thing in his company. Like, I was so shocked! I thought I was just being nice! The girls who worked with me just whispered and wouldn't look at me and giggled when I went to pick up my things.

Anyway, here is my question. I am going to an interview in a week. Do you think it's wrong for me to be that 'nice' to the man who is going to be interviewing me? And please don't make fun of me being blonde or anything. Please give me your best advice, but don't be too blunt, okay? Okay?

Jobless and Confused

> **Dear JC,**
>
> **First of all, I'll be as blunt as I goddamn want to be, Little-Miss-KY Jelly-for-brains. Second of all, Brittany silicone-on-a-stick Spears only looks good bent over with a bag on her head...at best. Why you hula-hoop around, deliriously happy to resemble her, is beyond me. Anyway, as I'm so fond of saying, there is nothing wrong with being a slutty little tuna melt as long as you're coiffed, clean, and lipstick is applied evenly. One more adjective I should add here: intelligent. At least smart enough to tell an uncut dog dick from a tube of lipstick, and frankly I don't think you could.**

Straddle as many fellow employers as you want, but if you're doing the boss too, then for crying in a freakin' bucket, use your flea brain for more insightful thoughts than, "Should I favor all men because, um, I'm alive?" Have some stinkin' dignity.

You can sue your boss for sexual harassment or try as you might to get a job without blowing anyone, however it may be all you've got. Please just shave your head and stop giving even us bleached blondes a bad name.

Dear Mz. Conduct,

How do you go about asking someone if they would like to join you in a threesome? If it's a couple pursuing a third party, should both members of the couple approach the person or only one? Hell, how do you decide how to pick a third person in the first place?

Three's Company

Dear TC,

The threesome selection task is not always easy, let me tell you! Not simple if you are selective. If you don't mind that the person doesn't have teeth, can't spell his/her own name correctly and smells of yesterday's lunch, then it'll be a breeze. Otherwise I'd suggest talking it all out with your partner first; what you want, what they would want, individual turn-ons, etc. It's fun to fantasize with a partner about inviting another in, and sometimes that can be enough. When you're out with your partner, do some people-watching. See how that curvy chick sidles her hips onto that barstool and imagine the positions you could all be in, with and without the barstool involved. The imagination is fabulous baby, and the positions are endless. Look at your waiter, yum, can he really be of age? This way, along with sprouting boners and/or wet panties, you can get an idea of you both want, if you did decide for sure to do this.

There is in fact a subculture of people who swing, or singles who are interested in getting together with a couple. Unless you search out a club that tends to cater to that subculture (and there are plenty of those around), you could put an ad in the personals, as it's a great way to weed out undesirables. Ask for correspondence via email and request recent photos. Get some information on the person, etc. You can go from there, meeting people, finding out if there is any chemistry and making an informed, intelligent decision. Be sure you have a stable relationship with your partner and set rules to respect and stick by. Be safe always, and have fun!

Dear Mz. Conduct,

I have a girlfriend who has three dogs. Two are pretty big and one is even unfixed. When he gets excited, his penis comes out and it's enormous. I've teased my girlfriend about not needing me around when she's got that dog, and we laugh about it.

Lately I've been thinking how it would turn me on to see her getting the bone from her big dog and I've even masturbated to that thought…a lot. I want to suggest this to her, but wonder what you thought about it?

Doggie Style

Dear DS,

This is what I think; I'm reporting you to the Humane Society as soon as I get through telling your girlfriend what a freak you are and that her poor poochies aren't safe around you!

Personally, I draw the line with poo play and animal sex. Hey, here's an idea, how about all three of your girlfriend's dogs hump you senseless after taking a

Mz. Conduct's House of Sin

big steamy poo on your face? Have your fantasies if you must, you sick boy, but keep this one to yourself! Here you go, you twisted nutcase, www.bestiality.com and Merry Freakin' Christmas!

Oh, I Just Knew I Had a Gee Spot!

"Life's a rash, and there's death and the itching's over."
—Cynthia Kraman

Oh, what a wacky few weeks it's been. I haven't seen the Lil' Princess, as she's whooping it up in Disneyland, probably feeling up Goofy as I write. The Transient Trollop, my oldest bosom buddy, called me from an undisclosed state (of mind), to tell me that she's now a redhead, and, by the way, marrying an uncircumcised migrant worker, or something like that. She did inform him that if I came to town, he would politely introduce himself and then be promptly dismissed. He readily agreed, so hey, he can't be all bad. Believe me, he wouldn't want to stick around after we've swilled several bottles of good wine (and a couple of cheap ones), and heard our never-ending "perils of the penis" stories.

So, other news, the Catholic, ultra conservative in-laws were in town, ordering deep-fried everything and looking down their large pored noses at my vegetable stir-fry or spinach salad entrees. As much as I wanted to say things like, "I'm trying my best to avoid looking like you," I kept silent, napkin in my lap like the good little evil-thinking girl that I am. While we drove around the city in their rental car pointing out sights, my mind kept screaming bad girl things. As we passed the green glass towers alongside the river park, I wanted to point and say, "Look, there's where I got my last abortion!" Instead, I just smiled, discreetly fingering my nipple rings, and pointed to the skyline or the new ship in the harbor.

My husband, at the time (a decade and a half younger than me), was whining that he couldn't keep up with me in bed anymore and that perhaps I was the one with a problem...and overactive libido. Ha! To appease him, he made an appointment with a couple of therapists (in training) the next week. I had PMS and was hankering for a cocktail, but there I sat trying my best to be open and honest and receptive. This is where that landed: one wannabe doctor of the brain sat clutching her notepad to her chest each time she spoke,

"Does sex fill a looonely spot inside you?"

She would draw out each breath, "Do you have a constant craaaving for sex?"

"Do you feel a compulsion, an obsession, an overwhelming need to have sex all the time?"

Holy hampers of chutzpah! I thought I was going to pee my panties and start laughing right out loud. I wondered if it wasn't she who may be feeling these things. After excusing themselves for twenty minutes, they walked back in the room with frowns on their wrinkled-up faces. The other grad student looked at me and in an annoying, whispery tone said, "We have discussed this with our supervisor and with each other, and think you may have some neurological disorder. We recommend you see a specialist and get some medication to help!"

I'm thinking, 'you gotta be freakin' kidding me, right?' and immediately smiled as I envisioned them both stripped naked and set loose in my part of town…at midnight. Then I told them that this so-called affliction they're pegging me with is only a problem to them and please, do not inject their morals into the mix. It's not a therapist's job. I continued to explain that in their chosen profession, they most likely—though not typically—would come across certain individuals that do not fit into any profiles or textbook cases they've ever studied. This does not necessarily mean there is any sort of 'affliction'. Besides that, medication is not the answer to everything in this world. I smiled calmly and explained, "I am very secure and comfortable in my own skin and my sexuality. I sincerely hoped that they learn from this session. Oh, and by the way, I won't be returning either. Now, if you'll both excuse me, which way to the nearest cocktail lounge?"

Good Advice from a Very Bad Girl

I thought I heard them desperately leafing through manuals for alcoholism as I sauntered down the hallway feeling better about myself than ever before.

Dear Mz. Conduct,

I've read about the supposed famous G Spot, but it's confusing to me. Is it possible I don't have one at all? My gynecologist and family doctors have both informed me that maybe I am just not finding it. They have told me to try different positions and where it should be located. They have instructed me to search for it MYSELF, which I have done. Nothing works. I can't find that little spot no matter what I do.

As a matter of fact, I find it odd that I can't really feel anything but pressure when I am having sex. I don't get any sensation whatsoever, except pressure.

Is it physically possible that there is something wrong with that? Is there some reason this would be happening? The only time I have ever "gone" while someone was in there was because he was also getting the little button on the front at the same time. But I thought I read somewhere that they are connected somehow (that and the G spot). I might be wrong.

I am getting really tired of faking it. I would really like to have one of those wall-banging, screaming orgasms everyone else seems to achieve. I have had some great men in bed and they do all the right things, been perfect sizes etc., but as soon as they are in, I feel nothing but pressure.

Ok Mz. Conduct. I'm ready. What the hell is wrong with me?

OH "G" I Can't Find It

Dear OH,

Hmmm. I was reading and waiting for you to actually say 'orgasm,' but you did at long last, thank the stars and stripes forever (insert big band music here.) First off, there is nothing wrong with you a date with me wouldn't fix, complete with scuba gear and lipstick. Seriously though, a lot of women have never found their G-Spot. I think it's mostly due to a lack of self-exploration and knowledge, but that's something that can be changed easily.

Good news honeybee, every single woman has a G spot! It's actually a spongy tissue found beneath the surface of the vagina, accessible from about two or three inches from within the front of the vaginal wall (between the cervix and the vaginal opening.) I have heard that some women actually feel an irritation when it is hit, however most of us find that they can have a most definitely divine orgasm. In any case, it's sure worth the discovery. Oh, when that beautiful, fat-mushroom-headed-wand o' flesh hits me from behind, that breath on my neck and nasty talk oozing from those wicked lips, it just rocks me right over the slaphappy rainbow. Oops, I drifted again. Now that I'm as moist as a snack cake, back to you.

Masturbate a lot and try to explore your realms of pleasure. It's hard to find the G-Spot with your own finger; they usually aren't long enough, but there are dildos that are slightly curved made just for hitting the spot. Hop on down to your local Weenie Mart and treat yourself to a new toy. Can I go, huh, can I?

It is better when you're all worked up like a bowl of chocolate frosting waiting to be licked. When you're with a comfortable partner, and after you've both had a good amount of foreplay. Work yourselves up, have them slide their finger (skip the Lee Press-On-Nails here) gently, yet firmly up inside your vaginal wall. Your partner should try circling around the wall and putting a bit more pressure towards the wall facing your belly. If you're on your back, then put the pressure towards the heavens. A good reference point is the pubic hairline. If and when you do find it, and you should be patient with yourself, the G-Spot lies roughly behind that hairline. Once it's hit your partner can crook their finger—like a come here gesture—and the tissue will swell up to the size of a quarter. You may feel an urge to pee, much like a man when his prostate is stimulated, but it'll pass in a matter of seconds…the feeling, not the urine. Sometimes when the probing is right on, women can ejaculate a milky fluid, much like the seminal fluid of men (minus the sperm of course).

Mind you, don't expect to hear Ethel Merman singing "I Love a Parade" the first time you find your own personal G-Spot; you may have tried to focus too much and not been fully relaxed. Next time honey, next time. Anyway, if you're anything like me, Ethel Merman won't have a chance to be heard over your own vocals.

Here are a couple of positions that Mz. Conduct likes best for rainbow racing orgasms:

1) Reverse Cowgirl: straddle you partner, facing away from them towards their feet. It conveniently puts the penis right against the G-Spot. You can try a variation where your knees are between his legs and you control the thrusting. Oh sweet mama, the view from both ends is absolutely yummy. It also makes for easy access for anal play that way.

2) Bend way over Grandma's kitchen table and have your partner take you by the hips and plunge. You can push your clitoris against the tabletop at the same time, and soon you will know that nothing on Grandma's table will ever taste the same.

Stop faking it. I think it's a bad habit to get into and will stand in the way of you achieving an actual orgasm. When you do find it, don't be afraid to share this new information with your partner. Be a greedy bitch and ask for what you want and where and when. Men appreciate that. Besides, you deserve it. We all do.

Dear Mz. Conduct,

I recently and finally went out with a woman who I had pursued for quite awhile. We were having such a good time until she asked if I liked to get done up the butt! I couldn't believe she asked that, and of course I said an emphatic no. She seemed instantly turned off and although the rest of the evening was pleasurable enough, I don't know what will be. Am I wrong to hold on to my masculinity like that?

One Way William

Dear OWW,

Water weasels in a wheelbarrow! What the hell does masculinity have to do with exercising your prostate? I swear, some men should never mingle with the public sector. I would join her in being turned off. Men brag about hiking up the Olympic peninsula and sea kayaking next to sharks, but they cross their legs when it comes to a question of anal stimulation. That's just repressive and goofy, and I personally wouldn't hold my breath thinking this girl will see you again. Oh go ahead, hold your breath. When you're dead, she and I will both strap on, and ream your pucker in front of all your co-workers and the local football team, so there!

Okay, cutting you some slack, some straight men think that they are somehow turned into homosexuals if they have any sort of pleasure with anal play or penetration. That's just dumb (except sometimes it's right). Isn't that just life though? There are hidden jewels to be discovered in our bodies; try to be more open-minded.

The perineum (the stretch of skin between the balls and the anus) is very sensitive and can be played with during sex for an even better orgasm. If you do this by yourself then you can be man enough to show a partner. Now, a man's prostate gland is his G-Spot. That extreme deep tingle you get in your crotch when you are turned on is actually your prostate gland. It can be found about one or two inches within the anus, towards the penis, like a little dome. Try inserting your finger up your ass just a bit. If you are feeling brave when you go where no man—or woman—has gone before, you should use a little lubricant to ease it along. You don't have to go buy anything either; olive oil (extra virgin in your case) makes a nice lube. If you feel the urge to pee, it's a natural trigger, but will pass in about ten seconds, give or take. If you stroke your penis while your finger is there, you will thank me forever. And of course you will try this, and you're welcome. Think of it as preventative medicine if you must. Prostates that get prodded have less chance of acquiring prostate cancer. Explore, and if it feels good, continue. Share the love and evolve damnit!

Mz. Conduct's House of Sin

The Perils of the Personal Ad

"The only way I would take up jogging is so that I could hear heavy breathing again."
–Erma Bombeck

I have come to the ultimate conclusion that many men are just plain misinformed as to how to initially communicate with women. Now, women aren't excluded in this area, but men seem to really be clueless. To help you men out, I've composed a top ten list of what NOT to do when responding to a personal ad. If you're considering finding someone you want to actually meet, and not send screaming into the streets, then this may be of help.

I deem myself worthy to do this because I have my very own tiara and porn star lipstick and because I can!

Mz. Conduct's Top Ten List When Responding To a Personal Ad

1) Speak clearly, preferably in English, although throwing a little French in—only if you really know it—is always acceptable. Refrain from whispering and/or trying to sound sexy. It just sounds like you're jerking off or something. Yuck.

2) Be sure you READ the ad. If the ad says that the person is an adrenalin freak and likes to bungee jump and sky dive naked, do not tell them you are hoping for a bridge partner.

3) This is a biggie, boys. Refrain from saying that you are "attractive" or how many others think you are. That's entirely subjective. I mean it's nice that YOU think you're attractive, but Christ on a crumpet, the girl may think you look like poo-on-a-stick. Plus, it's just freakin' annoying.

4) There is no need to give a complete résumé either. It can be somewhat interesting that you have spent the last six years working in the Yukon with only a box of toothpicks and a hand warmer, but we don't need the entire experience.

5) Keep it fairly short and do not keep repeating the same thing. Practice your speech beforehand so you don't seem like an Alzheimer patient.

6) For the love of labia, do NOT explain how big your penis is! Don't say things like (and I have absolutely heard every one of these)," I'm extremely hung and have never disappointed anyone" or " I am nine inches of love muscle" or "I am very well endowed." UGH! It doesn't really matter how big you are if you look like you were just cast in an alien movie.

7) Don't try to sell yourself; if we women wanted a sales pitch we would go to Sears and hover around the appliance section. One guy who answered my ad actually announced—after saying he was five feet, six inches tall— that he was better for stand-up sex. Oh bouncin' buttplugs, like that's what I've always been waiting for, some damn good stand up sex, just looking for that short guy, and voila, here he is!

8) Please, oh please do not say that you like "long walks on the beach" for gawd's sake. Again subjectivity enters. I'm sure you would definitely wish to be elsewhere if you were on a "long walk on the beach" with a chinless, zit-faced creature whose snatch smells of a washed up mackerel, right? Well, the same goes for us.

9) Go easy on the cologne and only apply if it costs over sixty dollars...we can smell your cheap ass even over the phone.

10) Lastly, if you have a freakin' comb-over, don't even bother calling. Go directly to a barber and have him shave your head bald. There, so much better! Do you honestly think some woman would want to run their fingers through your four strands of greasy, foot long hair? I think I'm going to hurl just think-

Mz. Conduct's House of Sin

ing about it. You should know that comb-overs just scream: Bowling Champ of the Seventies, Trailer Park Janitor and/or Kiddy Diddler from Des Moines.

Okay, now I need that girlie with the onion ass and knee socks to skip on over to the bar and whip me up a stiff one. Are those olives in her blouse or is she just glad to see me?

Dear Mz. Conduct,

I've been married for almost one year, but my husband and I have been together for a total of four years. The problem is that my husband masturbates all the time. He has done this since I've known him, and at first it was kind of a turn-on, but now I'm repulsed by him and it.

He masturbates when he gets up, after work, before bed, and sometimes in the middle of the night. The worst part is that he does it right beside me in bed. This hurts me on so many levels. I've tried to talk to him and explain how this is affecting me, but he says I'm the one with the problem.

Otherwise, he treats me great. And besides this problem, our sex life is fine, and we really do get along well. But I'm finding that whenever he touches me, I cringe. I am at my wits end. Part of me is thinking about a divorce over this. Can you help?

Ill in Illinois

> **Dear Ill,**
>
> I wish you had explained to ME why your husband's schlong-stroking "hurts you on so many levels." I almost launched my good gin across the room and if you were here, I would feel compelled to slap you until you loved it. Semen on a saltine woman, he's not whacking his weenie in the kitty litter isle of the supermarket, or pounding his palm at your auntie's dinner table, so what's the deal?
>
> It sounds like your hubby has a good strong sex drive and if I were you, instead of laying there next to him in the middle of the night, sobbing with self-pity for whatever reason, I'd jump on that thing! Why do women take it personally when a guy masturbates? Yeesh, it's just what guys do, and if I had that hunk of sensitive flesh hanging between my legs all day, well, let's just say I'd be dangerous. I agree with your husband, it's you that needs to shape up. If you don't want sex that often—some of us have more libido in their loins than others—then maybe you should help him masturbate. You should try masturbating more yourself and relieve some of that pent up stress you seem to be carting around. Maybe you're taking medication that hampers your sex drive, and you might look into alternatives, I don't know. Is his penis getting more attention than you are, doesn't sound that way, geeze.
>
> Contemplating divorce is about the goofiest thing I have ever heard since Dick Cheney auditioned for the tin man in the Wizard of Oz. Worship that working appendage for all it's worth and quit being "repulsed," or you may turn into a frigid, blow-up doll.

Dear Mz Conduct,

The last party I was at, I was helping my girlfriend's roommate puke outside at three in the morning. When I ran back in to grab my girlfriend, I saw her in some other

Good Advice from a Very Bad Girl

guy's arms, making out like crazy. Later she tried to apologize and said that she was just trying to get back at me. Earlier that night, I overslept because I'd been out drinking with my buddies and I was late to the pre-party. The problem is that I still love her. Whenever I see her face, I just melt. I want to forgive her, but on the other hand when I think about what she did, and more importantly, why she did it, it makes me sick. I don't know whether to forgive her or not. What do you think?

Forgive or Forget

Dear FF,

Perhaps a week without alcohol would clear your housefly infested brain. Do you realize just what a childish ordeal this was? "Oh no, should I forgive her... oh I can't believe she did that...oh boo hoo sob sob." Kill me now! If I wanted whine, I'd order a bottle of French red and have you pay, but it's morning and coffee is all I have to fuel me, that, and what a dolt you are.

So your girlfriend smooched up someone else. You were all at a party and having fun. Lots of alcohol will loosen the inhibitions. I mean, she couldn't smooch you, you were helping out the puking friend. She couldn't smooch the puker either because that's just gross, so she smooched someone else. Get over it! Sometimes a girl just has to smooch, besides you'll have 'one in the bank' to use for yourself if you're ever in that position. Of course you will be in the same boat at some point, because you're HUMAN! Personally I'd like to smooch your ass with a telephone pole just for being so high and freakin' mighty.

I suggest that the two of you watch one of my favorite movies (do it, I said so!), *Breakfast at Tiffany's*, and see the fabulous parties that Audrey Hepburn continually throws. Absolutely everyone is smooching everyone! Move on mister.

Mz. Conduct's House of Sin

Gas and Giggles

"We're all in this alone."
–Lily Tomlin

My last column, Top Ten List of Things To Do and Not To Do When Responding To a Personal Ad, seemed to go over well with folks. I came up with two more important facts, in light of the responses I received this week. I've edited to a Top Twelve:

11) Use your freakin' spellchecker! Compose a proper sentence. Have enough respect for the woman to expect that she is a literate, intelligent, goddess. Even if she only has three good teeth, smokes camels in a tattered muumuu, and resides at the Twilight trailer park, she still deserves your efforts. If you are not of this caliber, then just whack off to the idea of a meeting, and don't even bother responding. When I get mail like this; " I [sic] should be a porn star. you [sic] will love my big cock and i waon't disapont u, call me soon hun," well, it just makes me want to up-chuck my good gin, damnit!

12) I've also heard, "I know you like younger men, but I'm a very young fifty-five year old." Yeah right. Please, the crows feet alone could create a full-fledged flock. It's nice that you FEEL younger, and good for you, but guess what? You're NOT! Let's face it, I FEEL like I'm a twenty-something Jean Harlow, but guess what? Close, but no cigar. Leave out the fountain of spewing testimonials.

So, on another note, The Transient Trollop called from a state of southern exposure and blurted, "Guess what I got?" And I guessed, "An STD?" Not quite, instead she got a marriage license. She and the man of her dreams stood in line for hours to obtain the thing, chatting with folks getting landfill permits. Friday the thirteenth is the big hitching day, the T.T. replied, unless of course they're having a sale at Wal-Mart. Congratulations my dog-eared bosom bitch, and if you end up at Wal-Mart, would you pick me up a gallon of bleach?

Good Advice from a Very Bad Girl

So, like my bumper sticker says, "Everyone is entitled to my opinion." Here it comes again!

Dear Mz. Conduct,

This is so embarrassing to even write about, but if anyone could give me a straight answer, I know you will. I've been dating this adorable guy for a few weeks now and we have the best sex ever. The last time we had sex, at the exact time I had an orgasm, I passed gas at the same time. I thought I was going to die. Of course this guy heard it and started laughing. Needless to say, the moment was lost and I ran out of his place completely humiliated. We haven't seen each other since, but he has been calling. I can't even talk to him right now and don't know if I ever will, out of sheer embarrassment. How do I get over this?

Red Faced in Reno

>Dear RFIR,
>
>My drag queen Jesus night-lite hasn't worked for over a year now, but suddenly flipped on when the Catholic in-laws were here. That's some religious irony, eh? Hey, such is life, and that's my response to you and your goofy predicament. You're being a nincompoop (only slight pun intended) for making more out of it than it is. I'm reminded of a line in a book I once read that said, "When grandma breaks wind we beat the dog."
>
>When you are in the midst of a rocking orgasm, sometimes everything just breaks loose. This shouldn't be a big deal. It's not like you had an attack of explosive diarrhea and sprayed your sweetie in the snout. You should have just laughed along with him and that would be that. Instead, you've analyzed this too much. You need to just call up this guy and tell him you are sorry and you were just really embarrassed, but you're over it now. Life is hilarious and if you can't laugh at yourself, well then, everyone else will.
>
>I crack myself up sometimes just thinking about the little social blunders I've had, such as having seventeen too many cocktails and falling out of a car—in a short black dress and do-me pumps, no less. Right when my ass hit the ground, the biggest fart in the whole world emerged and echoed through the entire parking lot. That was lovely and laugable. Another time, my boyfriend was orally pleasing me and when I came, I farted at the same time. Guess which one he didn't particularly like? We both laughed like crazy (me, especially.) My point is, these things happen. Are you over it yet?

Dear Mz. Conduct,

I've lived with my boyfriend for four years now. We used to have a very hot relationship, but since we moved in together the sex has dwindled to two or three times a year. I've tried different settings, vacations, cocktails, lingerie, baths, etc., nothing can perk up my/his desire.

I've had a physical and the doctor says there's nothing wrong. I realize I'm pretty bored with my partner and that he doesn't stimulate me mentally at all. But I'm too young to give up on my sex life altogether. What should I do—get a lover? Move out? Masturbate?

Empty Nest

>Dear Empty Nest,

Mz. Conduct's House of Sin

All of the above, honey! That ought to perk up your desire. I'm curious as to what you considered a hot relationship was, what, maybe six times a year? Although people so have different ranges of libidos, you sound like you have about as much self esteem as a side of cole slaw. Christ with a cock ring, you give women a bad name! Where oh where is my hairless sweetie, with my gin-n-juice, when I need him?

Let's see, you're not married so there won't be any messy paperwork or lawyers to deal with. Since you don't get much use out of his dysfunctional penis, you may want to tie him to a chair, sprinkle lighter fluid all over his crotch and then flick matches at it. You know, just for fun. He's obviously an oblivious dolt not to realize that you're not happy, not getting it, and just letting things go on as they are. He may even have some burger slinging, knocked up, teenybopper on the side. Men do like to avoid conflict whenever possible. It surely is time to take matters in your own hands. Tell him you need more from a relationship than what his lame ass is contributing then pack his stinking bags with all his skid marked underpants (because we know he's that type), and toss them into traffic. You said it yourself, he's not stimulating you mentally or physically, so what the hell are you sticking around for? Quit being a whiny wench and wave bye-bye. Better things (canned meat for instance) await you, my dear, I promise.

Divorced and Dickless

"Enemies are so stimulating"
–Katharine Hepburn

Friday the thirteenth has come and gone, but not without dropping its twisted little hexes on some of us. There has been a tad of pyromania in the House Of Sin this week. It's the end of the line for some things and the beginning for others, but isn't that how it always goes? Congratulations to the Transient Trollop and her man for hitching the wagon to the horse, so to speak. May you stay clear of the potholes and ride smoothly through the manure free valley forever. Remember, when the going gets tough, use the freakin' whip! Divorced and dickless is no way to travel.

So, the spiral continues, the phoenix rises, and life goes on. I had quite a handsome boy croon, "My Funny Valentine" for moi when the Lil' Princess and I were celebrating the day at our favorite dive karaoke bar. Although he didn't come close to my favorite Elvis Costello version, his rendition was intended just for me alone, and that's what it's really all about, isn't it?

I'm certainly going to hell on a sex scholarship. I have been an extra bad girl this week but damn it all, not without my proper discipline. Spankings by my Wise Ol' Yippie Mentor, tongue lashings by a new found, brilliant old coot, and engaging aggressiveness from my submissive boy toy. I deserve it all and so much more. However, as The Transient Trollop and I always say, 'if I'm run over by a beer truck tomorrow, by Gawd I'm going having a good time today!' As always, bottoms up!

> Dear Mz. Conduct,
> For the first time ever, I've been having lurid fantasies about a boy/man half my age. He IS legal, over the age of consent, so this isn't the crux of this annoying little brain drain. The problem is how to delight in his very being without his parents running me out of town, which by the way, is very small. He, in his innocent way, makes peewee moves and gestures in trying to show me he is interested in whatever I want to do, but I refrain. Not sure of the appropriateness, and his more than likely irate parents.

Mz. Conduct's House of Sin

I have heard from some men, their fond memories of 'that older woman' that introduced them to the pleasures of the pleasing. Now you never hear of these older women, and what backlash they endure, right? Oh, he's so delish, it's almost worth the risk, but I come to you for your pearls of insight and wisdom. So? What say you?

Twitching in Anticipation

> **Dear TIA,**
>
> Oh my lips and lashes, this is right up my alley, honey. Or what I wish was right up my alley, anyway…hmmm. Now, Mz. Conduct just loves those young spring chickens and although I've gotten myself into a wee bit of hot water with that fetish, what the hell! I say the same to people stressing about trying to quit smoking; we'll all be smoking in hell honey, do what you want.
>
> Since he isn't underage, you aren't a kiddy diddler, and it's his unfortunate problem that he still lives at home. If you are friends of sorts, you may want to suggest that he look for a place of his own or one share one with friends. This would be just a friendly gesture, a helpful hint, a wise piece of advice, and an intent direction for throbbing lust. Until then, holy handbags on hold, don't you have your own place?
>
> Those young boys are so willing and wide-eyed with appreciation. Memories of that youngster from out of town, who in the middle of an enthusiastic cunnilingus chokehold, looked up and said with matched enthusiasm, "Wow, you have a killer pussy!" Well, you know, sometimes, it's best if they don't speak. It can become a bit of an ego trip, for they honestly will never forget you if you rock the holy snot out of them. Just be careful as to what happens afterwards. If you want a relationship with him, it will be tricky. I don't recommend it. They may get attached to you and you will have to scrape them off gently (or not so gently, depending on their IQ). However if you are honestly straight away about everything—my motto in all of life—then there shouldn't be a problem.
>
> As for his parents, oh well! It's none of their damn business what their son does in his sexual life. It's not their place to run you out of town, Mrs. Robinson. Where are you…Mayberry circa 1902? He's an adult and can do what he wants, as can you.
>
> William Blake once said, "Those who restrain desire do so because theirs is weak enough to be restrained." 'Nuff said.

Dear Mz. Conduct,

I am a thirty-two year old man who likes to be nude whenever possible. I not only like to be free of all clothing, but I like to be seen nude as well. I have an office job and am pretty "normal" in every other aspect. If it were legal, I would spend every minute nude, even public. I love going to the nude beaches where people are just going about their business: having picnics, playing volleyball, swimming, etc. all in the nude. It all started when my exhibitionist neighbors would walk around their house naked, even having sex in full view of the window with the light on.

I wonder if this is a condition that I should seek help for?

Baring It In Boston

> **Dear BIIB,**
>
> A man after my own heart! I also despise wearing clothes unless need be. The exhibitionist part is identifiable as well, and not that uncommon. I don't think it's a "condition" that needs any sort of treatment although I'm sure some shrinks would disagree. My latest experience with shrinks was that they wanted to label and medicate anything that didn't fit a certain textbook profile.

I have a big problem with that. When my son and I used to march in the Gay Pride Parade and the Walk for AIDS, we used to carry a sign that read, "Ignorance Equals Fear" which I believe still holds, unfortunately. The feel of a warm breeze blowing across your body, the tingle of the fresh air on your skin, the way we were born, the way we should be…yeah, I'm with you there. Some folks just have a problem with nudity for whatever reasons: "Oh my thighs are too large" or "Those parts are private" or "No one will know that I shop at Saks!" Whatever socially repressed and ingrained goofiness plays into it, it's their option and you definitely have yours as well.

I would just caution you on one aspect. On the nude beaches, as you say, people are playing volleyball and having picnics and whatever. Women can be sexually aroused without showing a big waving boner, but you cannot. Even if you have a cocktail wiener for a penis, you cannot get away without notice. Just be respectful, stay away from the freakin' bushes for instance, and be sure that it's not the only reason you're on the beach. Otherwise you may get arrested and that's just no fun.

Mz. Conduct's House of Sin

Happy Hoyden in Heels

"If I don't drive around the block, I'm pretty sure to make my mark. If I'm in bed each night by ten, I may get back my looks again. If I abstain from fun and such, I'll probably amount to much. But I shall stay the way I am because I do not give a damn."
–Dorothy Parker

Topless housekeeping, yes, my newest endeavor, has been a powerful and exciting way to make lots of loot. My fab new roommate, the Distinguished Deviant, is my agent, or pimp if you will. Or will not! So, not a surprise, but most men like to watch me bend over in my tiny, black skirt and shiny heels. With my pierced, bare breasts bobbing and swinging in time to the feather duster, the ogling begins. They talk about their wives that left them, how they were laid off their jobs, the dog that died, and every sad thing known to man. They cannot touch me in any way, shape or form, and sign a waiver in agreement of this when I arrive. One guy asked if I could clean his bathtub without my panties on and I told him it would be an extra thirty dollars an hour. Not a problem. It was a ninety degree day and I liked the breezy bending much better anyway.

After a week of blubbering, blathering, inhaling oodles of ciggies, and upchucking Chardonnay, I've come to realize one thing; you must be your own true self and that true self should be cultivated, cherished, and celebrated no matter what.

The other day, I was forced to sit next to a beer soaked individual, in a sticky, crowded government office no less. He had his Hawaiian shirt unbuttoned exposing his protruding belly and was scratching and burping simultaneously. It took forty-five minutes for them to call my name.

Another day in the same week, wanting to do a good thing, I gave two toothless transients a ride in the back of my truck. I was feeling camaraderie of sorts, but I bet myself a martini that when they baled out, they'd ask me for cash. I was overdrawn, penniless and fridge-bare, but that's beside the point. I won the bet but couldn't afford the martini.

Yet another day, same week...I was driving home one late afternoon when an enormous tree branch fell and missed my car by about two inches. I screeched on my brakes and got out of the car in wild disbelief. By this time, a line of traffic was behind me and I was trying to wrestle and drag this twelve-foot tree limb to the side of the road. Finally some slow-witted men came and took over, mumbling macho threats about calling the city and such. Then it started hailing, yeah.

Things did pick up, as they do eventually. I had a sexy intruder at two in the morning, although he did call first, does that count? (Hey, role playing is fun.) Wild Bill and his Amazing Appendage came over to cheer me up. I wasn't much of my usual 'hostess with the mostess' with the week I had, though he became the host with the most and banged me blissfully until the sun came up and yet again, it was a new day. Yes, I am an inevitable gutterslut.

The Transient Trollop and I have already perfectly pictured ourselves as eighty-year-old lesbians. We'll end up living together, sitting around in our ripped fishnets and fuzzy slippers, chain smoking hand rolled ciggies and screeching at each other over who drank all the booze. Que sera sera. This week calls for martinis by the score and lots of young, supple tramps in Betty Rubble attire to serve them to me, don't you agree?

Dear Mz. Conduct,
My husband and I have been married for fourteen years and we just don't seem to have any time for sex. I don't know when it started going downhill, but our busy schedules keep us from having any intimate time together. We don't have kids, but we have our careers and on top of that: yard and house work, various and ongoing projects, and our volunteer work and community projects. Do you have any suggestions?
Busy Bee

> Dear B.B.,
> Lop off my labia and call me Dick! I can't personally even imagine this scenario although I realize it's likely a common problem, especially in this day and age.

Mz. Conduct's House of Sin

Good gawd woman, how can you cheerfully volunteer and be a productive part of the community when you're all sexually bottled up and ready to release about a pound and a half of fluid at any given time? Listen, if you have time to chop a cucumber for a salad, you have time to bend over the kitchen sink. Let your husband use his cucumber for sexually nutritious explorations.

It doesn't always have to be a romantic, candle lit, all-nighter. Lollipops and Lincoln Logs, you don't have kids banging on your bedroom door so while you're planning the weeks corporate meetings, pen in an hour for a romp. Call the hubby on his cell phone and ask to meet him somewhere, do lunch, do him. You can also slip into the shower with your hubby and kill two birds with one bone, so to speak. Maybe sit on his lap while he's filing reports or polishing off the lasagna. He never even has to get up! Sit on his lap and talk about the first thing that pops up. That's what we used to say in grade school before we knew what it meant. Well, maybe I knew, but at the time I felt it may be premature to be outed as the gutterslut that I am.

Anyway, my point is that if you want it badly enough you will find time. If you make the time, it will be a healthful and helpful aspect in the rest of your daily life. Just think how much better you'll feel, the endless blush on your face as you deliver those geriatric lunches, bake those cakes for the neighborhood sale, or what ever floats your altruistic boat. Take care of sexual self, even if you are an over-achieving housewife. That should be a motto for life.

Mullets and Make-Up Sex

"Sex is never an emergency."
–Elaine Pierson

I bought myself flowers this week mainly because no one else did and you know what? They're just as beautiful! It's been a trying time, so I'm listening to PJ Harvey and she gives me strength. It's the sureness in her voice, nothing ethereal, just guttural moans and cries of painful passion. Right there in your face. Strength is food right now and silly as it sounds, I also get strength from my Eloise books. Eloise is the story that Kay Thompson wrote over forty years ago about a precocious six year old girl who lives at the Plaza hotel and has a nanny who drinks pilsners. Eloise says things like, "Oh my Lord, there's so much to do, tomorrow I think I'll pour a pitcher of water down the mail chute. Oooooooooooooo I absolutely love The Plaza."

I may have a multiple personality man picker this month because I am feeling like Scarlet O'Hara, Dorothy Parker, Anais Nin, and the aforementioned girls above. Maybe we all gather and shift from time to time. It is indeed a full moon and gawd knows the feces is flying. One more martini and I should have a handle on it all.

The Transient Trollop is now divorced, and motivationally speaking, living in a van...down by the river. I reminded her that just because you love someone, it doesn't necessarily mean you have to live with them...or in a van down by the river. Something better is just around the bend.

The Lil' Princess and I went to visit our friend, the Glamour Girl at her place of business. Glamour Girl poured us some heavy-duty cocktails and I ogled her ass for a few minutes. Casually, I mentioned my strap-on and it scared the boys sitting next to us right off their barstools. I'm sure they were off to see their ancestors in the Planet Of the Ape movie anyway. I'm such a brazen bimbo and one wish of mine is to ride the Oscar Meyer wiener mobile right through the swankiest part of town. Oh yeah! I would have my tiara on of course, and wear my shirt that says, 'Queen of Fucking Everything'. Oscar Wilde alluded to a relatable line; I may always have one foot in the gutter, but will always be reaching for the stars. And preferably straddling the wiener mobile.

Dear Mz. Conduct,

I haven't been laid in so long I'm starting to experience hallucinations and I'm not even smoking anything. I'm seriously considering lesbianism because the women in my life are much more in tune with their own needs and the needs of those who they love. Meanwhile, my purple, plastic vibrator is going through batteries like you wouldn't believe. I do enjoy the feel of a penis being shoved inside of me, but I could happily give that up for some real, human passion. At least I think I could. Should I give girls a try?

Girl Crazy

> Dear GC,
>
> I think you should continue to treasure your female companionship for what it is. If something more develops then go with it, but your friends are already in position. When/if you want to actually seek out a woman for sex, that's a whole different story. There are plenty of bi-curious women out there and if you're serious about pursuing this, then check the personals. Put an ad in of your own. If being with a woman really makes your panties moist then I'd say pursue it, if it's just the fact that you're sick to death of the minnow-minded men in your life, I'd say, join the millions of women who feel the same. Think it out first, what do you really consider a thigh throbbing thought? Is it a girl in a tight skirt or a girl slapping the shit out of some guy who you've been doing laundry for ten years running? Get it straight, and if you decide you are anything but straight then give me a call honey.

Dear Mz. Conduct,

I love my girlfriend, but whenever we get ready to go anywhere, and I mean anywhere, she takes forever to get ready. What is that all about? I guess I don't understand the importance of re-applying layers upon layers of foundation just to go to the grocery store, or at all for that matter. I've asked her about this and we always get into a huge argument so now I just sit, wait and fume in silence. Then I'm irritated when we do finally leave and it makes for an unpleasant trip wherever it happens to be. This has really become a problem, at least to me, but is this MY problem that I need to get over or perhaps there is a compromise that you can suggest?

Make Up Or Break Up

> Dear MUOBU,
>
> Christ on crusade mister! Your girl may have some insecurity hang-ups big time. I personally wouldn't even look at a chickadee that wore layers of gunk on her face. Okay, a tad of waterproof mascara (for watching Spanish films), and always, but always THIS girl must have on lipstick. Other than that, I see no need for any of the garbage that turns your white shirt to an abstract painting when you hug, or that stains your pillow and announces that maybe a drag queen just spent the night. Now there's a new meaning to make-up sex, ha.

I suggest that you get under all those layers and see why she feels it necessary to wear all of that gook. Let her know that the rawness of her skin turns you on. Tell her how beautiful you think she is without it and blah, blah, blah. If she refuses to listen to you then inform her that you will now be sporting a mullet and calling yourself Jethro. This way you'll match each other more evenly. You can put a ratty couch on your front porch, sit on it (near the exposed springs) with a jug of booze and a pellet gun and really get into the whole white trash experience.

On the other hand, if that's an unreasonable task, then just deal with it. It's her thang. Go do something useful while you wait and quit stewing. You know, I would just bet my bug spray that you have qualities or lack thereof that equally annoy her. Now, even I'm annoyed with you.

Mz. Conduct's House of Sin

Break Up and Suck Up

"Imagination is intelligence with an erection."
–Victor Hugo

I think I may change my misnomer to Ms. Knowmer or even Helen Back after this week, Yeesh! There are just way too many men out in the world awaiting a spinal transplant, a self-security deposit or just plain old testicle transaction. I should start a crusade, a telethon, that's it! I could call it, 'Mz. Conduct's 24 Hour Thrash 'n Lash Telethon.' Good gobs of Gonads, weeks like I've had make for grateful sisters in sin

I did have a date this week with mister television man. He was nice enough to bring along his shaved and sassy sausage. While getting ready, I was thinking how long it's been since I had an actual date. A date defined as someone coming to pick you up in a sporty, little, bachelor car, complete with wine in hand instead of just their wiener and a cigarette. I changed outfits, on that ninety degree evening, about four times, all the while talking to the Lil' Princess on my giant, red lips telephone. The first ensemble looked great except for the fact that certain areas were screaming, "liposuction!" I couldn't foresee trying to carry on a conversation with that interference all night…so that dress came off. The next dress accentuated the negative and that I immediately ripped to shreds. The third dress seemed okay, and although resembling a sleazy nightgown, was loose enough that I didn't have to worry about holding my breath consistently for six more hours. The next question, it's freakin' hotter than Georgia asphalt and should I even wear underwear? Yeah, I'll be a good girl, maybe a thong. Yanking a thong halfway up my thigh, the black lace snapped and flung itself across the bathroom, landing on the back of the toliet. Okay, so that answers that…to hell with the undies.

I did sell an erotica story this week, and although I won't be putting a down payment on that '57 T-Bird, I will be able to afford a couple of gin and juices and a new thong. Bottoms up baby!

Good Advice from a Very Bad Girl

Dear Mz. Conduct,

How can I ask for a break up with my boyfriend that would not hurt him? I want to tell him that I still love him though. He can be really sensitive and I worry. I just want to do more things with other people and he's not usually interested in the stuff I do anyway. So how do I do this?

Heartbreak Hoopla

> **Dear HH,**
>
> Tell him just what you told me, Duh! At least mention where things went downhill so he has a friggin' clue. Be honest, not only is that the best thing you can do for someone you love, but you will help him in his future relationships too. Look how thoughtful you are!
>
> If the wimp starts sniveling and his tears are spraying all over your blouse, then maybe you can taper down the relationship a bit. Tell him you'll see him once a week, but that your dance card will be more than likely full of others as well. If he can't handle that and threatens to throw himself off the footbridge at the Japanese gardens, then tell him that if he's not careful he'll lose your friendship as well. Hopefully you two can remain friends and if and when you want to have sex with him again, he'll think he's got some power over you. Boys like thinking that, we all do to some extent. Girls still rule!

Dear Mz. Conduct,

I'm about to be married and have never given oral sex before. I want to do it well and give my husband what he desires. I thought that of all people you could tell me how to do it.

Oral Virgin

> **Dear OV,**
>
> Bravo for having an enthusiastic approach to this. There's a dumb, old joke which says that a bride is only smiling when she's walking down the aisle because she knows that she'll never have to give another blowjob. I suppose there are women like that, but to me, it is a damn shame. I might have a gag reflex after all!
>
> As with women and oral sex, we're all a little different. Men tend to be more single minded when it comes to their penis. Big surprise! Remember it starts in the brain, so work that area first. Explain what you want to try and tell him how beautiful his penis is. You can pour it on thick, explaining that you can't sleep nights with the pestering penis visions dancing in your head, and so on.
>
> A decent percent of giving good head is in the attitude. If you're squeamish or worried about swallowing his cum, it'll show. Let's face it, if you're in the middle of a mad romp and your partner screws up their face with concern over an unpredictable spurt of body fluid, it's not such a turn on. If it's a chore or you're doing him a favor, schlong smooching can take on all the charm of him sticking his dick in the vacuum cleaner hose. Hey, it's Mz. Conduct you're asking remember, not Ann Landers.
>
> Learn to love it, honey. Start by admiring the beauty of the penis. Generally they all have something beautiful about them, for the most part.
>
> Look at it, touch it, run your fingers over the ridges, veins and folds. Kiss it lightly on the head, a little licking and wetness. Don't forget about the testicle twins, most guys like their balls cupped, squeezed lightly—and sometimes

Mz. Conduct's House of Sin

hard—and sucked on too. Underneath and between the ball sack and the anus is the perineum. That's a highly sensitive area as well. If you run your finger along there and then your tongue, and then run your tongue around their asshole, this should get the juices flowing, literally. Try doing this while stroking his penis slowly. Each time you bring your hand up, cup it, brushing the head lightly. Cover with foil and bake at 350°. Sorry, all of a sudden I had visions of a turkey baster and oven mitts. Yeesh, unless I have a penis, dangling on a piece of string in front of me, I get sidetracked, okay?

You can use your hand while you kiss the head of his penis, stroking the base of the shaft and gradually slide what you can in your mouth and suck it like a tootsie roll pop with a four-carat diamond in the middle. I've heard that some girls have problems with fitting the whole thing in their mouth however I am not one of them, but then I've been refining my skills for decades. Anyway, back to the task at hand; alternate using your hand and your mouth and for the love of little leather boys, pretend you just don't have teeth. Use your tongue on the head and up and down and round and round and worship it honey. Whew, okay I now need a cold gin and tonic and a boy in his birthday suit…and fast!

Each time you do it you'll learn more about your partner and what he likes. I recommend watching my personal porn hero, Ms. Jeanna Fine in any film she does. A good choice is one called *Erotic Obsession*. Hmmm, I think I should probably go review it again myself. Good luck and happy Hoovering!

Good Advice from a Very Bad Girl

"If the world were a logical place, men would ride side-saddle."
–Rita Mae Brown
The Good, the Bad and the Better

Slap my ass and call me Polly. Polly Theist that is. After this wacky week, I've come to realize that I worship many Gods. The Goddess of martinis, for instance: the God of "it could always be worse"; the Goddess of guts and gumption; the God of razors and romps; and the list gallops endlessly into the Goddess of sunsets.

Driving downtown this week on fumes and a prayer, I put my last forty-five cents into a happily discovered parking meter and walked the six blocks to the Old Town Clinic. It was just this red tape thing I had to do. I'll leave it at that. Up the stairs and into a dingy hallway, I swallowed my pride, inhaling what I imagined to be stadium full of second hand smoke. Looking around, I understood the odor was just on the clothes of the toothless, raspy voiced people waiting in line. I had to pee like a plugged up fountain, but was informed briskly by a pimple-faced lad that the restroom was out of order. Swell. I stood cross-legged in the waiting room, which was actually just a filthy hallway resembling the waiting room to hell in the movie, Beetlejuice. I stood, using those Kegel muscles for fifty minutes before Dr. Bitchface finally saw me. She was a nightmare with no bedside manner to speak of. Skedaddling out of there as fast as I could, I got to my truck to find a freakin' parking ticket...of course. After blurting a few well-chosen expletives, I zoomed off to work...and a bathroom. Halfway there, I ran out of gas and chugged to a stop in mid traffic on one of the busiest streets in the city. All I all, it was a day I could have very well done without.

Later that day, I had a blind date with a girl. Although she was nice, she was built like a boxcar. I hate to be superficial, but my personal ad wasn't advertising a walk on the beach type relationship, it simply asked for a girlie romp with a naughty lipstick lesbian. For the life of me, and after three glasses of Merlot, I couldn't picture her and I—as hard as I tried—in any sort of naughty scenario.

Mz. Conduct's House of Sin

She was definitely smitten with me, but I politely wrangled out of seeing her again, faster than you could say booty call.

I ventured out on a fun date to the comedy club. Lord knows I needed to laugh like a hyena for a couple of hours. Now, you can be amused, alarmed and downright petrified at the crowd in line. The comedy club in this city is like Velcro to the mullet heads and morbidly obese, who marinate themselves in Walgreen's perfume and hairspray. And Christ on a call girl, what's with the buttpacks! The fashion police were undoubtedly at some convention for middle aged men in bicycle shorts this week and weren't available on this evening. The comedian was hilarious, and did a mean impersonation of Christopher Walken. He had me coughing up my cocktail when he told a story about his girlfriend licking his asshole unexpectedly, saying, "All I could think of was, did I shower or shit last?" His routine was wonderfully nasty and just what I needed. After the show, in the smoking corner of the parking lot, I spotted him with his fifties-tough-guy look and felt compelled to have a conversation. After our brief chat, another enamored audience member came up to give him kudos. The fan was a cute New Yorker boy who had his mother and grandmother visiting. They adored the comedian and his filthy act and came screeching out waving their hands in the air. Video camera in hand, they proceeded to sidle up to the big comic saying, "Get our picture, get our picture!" Little old grandma was cute as could be; about as tall as she was wide, and smelling of gardenias in a loud floral dress. The comedian leaned over and flicked his tongue lewdly, like he was licking a bottomless pit. Grandma just giggled and SNAP went the picture. Too freakin' funny. These are moments that make my life worth living.

My neighbors had about seventy thousand pre-schoolers over for their kids' birthday bash, complete with the bizarre Mister Reptile Man. He drives a safari painted truck and carts around all sorts of reptiles and dresses up like a giant lizard. My neighbors are very nice and saw me sitting on my porch swilling alcoholic beverages, so they politely invited me over. I thought about Mister Reptile Man and wondered what his real lizard looked like, thought about all

Good Advice from a Very Bad Girl

the screaming children, about all the booze I had in me, and then I sensibly declined the offer. I could just see the headlines in the local boring newspaper, "Horny Harlot From The Hood Sexually Attacks Giant Lizard Man—Children Were Screaming!" Probably not a healthy scenario, I decided, so I just spruced up my cocktail and went inside.

Dear Mz. Conduct,

My fiancé and I met online and he moved here to Canada from Texas. At first we made love regularly, but now it is a rare occurrence. He says he loves me, but I am always going to bed alone…I feel I have to compete with this computer and the TV. What should I do?

Don't Feel The Loving

> **Dear DFTL,**
>
> First thing that comes to mind is, kill him in his sleep; but then there is all that messy clean up. Men can be such dim bulbs, but we can't read each other's minds either, you know. I would tell him just what you told me. Relationships require paying attention and constant work. The big lug from Texas may not have a corral full of cattle, if you know what I mean, so this may require careful explaining. Talk slowly, use pictures and a pointer if need be. Remember that George Dubya is a Texan too.
>
> If he's not willing to make an effort, just too stupid, or thinks you're asking too much—the well deserving princess that you are, no doubt—then go straight to your bedroom, get down your hatbox and all your best luggage and pack it full. If it's more important for him to get his fat, hairy assed, ya-ya's out by blasting aliens or sucking up cathode rays then you really must leave his sorry ass. Do it now before you screw up your life by marrying him. Honey, no meat whistle is that good!

Dear Mz. Conduct:

I have the hots for my roomie, but he has a girlfriend. She only comes to visit once a week and the rest of the week he and I spend late nights up talking and goofing off. The weird thing is, we never touch each other. No hugs, no patting shoulders, nothing. Then when we are sitting on the couch together watching a movie or something, if his foot touches mine accidentally (on purpose for me…) he jumps like I have electrocuted him. Does that mean he WANTS to touch me too, but has some guilty conscience thing about it? My mother told me she thinks there is some kind of weird sexual tension between us. I have no idea what she means. Does it mean he wants me, but has that guilty conscience thing about his girlfriend going on? So when I do touch him accidentally (or on purpose) it arouses him? I haven't ever seen a guy so jumpy and paranoid about touching feet or arms etc.

He asks me to stay up late with him, asks me to go see movies with him and we share so much in common. Half the time he is just freaking amazed that I like the same things he does. Art, music, books, all the things he loves, I love too, and we have the most incredible conversations. We talk for hours at night, until 3 a.m. sometimes. Sometimes he just pops into work and says hello. We work at the same place, along with our other roommate. He will ask when I am coming home, will I be home in time for a certain movie to start so we can watch it together, etc. Is this

Mz. Conduct's House of Sin

something I should pursue or just see what happens? He confuses me. He's a man, it's in his genetic code to confuse the opposite sex, I know.

Should I just wait on him? I try not to show interest, like obvious interest, but I find myself missing him when he isn't here, or staying home instead of going out just to spend time with him. I enjoy our talks and such. I am in the middle of getting a divorce and wonder sometimes if it's not just a rebound thing. I guess I really don't know what I'm doing. So maybe you can tell me what you think.

Thanks Mz. Conduct, you're my heroine…a naughty one, but a nice one too.

Romping Roomie Dreams

> **Dear RRD,**
>
> If you can say cum, you can say communication. Chimps in Speedos girl, you need to speak! This is ninety percent of everybody's damn problem, if you ask me, and you did.
>
> You're playing games and I feel the immediate need to bend you over my knee and spank the Cheez Whiz out of your brain. First of all, YES when your leg touches his, it sends a jolt up his spine and then back down again to his cock-a-doodle-doo. YES he feels guilty because he does have a relationship with someone else. He obviously has an equally fun time with you and has made you see that. No you should not "wait" for him. What you should do is sit down with him without touching any of his body parts, as that will distract him. Many men are visual creatures and have a hard time verbally expressing their emotions. For the most part, women seem to be blessed/cursed with a greater ease in this area. Ask him about his relationship with this other girl. Your mother is right. there is a lot of sexual tension between you. You have someone giving you attention and especially during a divorce this is a good thing. Just keep it in perspective. This could be balls o' fire or it could burn the freakin' house down and you'll be rooting around in ashes looking for your dildo. Tits on a timecard girl, you already work with him, so I caution you as a roommate to be careful.
>
> If it were me, I'd run my foot up his thigh and massage his bulging gristle, pin his wanton ass down and ride him into the sunset. But that's just me. If you really care for this guy then talk to him, see what he wants. Communicate verbally. If he is trying his best to be faithful to the girlfriend, but ridden with guilt of thoughts of being ridden by you, then get over it, respect that, and just be his pal and enjoy his company. Go to bed and beat off every night and leave it at that.
>
> Don't pass up any dates that come your way, force yourself to go out with mister bald spot even if you'd rather hang out with roomie boy. He may see you going out and eventually have a surge of testicle power and ask you out himself. Time will tell, and remember that tomorrow is another day as I puke up one cliché after another. My point is, you just don't know what will happen, that's the beauty of life.

Good Advice from a Very Bad Girl

"Sex is an emotion in motion."
—Mae West

Hickeys on a Hussy

After two French movies and a handy little house painter giving the House Of Sin a fresh new glow, this week has still been like a hangover at a church bazaar. I've been presented with tempting offers from suitors such as: "I've shaved my ass, can I show you?" and "If I promise not to leave a used condom on your floor, can we get together again?" Lord on a Longhorn, I swear some men don't have a clue. Even the Lil' Princess, having three too many cocktails at the Karaoke bar, jumped me and sucked my skin, leaving several high school hickeys on my neck and boob. What's a bad girl to do?

Mz. Lula la Paintbrush and I went to a favorite, dark, and crowded hang, where we swilled martinis and smoked ciggies, but ate healthy vegan entrees of course. Scanning the locale with disgust, we had a blatant realization that, ages ago, we had both been like the young spring chickens clogging the joint. If those boys only knew that we would break them in half. Now, Mz. Lula has been shtuping a Catholic priest for the good part of a decade, and I do so like to hear the sordid stories. She lassoed him with a pair of rosary beads and dipped him in her hole-y water; it's all so wickedly hilarious. I was raised by psychotic, flying nuns so, for me, her tales provide just one more olive in the martini, ya know? Bless me father, for I have sinned, it's been sixteen days since I gave my last blowjob. We also realize we'll be traveling to hell in a handtruck.

The Lil' Princess was looking through the community college catalog, deciding on which home improvement class to take. Enough of depending on men to come clean the gutters or repair that window, she's taking matters in to her own royal hands and I give her kudos for that. There were a whole slew of classes just on dating. Some of the classes were hilarious, and obviously geared at those poor helpless souls that haven't got a clue as to who the hell they are.

Mz. Conduct's House of Sin

There were class names like, "The Art of Being Single", which I guess, makes people feel better if they call it an art. Makes you feel like an artist in some dire respect. One class was called, "How to Make a Great First Impression." Ugh, Jesus in a jumpsuit, I should teach that class!

"Welcome class. Be your total self, nothing but yourself, so help the Goddess of Guttersluts, and if someone doesn't like it, then to Oz on a hotdog they go! Class dismissed, now give me your thirty bucks and I'll be at the bar."

PMS is biting at my heels again and at an inopportune time when I'm forced to re-plan all my dreams. Damn it all to hell, all the Billie Holiday tunes I can absorb, all the hair bleach I can apply, and all the gin I can swallow without getting alcohol poisoning just isn't working. Not this month. On the wee bright side of things, I do have a crazy plant in my garden this year. It's a climbing squash that has grown two-foot long zucchinis that hang down off the fence like giant green snakes. Perhaps they'll have more uses than one.

> Dear Mz. Conduct,
> My girlfriend is rail thin, and I like my women with some meat on their bones. I've often thought about asking her to gain weight, but I thought this might be overstepping my bounds. I love her personality, but I'm not attracted to her. Should I make a break for it and find a girl who is more my type? Should I tough it out because she is cool to be with? Or should I dare to step up to the dinner plate and ask her to gain a few extra pounds? What is the best thing to do?
> Confused in California
>
>> Dear CC,
>> The fact that this subject is bothering you enough to write to me about it says something about your character, and it's not a lot. You could point to Bettie Page posters and tell her that's what you like, and how she could really pull that look off if she'd just put on a few pounds. Who knows, maybe she can't gain that easily and you'll get slapped right then and there. I want to slap you too, just on principle (feet stomping up and down, tiara sliding off!) Honestly, you're probably some California surfer dude that wants all her weight gain to be in her 'rack.'
>>
>> I suppose I should be more compassionate towards you for not spouting the opposite complaint. I do agree with you for the most part; I like people with meat on their bones, muscles in their arms, something to not break in half when you're rocking the rodeo horse. I have madly loved big and beefy men and Amazonian women. I have loved skinny, little men, and drooled over petite little girls. It really is all in the attitude and the chemistry of the said person you love. Then again, you never used the word love, did you?

Good Advice from a Very Bad Girl

So, your relationship may not be that serious. Most likely not, or you'd be blinded by love and saying things like, "Oh baby, your shoulder bones sticking out remind me of angel wings," or "Damn, your skeletal profile makes for easy lifting," because that's what happens when you're truly in love.

I remember the Transient Trollop and I walking ninety-seven blocks in the pouring rain, to the shop she insisted on dragging me to each week, just to get her precious imported cigarettes. Well, lo and behold, as we walked, bitching profoundly, up popped the guy in the band that we had been slobbering over from afar for a goddamn year! Just drop dead gorgeous with the look of Elvis slathered all over him. We caught up to him, one of us on each side, and proceeded see what he was about. Close to ten moronic sentences later, we looked at each other behind his black pompadour and rolled our eyes. We said a prompt good-bye and screeched all the way home at what seemed his endless lack of intellect. My point is that beauty is in the eye of the beholder and if you don't like what you be holding, then off you go. Quit complaining.

Dear Mz. Conduct,

I'm a straight girl that has been thinking about being with another girl sexually for a very long time. As I get older I am feeling more comfortable with my own self and don't want to regret not trying something that I feel consumed with at times. I don't have a boyfriend right now and think this may be the right time, but how do I go about doing this?

Missing Piece

Dear MP,

You trot your ass over to my house and let me fix you an extremely dry, three olive martini. Seriously, you are not alone and that's a plus right there. Think of how many women there are in the world wanting to wrestle with the same issues and tissues. You could go to a club and hang out, be yourself and have a cocktail, which is my motto, by the way. You can always put an ad in your local rag, as that's been the most prosperous and interesting way to go, at least for me. Classify yourself as bi-curious if/when you place your ad and that gives the reader more of an idea of what you're about.

As I've said in previous columns, the Transient Trollop and I are forming the Old Lesbians Club. All my straight girlfriends are hankering to join the club and love the idea. At the end of our days we will smoke through long cigarette holders, drink gin from Dixie cups, mud-thick coffee from broken china, and Bloody Marys from combat boots. We'll shave our legs (maybe) at the kitchen table and paint each other's toenails with Rape-Me Red. We will always have lipstick on, pointed cup bras and men's boxer shorts. What little hair we have left on our heads will be bleached and coiffed to no end and on occasion, we'll bring home a penis to share. We will then ridicule it, reminisce over it, damn it all to hell, and pour each other a bit more gin. Amen.

Mz. Conduct's House of Sin

"Sometimes being a bitch is all a woman has to hold on to."
–Dolores Claiborne

B is for Bitch

Being sweet and wonderful to all living things can only get you so far in this world. There comes a time when you have to reach deep down inside yourself, grab that inner bitch by the scruff of the neck and piss her off enough to take control. Everything cannot always be peachy, as I told Cinderella Cyber-twat this week. As a matter of fact, I feel like puking up peaches when I hear voices too chipper. Speaking of which, I'd like to throw those high-voiced cha'chas into a wood chipper and yell over the grinding, "Things still freakin' peachy now, honey?" and then I'd have a cocktail. Love can be so incredibly blind, and without a seeing-eye dog, a girl can get screwed without even getting laid. This is when the bitch needs to come out and play. Think of it as a survival tactic that can save some sanity and bring back a little dignity. My thought for the day. The Transient Trollop reminds me: there is love and then there is reality. With a roof over her head, a cocktail in her hand, and the little Mexi Man ex between her thighs, she's content for the time. She's my amazing Amazonian, and together we put the fun in dysfunctional.

My son comes back from Spain this week and I'm almost beside myself with anxiety. The last time I spoke with him he was in Paris arguing with some French woman about his self-allotted pay phone time. By the time I hung up, I imagined them sword fighting with baguettes. I'm sure I'll be a blathering mess at the airport in my heavy lipstick and heels. He'll be so proud. I can rest assured with at least one accomplishment in my life. I know for a fact that there is one man out there, who not only is brutally honest (let's face it, that's the most respectful thing you can be), but a man who knows how to treat a woman. After all, he grew up listening to the Transient Trollop, the Royal Diva, and I continually screeching—over cocktails of course —about the subhuman swine that men can be. My son is one man I won't ever have to loan my testicles to.

Good Advice from a Very Bad Girl

The Lil' Princess has slipped in to some sort of functional coma and has literally lowered herself to some undeserving men. The Mz. Conduct bitch speech has been vigorously applied and she is honing a proper perspective. She did give one fellow a blast of what he deserved as she was releasing her gasses in his pathetic face…and I am proud to be a sponsor.

I'll be going up to Seattle next weekend for the Royal Diva's wedding bash. She is a celebrity up there with her jazzy bad-ass self so there should be some yummy tidbits to nibble on at the reception…and probably good food too. Needless to say, I bought her and her man a fabulous vintage cocktail shaker with glasses to match, and a hoochie mama dress for her to slide her beautiful brown form into when she's performing in her Ms. Kitty Wampus gig.

I had flowers sent to me, as I should, and if all men realized what this does for me, they'd be sending them by the truckloads. They weren't sent for a sympathetic "Oh you're all alone now after your divorce" but for a celebratory "Kudos, you're strong and man-less in mid-life" occasion. That sentiment makes my voracious vulva all aflutter. I'm also expecting a Sapphire gin care package from a wonderful couple that will surely tickle my fancy (my fancy? That's right next to my uvula). I suddenly seem to have more porn star wienies than I know what to do with, but unless one is strapped to an Amazon bitch, I am not remotely interested for now. So onward and upward goes life, as I sit in my men's pajamas on a freakin' Saturday night, stiff cocktail in hand, tiny penis ice cubes floating inside, I will sign off like the Transient Trollop does…'fuck me running.'

Dear Mz. Conduct,
I know that having a large penis is supposed to be every man's dream, but it has been nothing but trouble for me. I have problems keeping a girlfriend because of it. Many girls have said it hurts them, and as far as oral favors, well most don't even want to attempt it. It's pretty long, but really wide too. What am I to do, and please don't tell me to date whores.
Big Bad Johnson
   Dear BBJ,

Mz. Conduct's House of Sin

Christ in a cocktail, what's your freakin' problem? Oh, you just told me didn't you? I must've drifted while reading and now my naughty reverie has been interrupted by a need for response. Literal, that is.

Okay, so you have a porn star scrumper wand. Hey that's it! You can make a fortune by doing porn films! Seriously, it is an area you may want to look into, or you can decide you're gay. I have never heard a gay man complain about a big ol' wienie.

Now, some fellows have such wide weenies that it does hurt us tight-twatted tramps after hours of pounding. Other lads have extra long schlongs that can bang the cervix and cause some pain, especially if the girl has a tipped uterus, which by the way isn't that uncommon. So, cowboy, go easy. Be gentle and thoughtful and get her wetter than a Slip 'n Slide before you introduce the big boy.

My thought is that, hmmmm...bite sized people come out of that very same hole so, my advice to all your past girls is: pain heals fast, quit your whining, take it and like it, oh and practice your Kegels afterwards. In the meantime make some movies and send them to Mz. Conduct. Don't worry, baby, you will find the right partner someday, I promise.

Dear Mz. Conduct,

I work in a professional environment and this one man and I have been having little meetings after work. We'd been flirting friends for years, but recently it's gotten a little steamier. We meet in the coffee room and sometimes in one of the exam rooms. I always unzip him immediately and devour his beefy penis right on the spot. It doesn't take him long to orgasm, which is fine by me. I know he must like what I do. I'm also aware that part of the thrill of doing this is that we could get in hot water if discovered.

Lately though, I feel the need for more from this guy. He does have a woman he lives with, but I know he's not happy. The other day he was driving home and left a message on my phone telling me, "my dick is throbbing for your mouth and I'm heading to your house." I couldn't believe he'd just leave such an assuming message and am sure glad my kids didn't hear it! What should I do now?

Bottom Feeder

> **Dear BF,**
>
> I can surely relate to your oral fixation of the male appendage, as Mz. Conduct has a wee bit of a monkey on her back with that herself. A monkey with an erection at that! Be sure you want to do what you're doing, and if there are strings attached, on either of your ends, then curb your urges, honey.
>
> You've known this guy for years, so he should respect your friendship above all. So when you tie his arms and legs up with rusty, wire hangers on your front lawn and have the neighbor dogs line up to do their business on him, he should understand.
>
> Hey, if you get yourself on the same page, let him know what an assuming, asinine, prick he was to leave such a message at your home. If you don't mind that he'll stay with the woman he lives with no matter how much you polish his knob, then keep on keepin' on. Sure he likes what you do to him, his woman probably hasn't touched his penis in years, let alone admire it, but remember that if you want more you may not get it. It's a thrill thang, as you said. He obviously has no real respect for you, and if confronted—which is what you should do in any case—he'll probably pour out the apologies. He'll be sorry all

right, as the front of his pants expand and "throb for your mouth." Sorry, yes he is, move on.

Mz. Conduct's House of Sin

"From the moment I was six I felt sexy. And let me tell you it was hell, sheer hell waiting to do something about it."
–Bette Davis

The Museum of Erotica

Oh, how I wish Mz. Davis was still alive. I can imagine us having cocktails and discussing our shameless sameness.

What a wild couple of weeks it's been. After 9/11, I think it's time we all get back to it, as sickening and sad as the loss of lives continues to be. Falling prey to demons isn't my cup of tea. And by the way, I think it's just dandy that everyone wants to have American flags splayed across their foreheads, but some people should use that room for brain cells to expand. The other day there was a Buick in front of me, spewing out black smoke and driving along with a huge flag in the back window. The driver tossed out what looked to be the contents of his ashtray. A lovely, non-biodegradable, show of patriotism there. I heard another proud American say, 'every Middle Eastern person that lives in this country should turn themselves in.' To me, these people are an absolute embarrassment. I immediately needed a double martini along with several Spanish olives that my son brought back from Spain.

Speaking of which, the prodigal son returns with viciously delicious stories and gifts from afar. He brought me a brochure from the Museu de l' Erotica in Barcelona that was right up my alley. He told me it was a good thing I wasn't at the museum, they might of hauled me out of the place for lewd and lascivious behavior. There happens to be a beautiful, ten-foot tall, carved sandalwood penis that I surely would've loved to throw my arms around in glee, as the girl in the brochure photo was doing. Another photo from the brochure depicts an eighteen-century sadomasochistic contraption that holds a person-using metal and leather straps—face down and arched up and ready for a thrashing, pounding, or caning. It sits in a real dungeon with stone walls and a cold cement floor. Not the warmly heated dungeons I've seen with plush carpet and swanky décor, this was the real thing baby! Of course it is a more civilized age now, in some respects anyway. Oh, and the best thing in the brochure is called, "the pleasure chair" which is a huge, entirely metal chair complete with ankle and wrist restraints. It has several enormous, fleshy penises hanging from it. One of these beauties is under the seat of the chair and attached to a mechanical device that gets it cranking. It looks deliciously wicked, and I am dreaming of such devices each night.

The next week, I went up to Seattle to see the Royal Diva and her man get hitched into an abyss of matrimonial bliss. It was smack on the oceanfront, an eighty degree afternoon with sailboats lacing the Sound and Stevie Wonder music in the background. Ahh, being the Royal Diva that she is, she had French champagne (that I had a difficult time getting enough of), and was therefore looped by the time the ceremony got underway. No hunky man tidbits to nibble on, although the food was marvelous. I had my roving eyes on the photographer, but gave up the thought of him in a loincloth when the Lil' Princess noticed him eying my son like a bowl of whipped cream. Damn, that happens a lot.

We all chatted up a yuppie couple who bragged about taking their sixty-foot sailboat out in the San Juan Islands. Their poor dog just couldn't get comfortable and it was such a hardship. I was wearing my twenty-six dollar outfit, overdrawn in my pathetic-as-always bank account, but what the hell, I just poured myself more champagne. The yuppies did however redeem themselves from having my nail file surgically removed from the woman's overly tanned forehead: they almost had a stroke when my son called me 'mom.' They thought I was his date and just couldn't believe my age. Well, that warranted yet another glass of champagne for moi. The Royal Diva, looking like a chunk of heaven itself, walked down the path of rose petals to Stevie Wonder's "Ribbon in the Sky." That did it for me, I turned into a blubbering heap of champagne soaked, rayon covered flesh. Her own mother was more composed than I was, but it was a day of special meaning for me so, again, what the hell.

Mz. Conduct's House of Sin

I partied in Seattle that night at a funky, little dive called the NiteLite. The Lil' Princess—chauffeur extraordinaire—was with me. We met a drunken, wide-eyed boy in overalls consumed in a dart game until he saw us. The Lil' Princess played darts only on a challenge, hitting a bulls-eye right off the bat, and humorously humiliating the corn-fed bourbon drinker. I decided he needed more humiliation, so when he started boasting about his large appendage, I told him I carry a tape measure in my purse just for these moments. I dared him, he took it and we stepped into the girl's bathroom...and as I figured, he was once again humiliated.

I spent some quality time with my ninety-year old artists/friends, and was given an amazing photograph of mister Mark Twain himself. It was taken but my friend's father when she was five. They were great friends I was told. Amazing. Samuel Clemens is in the house! I felt as if I had won the lottery. All my friend remembers of Mr. Twain is him laying on a chaise lounge in poor health and she begging her mother to take her home. I told her jokingly, "but this was Mark Twain!" And she sprightly replied, "I was only five, I didn't give a damn." With that said, she stepped outside with her ninety-three year old self, her ninety-year-old sister-in-law, and her earring wearing, ninety-two year old husband, and poured a small glass of red wine and lit up a cigarette. I knew right then that life at its longest can be a blast.

Dear Mz. Conduct,
I've been seeing a woman for a few months, nothing serious, just dinner every few weeks or so. The last two times we went out, she wouldn't stop telling me I need to gain some weight. I am a thin man, in somewhat good shape and like my body just fine. At first I just laughed it off, but the last time she wouldn't let up and it was getting on my nerves. I personally think she could lose a little weight, but being a gentleman, I would never say that to her, even in teasing. What should I do about this?
The Thin Man

> **Dear TM,**
> Since you've just dated this woman casually and for such a short time, I say have one more dinner, a farewell dinner. Maybe at one of those white trash, all-you-can eat, buffet joints. Pile up on all the high calorie foods and chomp yourself into a complete and utter frenzy, then casually look over and tell her that it's just a damn shame she can't put it away like you can.
>
> Barfing Barbie at the snack bar, most women are pissing over their man being too pudgy. You are who you are, and if she doesn't like it then she can hitch it

to hell in a hatbox. Also a point to consider; if she's trying to change your weight now then think of what it would be like down the line. Next year she may want your full head of hair to disappear or perhaps you'll be just too sex driven. Oh I can't even think about this anymore, gawd! Where is that skinny boy with that sweet talk and the mean martini?

Dump the broad like a hot potato smothered in butter. Then pick it up at eat it...because you can.

Dear Mz. Conduct,

I seem to always sabotage my relationships. I have met several great women over the years, but each and every time the relationship comes to a crashing end. It seems that as soon as one relationship gets going really well, I meet someone else that I pine away for. When the woman I'm with wants more from me I can't give it, out of fear that this new woman will be perfect. She inevitably gets mad and dumps me. When I pursue the new woman, it always turns out that she's not what I thought or that she isn't interested. Help me oh Goddess!

Greener Grass Gary

Dear GGG,

Remember, the grass is always greener because that's where the septic tank is. Besides being a dolt, you are going to have to learn some things. One, life holds no guarantees about anything and as John Lennon said, "The love you take is equal to the love you make."

Two, there is no such thing as the perfect woman. You keep experiencing this revelation over and over yet your skull remains thick and Neanderthal like. Of course the intelligent girls dump you because they can see straight through you. Trying to finagle your way into their lives when you already have a good relationship going isn't attractive.

You're going to have to realize that you are missing out on potentially good things by not focusing your attentions where they need to be. You are selfish and gluttonous and probably one of those kids who was eyeing the candy dish as you were polishing off the birthday cake at some undeserving kid's party.

Think of this as a disorder. It's going to take some effort on your part. No matter how perfect a woman is you will always find flaws in them. This is expected, and it is okay, this is life with a capital L. When you reach that point, and only you will know when you do, focus on all the things good in that person. How they make you feel, what they bring to your life, what and how you can make them happy. When you focus your energy on these things, it comes back to you ten-fold, I promise. Sure you can desire others, that's also a fact of life, but remember all of the things that brought you to the woman you are with and if it still feels good then work at it. If it doesn't, and there is some real problem with the way you feel, then you can move on. Don't expect things with the women you pine and pound away for, because you will almost always be disappointed. The next woman that you're with, and amazingly enough there will be a next time, deserves your respect and attention...more than you deserve hers.

Mz. Conduct's House of Sin

"Too much awareness, without the accompanying experience, is a skeleton without the flesh of life."
–Anais Nin

No Mints on the Pillow at the Heartbreak Hotel

Traveling through this life, I found the perfect metaphor for mine: There are no clean sheets at the Heartbreak Hotel. There are no mints on the pillow, no fragrant little soaps, and certainly no room service. Though if you look carefully behind the commode, you may find a plunger.

I've been reading a lot of Henry Miller lately and feeling a past life calling. I'm hearing stories of a friend's year-long stay in France and looking at pictures of Paris streets and cafes. I made a decision to become an expatriate at some point. If David Sedaris can learn French then so can I. He says you can even smoke cigarettes in the bank! Gawd, I'd go just for that. I'll ride down the cobblestone streets on my big, red bicycle, and have three things in my bike basket: my notebook, a baguette, and a weenie dog dressed in some hideous costume, no doubt. He may sport a beret, an ascot, and, just to confuse the poor thing more, a salmon-colored tutu. I was telling my dream to the Transient Trollop who, amazingly enough, is not planning on moving anywhere soon and seems devoted to her multi-talented man. Anyway, she said I should be careful after my many glasses of daily swilling, not to get the baguette and the weenie dog mixed up. Good point. It's important to keep dreams alive and if one goes down the toilet, then you find that damn plunger.

So I had a big, welcome home bash for the boy who's traveled the world. My son has ridden camels across the Sahara, slept in the middle of a Turkish train station, walked lost in the streets of Amsterdam obliterated into oblivion, jumped of sixty-foot cliffs on a Greek island, and climbed the Eiffel Tower at night, but he hasn't been to one of Mz. Conduct's parties in a very long time. I just live to throw parties, swirling around for days, as I dig out all my sixties hors d'oeuvres Lazy Susan trays, martini shakers, glasses and cocktail stirrers. Baking and feathering and blending and chopping…I love it all. Preparing for

Good Advice from a Very Bad Girl

the bash, I did defy death once, as the dogs looked on casually. They've seen this before. I teetered on a non-secured ladder, stringing tiki lights all across the backyard and in my tizzy, caught myself from falling and almost decapitated myself on the clothesline. I'm sure my dogs would've just played fetch with my head and looked at my mangled remains with a "Can we go to the park?" expression, as they do when they get a new toy. That would have ruined the whole damn party.

The evening of the party started with sizzling temperatures and a pink sunset and guests who seemed to gather endlessly. The glow of colored lights, BBQ smoke curling through the yard, overflowing ice buckets, and an eclectic array of music; Frank Sinatra followed by The Police, Al Green, and Johnny Cash. The shin-dig then slid into inebriated cross-gendered wrestling, annoying announcements of low self esteem, bitch-slapping, nasty girl dancing, sex in my bed (without me), gay boys from another planet, and me booting out my guest from Seattle when he asked me to marry him. He didn't like my answer and started some uncalled for drama. It was nothing out of the ordinary for a Mz. Conduct party. No matter the clean up: condom wrappers in my bedroom, empty bottles of gin with golf tees in them, toppled over lawn chairs, and the various pairs of non-matching shoes found throughout the house, it's always worth it to me!

Dear Mz. Conduct,

I met a woman, a very attractive and sensual woman. She pointed out to me that she considers having her pussy sucked to be an annoyance. She further explained that "penetration" as she calls it (I prefer the word fuck) is what a man should focus on.

Upon hearing this, I thought to myself, "How boring." I'd prefer the complete opposite: a woman who wanted her pussy sucked many times a day.

My question, Mz. Conduct, is in your opinion, what do women really want? Am I confused here? I enjoy reading the past stories from your column. It seems to me that men should back off on the ego talk and practice applying their mouths appropriately.

Mouthy Man

Dear MM,

Mz. Conduct's House of Sin

Yes, you are confused, but I won't hold it against you. It's very difficult for men sometimes to know what women are thinking, feeling, and wanting. It goes back to that hormonal difference that our species possess.

Each one of us differ in many ways, as well as in what we like. One thing I think we can all agree on is that we like a man who takes enough of an interest to find out exactly what that may be by asking. Some women don't tell you, and haven't any idea what it is they want either, and that always poses a problem. You really have to be patient and figure it out with those women. You would get Mz. Conduct's Purple Weenie Award for that! Or you can choose not involve yourself with a woman who is confused herself, it's up to you. Let some other poor slob take them on.

Some women just don't like the stimulation from oral sex. It's the same confounded conundrum that makes me wonder why some men don't care for their penis to be swallowed. Those men are few and far between, but exist nevertheless.

One reason for a woman not wanting her snatch to be devoured may be because of a medication she's taking. Some anti-depressants, which everyone seems to be popping these days, can cause the nerve endings to lose sensation, sometimes creating numbness, or what your friend may call "an annoyance." We all have our preferences and some of us are just more orally driven than others. It's sad to me that your friend wants to "focus on penetration" when so many men get verbal abuse for just the opposite. Bottom line is that each woman is different and hallelujah when we can find someone that we connect with or compromise with.

Either respect her wishes or continue your search for a sexually compatible woman. I believe I saw some on sale at the local Blow-Up-Doll Mart.

Dear Mz. Conduct,

My boyfriend is great in every way, but one. He takes me out and treats me like a lady and we have amazing sex. The thing that bothers me is that he knows how much I love flowers—I was a florist for many years—yet he has never in the seven years we've been dating, bought me flowers!

When my birthday rolls around or our anniversary comes along, I think maybe this time, but no, never once! What should I do?

Flower Girl

> Dear FG,
>
> Well, you are a woman after my own heart, I must say. Meaning, along with reeling from a bouquet, we also feel compelled to bitch about something just for the sake of bitching. Why don't men understand that flowers can heal the heart, soothe the soiled soul and make anything just that much better? Well, maybe it's because roses don't have football scores printed on their petals, or hyacinths don't smell like cigars, I don't know. They're just dolts in this area, unless they're gay of course, in which they still wouldn't bring us those meticulous arrangements. They bring those to the guy in the Prada suit and the perfect freakin' sideburns.
>
> It's a rare man who can understand this flower power, but here you are enveloped in all his other charms and you're complaining about the lack of lilies. Marigolds on a Maxipad woman, as you go fuckety-fuck in la-la land, realize that at least you're getting the mighty stiff one, you're being treated like a lady as you seem to enjoy, so my advice is learn to buy your own damn flowers and shut the hell up!

Good Advice from a Very Bad Girl

"Imperious, choleric, irascible, extreme in everything, with a dissolute imagination the like of which has never been seen, atheistic to the point of fanaticism, there you have me in a nutshell, and kill me again or take me as I am, for I shall not change."
–Marquis de Sade, *from his* Last Will and Testament

Don't Hose Without a Hat

This week has been one vicious cycle after another, the men without testicles syndrome has been prevalent again. Why don't we women stop trying to change this fact? We are relentless, but we sure have spirit! We can juggle, jiggle and work things out and for the most part, in a sensible manner. And we have balls! They're just really tiny and hide in our clitorises.

The Transient Trollop caught her man lying through his ready-to-be knocked-out teeth about dipping his stick in his ex-girlfriend. The Lil' Princess is confronted by a higher authority about sneaky snacking with her married man after hours in the workplace, but when it comes to accepting an invite to her house, well whoa Nelly, that won't fly for him. Mz. Lula La Paintbrush can't get her Catholic priest to leave the priesthood even after ten years of showing him a real religious experience. Wonder Waitress has been deceivingly put on hold by a Canadian goose who has to "think things out for awhile" as his wife tightens the shackles. Cinderella Cyber-twat has filed for divorce, but her also married boyfriend claims one excuse after another, as to why he has to hold off on divorce with his ball and chain. Mz. Conduct herself has decided to get a really big net and go lion hunting in search of the vertebrae voided Lion King.

These men profess their undying love to us, they are completely happy when with us, we rock their world and blah, blah, and freakin' blah, yet they misplace their backbone when it comes to making changes in their lives. They want their cake and to eat everyone too. I suppose they're afraid of confrontation with a wife that won't let go. They feel sorry for them, pity their being alone, feel an obligation that overwhelms them with guilt, and don't want to deal with the paperwork. Men think with their heads—both of them—and

Mz. Conduct's House of Sin

women tend to think with their hearts in these matters. I think it's admirable to hold on to something you love and fight for what's yours, but it's also important to know that you really can't own a person. Indigence is so unattractive. Do we really want spineless men like this, girls? If they didn't come with those damn pretty weenies attached, we'd really have no use for them. Oh hell, life is short, and titties on a Triscuit, I just hope we all don't get anthrax by Christmas. That'd be such a buzzkill.

Dear Mz. Conduct,

I have a question about birth control. I'm on the pill but I want to use another form of birth control just as a back up. I don't want to use condoms. I was thinking of spermicide, but I was just wondering if there are any interactions between the chemicals in spermicide and the chemicals in orthotricyclen, my pill, that I should know about. Is there any reason that I can't use both at the same time?

Wondering in Washington

>Dear WIW,
>
>Garters on a gargoyle, girl, I suggest you avoid condoms with spermicide all together. Actually, I don't recommend using spermicide to anyone and think it can be quite harmful. There are so many uncontrolled toxins in our life already, why would you want to add any more? Nonoxynol-9 is a chemical detergent! It's a rather harsh chemical and can cause itching, burning, rashes, infections, sores, etc. Also, it was believed that N-9 was helpful against the spread of HIV (since it was shown to kill bacteria in clinical tests). Now, though, it seems that it actually makes the transmittal of HIV more likely. Because it can cause sores and goobers and such on the walls of the vagina (not fun honey), it makes the transmittal of HIV more likely (since HIV has more direct access).
>
>In 1994, *Out* magazine printed this article on Nonoxynol-9 that you may want to read, http://www.walnet.org/csis/news/usa_94/out-9402.html
>
>If you're taking the pill correctly, then that's a pretty sure-fire method. Of course you could always give your boyfriend Mz. Conduct's easy home vasectomy, especially if they've misbehaved, which inevitably they all do.

I've been dating this guy for the past 3 months, and we have not had sex yet, but we both want to. I have been saying no, but now I am ready. Does it matter if the guy or the girl buys the condoms? I have never bought them before. What are the best ones to buy? Is there any particular style, flavor or color guys prefer?

Courtney Condom Hunter

>Dear CCH,
>
>Yes it matters. You should both buy them. It's good to avoid situations where you're all worked up, sweatin' and dry humpin' and you start screaming for the big weenie insertion, only to realize that each of you thought the other would supply a condom. Personally I like to have a nice little box behind my bed (and sometimes in my bed…mmmm) full of several varieties. It's also a good idea to keep one or two in your purse just in case you have one of those bathroom encounters, but then that's just me, the gutterslut, talking. Hey, it doesn't hurt. People like different brands and styles, but I like the Lifestyles brand, Ultra

Sensitive with no lubricant. Also, the Kimono brands are nice. They have a Micro-Thin Plus that is strong yet very thin.

Oh, and despite their advertisements, ribbed condoms generally do not add any real sensation for either partner.

Check out this site as well, http://www.condom.com/index.html and happy humping honeypie!

Mz. Conduct's House of Sin

"Do you really think it is weakness that yields to temptation? I tell you that there are terrible temptations that it requires strength, strength and courage, to yield to."
–Oscar Wilde

"Please spank me, I really want you to, please," begged my cross-dresser comrade, Mister Bo Dangles, at the fetish bash I went to last weekend. I keep saying no, but since he shaved, I may change my mind someday. But I doubt it. "You're such a bitch" he pouted in a whiny, but nice way. We were watching videos of the famed fetish photographer, Charles Gatewood, www.charlesgatewood.com, who was the honorable guest of the party. The girls in the video were shaving and spanking each other and I pointed out that that's what I would spank.

Mister Wild Bill and his amazing appendage escorted me to the big Victorian house. He was looking quite fetching in his latex pants and black suit jacket. The evening was an interesting mix of SCA (Society for Creative Anachronism) members, obese drag queens, voluptuous dancing girls, beautiful punkettes in Catholic school girl attire, some of the D/s crowd, a tall beauty with a very tight corset and white contacts in her eyes, and a slew of other freaks like me.

I dressed conservatively naughty. As always, I wore all black, which consisted of my wet leather heels that are taller than most guys' dicks, my crotchless, lace body stocking under a very short, black, pleated skirt with a long and low-cut matching jacket. By the end of the evening I felt a little over dressed. I tore myself away from a salivating strip tease to go upstairs and watch two deliciously licentious girls using an electricity wand.* Oh I just had to participate! Wild Bill and I both like it, and all the assorted attachments. The wand feels like a million tiny, hot, glowing needles pulsating all over your body or at least the parts you choose to subject. It's a rather yummy sensation if you get off on a little pleasure/pain. Like the lovely and royal subject of the moment said, "It's easy to become an electricity slut!" Uh-oh!

Good Advice from a Very Bad Girl

After a nightmare of an outing the evening before, a death defying debacle, a never-going-to happen-again evening with the Wonder Waitress, and on top of sporting a gruesome hangover and three hours of sleep, it was a downright miracle I made it out again. My thirty-four a day vitamins didn't seem to help my motivation much. Perhaps a wee little electrical jolt would've helped me out. See, I can't get my mind off that 'current event'!

Dear Mz. Conduct,

Hi there. Love your writing and I have a conundrum for you which you have probably heard before. Basically, I love getting blowjobs, but my girlfriend has only given me one (perhaps two—I was drunk) in the last two years. It's getting to the point where I am really craving one. I realize I should talk to her about this, but can't seem to bring it up. What on earth should I do, aside from visiting a $40 an hour call girl?

Mr. Needs-One

> **Dear MNO,**
>
> **First of all, mister bobbing for boners, you will not get a call girl to suck your needy appendage for forty bucks, more like $200 at a decent escort service. You may however get that tube-topped, stringy-haired crack-whore that walks the main drag to blow your bulge for about that much.**
>
> **So, the two times your girlfriend has pleasured you orally, did you just cram your wad into her mouth and pound away until your stream of excitement released itself down her throat (Whew! is it hot in here or what? Hey not all girls are like me, ok?) Some women would not especially like that.**
>
> **While I do sympathize with you, you said it yourself; you should discuss your cravings with your girlfriend. Just don't force the issue. Ask her about her fantasies, her passions, and her secret fires burning below. Communication is the key to all healthy relationships, sexual or any other, keep that in mind. If you make her feel uncomfortable or pressured, it will only push her away. The idea is to make your lady feel like your absolute queen. Do all the things she requires and desires and the next time—this is after you have discussed your wishes and depending on her openness to it—devour her flower and then ease into asking if she'd try the 69 position with you. If she doesn't want it stuffed down to her uvula, then ask her to just kiss it, around it, under it, get familiar with the damn thing for gonads sake! Okay, I've gotten myself all worked up now. Where is that hairless boy with the ice bucket?**
>
> **Make sure you're trimmed and neat around your penis because I don't care how spectacular a man's schlong is, if it's all nappy and covered with hair, I wouldn't touch it, unless I have a razor in hand. That may be something she'd like and hasn't thought about. Groom your region and ask her if she likes it. It's start.**

Dear Mz. Conduct,

I have been going out with a woman for several months, but just as friends. She hasn't wanted it to go any further than a hug and a golf game. That's been fine with me, but then one night she made it clear she wanted more. I gave her more and it was great.

Mz. Conduct's House of Sin

She asked me to come over the night after that and when I told her that was fine, but that I had dinner plans with my ex-girlfriend to attend first, she blew up at me. She suddenly became a jealous and possessive woman. She's met my ex-girlfriend and knows we are, and have been, platonic friends only for almost a decade. I wouldn't change that for anything and I value my ex's friendship more than anything.

I guess I'm confused, I don't know why she's acting this way after such a long period of "just wanting to be buddies." She's asked me to not see my ex now and this upsets me because I really do like this woman, or did until she's turned over this side of her. What should I do about this?

Lost In Space

> Dear LIS,
>
> Cockring on a cannoli man, lose the bitch! I've been in a similar predicament myself and must say that there is no room in this world for insecure, indigent, possessive, women such as she. I could see if you were slipping it to the ex from time to time, or if you lied about your relationship with the ex or whatever, but you didn't. She wanted no sexual part of you until she felt she could control you, or so it sounds, and then thinks that putting out the pussycat will anchor you in. Ha! No woman is that good! Well, maybe me, but that's beside the point.
>
> Have a little tête-à-tête with the girl and tell her you will not be controlled and if she doesn't like it she can take her precious twat and hit someone else's bucket of balls. Mz. Conduct has faith in you conjuring up a set for yourself (yeah right).

*The toy known as a "violet wand" rather resembles a hand-held power tool with little glass bulbs sticking out of one end. When turned on, the bulb glows violet and crackles; touching it will cause static sparks to jump to your skin, with an associated "zap!" and a sharp shock. These do not send current through the body, and are safe for use anywhere except the eyes or major nerve clusters (i.e. the top of the spine) — though prolonged use will burn the skin.

Good Advice from a Very Bad Girl

"I've and got hampers and hampers of ironing and my diet pill is wearing off!"
–Divine (from Hairspray)

Mz. Conduct's ass is yummy, yummy sore and has delightful red and black stripes across it due to a fun play session with Mister Bo Dangles. We set out to find him a Halloween costume and wound up elsewhere. I'll leave it at that for now.

I was supposed to go to a Polyween/fetish party and had my gig already to go when Not Your Average Joe decided he didn't have time to go get the dress that he promised me. There was a major dress debacle that night, let me tell you. For some reason the boys that were going to the party with me didn't see the importance of me having that dress. Well, being the bratty bitch that I am, I wouldn't go unless I had that dress and stomped my vinyl-clad feet, pouting and whining. The dress, still on hold by the way, is a sheer, black, completely lace, slip type number and it's just screaming my name all the way from downtown. So, it got to be too damned late, and after such an unorganized mess, I pulled on my sweats and poured myself some gin and dammit all to hell and back, I was pissed. Still am, can you tell? Oh, but then I find out that one of my boys went without me! Ha! Can you say minced-up-monkey-meat? Mister Not Your Average Joe had a dildo dance with a hot chickadee and where was I? On the couch, sucking gin off my ice cubes, and in my freakin' sweats! Ugh! My bleached blonde hair is standing on end right now, even more than usual. You know what? I will get that dress and oh baby, sooooo much more. When I do go out next time, ready for a ravenous rendezvous, I will look as if I could eat the world and suck on the pit. Question is, who will be the deserving one to accompany me?

I finally got it through my thick skull, thanks to lectures from Ruby Liscious and the Royal Diva, that with some boys you really have to demand what you so rightly deserve. Okay, I did also watch the movie *Jackie Brown* for about the seven hundredth time, to reboot my empowered self. She is just so freakin' hot. A Goddess shouldn't have to ask for the proper attention, but lets' face it, unless you do, you won't get crap on a coaster. I've had a hard time with that because I'm so damn freakin' sweet, but oh yeah, I think I got it down now!

Ms. Lula la Paintbrush has done some demanding herself with the Catholic priest of hers. After her diatribe, he was promising her all sorts of unholy acts when next she sees him. Apparently he's discovered a bountiful sex shop to take her shopping at, and an appropriately swanky-sleazy motel to romp around in. I wonder when he found the joints, myself; probably in between fingering the day's rosary and giving communion to some devout and shriveled, little Catholic woman. The sex shop is supposedly a splendid shop full of merciful attire and ungodly toys, one that he's saying penance for even now, I'm sure. Thank God for that.

I was at my dear friend's, my very own spanking Yippie mentor, and happened to meet his long time buddy, distinguished Professor of Education at the University of Illinois and author of the new book *Fugitive Days*, Bill Ayers. He signed a book for me in special Mz. Conduct form and we yakked up a storm for hours. It was absolutely fabulous. I sincerely love sitting with a man who was on the FBI's most wanted list ten years ago, and my mentor, who among his zillion wild stories, used to hold Yoko Ono up when she was high on methadone. Sigh. Bill's book is described as such:

This memoir is by a '60s political activist who went underground after the famous Greenwich Village townhouse explosion in 1970. Ayers tells of the political and cultural influences that radicalized him, his life in the Weather Underground prior to the explosion, his life on the run, and what happened to him after he turned himself in, in 1981.

Anyway, he boosted my book idea and I gathered sordid stories for my memory bank. Ironically his book starts with the phrase, "Memory is a motherfucker". This may be the truest statement I've heard in a long time.

Good Advice from a Very Bad Girl

Mental note to self: don't eat Kalamata olives before bedtime. I most certainly don't want any more dreams of David Hasselhoff—the chiseled goof from Boobwatch —having his way with me in a bowling alley parking lot. No, mi lionito, he didn't drive a Landcruiser!

Dear Mz. Conduct,

The term "kissing cousins" is always affectionately used it seems, but what if you want it to go further, is that considered incest? I'm at this point with my first cousin and don't know how I should handle it. Help!

Family Man

> Dear FM,
>
> Technically, it would be considered incest if you gave your cousin a beef injection and a new meaning to the phrase 'family member'. If you can't seem to restrain yourself, as Mz. Conduct has had a time with this herself, just be sure to be discreet, especially if it's just something you want to get off your chest. Or out of your crotch. Unless you live in Arkansas and haven't seen a Wal-Mart in your life, I'd say just be very careful. You don't want the relatives whispering into their hankies and posting warning notices at the church functions. The age old taboo doesn't come from nothing, it comes from a fear of congenital defects in the children of people who are too closely related. If you get her pregnant and your kids have eight toes on their foreheads, don't come crying to me!

Dear Mz. Conduct,

My apartment is always trashed because I'm admittedly a slob. When I bring guys over, they act like it's a big deal. Some have even left without wanting to have sex! I would think they'd appreciate a girl who isn't all nit-picky and didn't care if they put the toilet seat down or not. What's the matter with them? Or do I have to become a Felix Unger?

Trashy Girl

> Dear TG,
>
> Flies on a footstool! No, you don't have to become an anal-retentive pucker head, but most guys are relieved when a girl's place is at least semi-organized. Just for the sake alone that when they have an unplanned, wanton-lust filled rendezvous, they don't accidentally slingshot their skivvies into something they wouldn't want to touch.
>
> Raise your standards, you filthy piglet, and consider that all the places you (should) clean, i.e., floor, countertops, bathroom sink, etcetera, are all potential places to have sex. Even the unshaven Neanderthals that I've know would rather hump away on a taintless towel rack than be trying to decipher what the green goo is on the heap you call a bed.

Mz. Conduct's House of Sin

"You better run me up to that hotel room, cuz baby, you got me hotter than Georgia asphalt."
–Lula (from Wild at Heart)

On a cold, clear, fall afternoon, one therapeutic thing I did was to bang the drum slowly, so to speak, after which I sauntered said voluptuous buns downtown and saw a movie. Something no one else wanted to see, it was either a foreign film—the people with overly relaxed brain cells won't tolerate those—or the latest, twisted, little treasure from the almighty David Lynch. *Mulholland Drive* is downright fabulous, especially when you watch it with a hand between your legs (just a tip for all of his fans and fellow moviegoers alike). Popcorn is another option.

The Lil' Princess and I went shopping at the biggest sex shop in the city. We carted home: black-seamed stockings, garters, camisoles and sultry, sandalwood oils. Then we went for much needed cocktails of course and wished for fairy tales to come true. You have to be careful what you wish for and in that bar especially. You ask for a fairy tail and you'll have a gay boy's ass sitting next to you in no time. That's all well and fine, if that's indeed what you're hankering for, but if you're sloshing gin and blathering about that knight in shining amour to come whisk your crotchless-pantied self onto a sleek steed, then forget it. Have another cocktail and focus on reality. That's what my own personal, spanking Yippie mentor would tell me, although most likely without the cocktail. Why? Because he's an old coot now and concerned for my health. Uh oh, I'm sure that warranted a series of paddlings on my big keister (works every time!)

Ms. Lula la Paintbrush and I got into some girl trouble. We were discussing how we had absolutely no desire to see any more penises, unless one happened to be severed by pinking shears and secured in a zip-lock baggie, that is. We got carried away on the subject and took advantage of the (she can't be twenty-one) new waitress. We had way too many martinis, inspected our boobs in the bathroom, and somehow drove home with hair-dos still intact. I dropped Ms.

Lula off at her house, stumbling up the stairs together in a never-much-of-a-lady type fashion. She—red freakin' alert—wasn't up to making dinner for the hubby and needless to say he, along with my demonic influence, won't be putting me on his Christmas card list this year. Ho ho ho, which by the way is what I think I heard as I left out their door.

Being the wicked brat that I am, I decided to see what flirtatious fiasco I could conjure up in the neighborhood while waiting for my date to arrive. I went out to rake leaves in a short, black, dress, my black lace stockings and garter belt, which was slightly visible when I bent over to scoop up leaves. Sure enough, the Christian couple packed up the kids and tore out of their driveway. Emergency prayer service I imagine. Then, Mary Magdalene with titty clamps, I notice an old coot across the street waving. He yelled over some amazingly intelligent comment like "Hey, looks like you gotta lotta leaves there sweetie!" to which I replied an equally clever, "Yep!" Just then, another never-before-seen neighbor came dragging himself down the stairs of the apartment complex next door. He was an even older, snaggle-toothed black man, and wanted to tell me he really enjoys watching me mow my lawn. Now, I do my gardening and mowing in the buff, always have, but this is the first year in this house and this neighborhood. My backyard is completely secluded except for the fact that there is that damn apartment complex on one side. At first I worried about this, but then realized that all the front doors to the apartments are around the other side of the building. I never saw anyone on my side so I kept gardening with the sun baking down on all of my cheeks. I adore it. Anyway, this old green-teeth curmudgeon goes on to say, "I be watching you out in your yard all nekked and uummm" —at this point he runs his hands up and down his whole big body—and continues to say, "I be having alllll kinds of chemistry for you, honey!" I doubt that chemistry is what he had, more like a handful of old man weenie meat. I told him, rather nicely, that it is my yard and that he needs to keep his so called chemistry to himself. My exhibitionist days over for the time being, I went back inside to wait for my date.

Mz. Conduct's House of Sin

I want to thank the very sweet fans, David and the Princess, who sent me a lovely bottle of Sapphire gin and a yum yum yumilicious jar of vermouth soaked olives, all the way from sunny California. I was extremely touched by the gesture, but of course I deserve it.

I must congratulate the winner of Mz. Conduct's best question ["I Just Knew I Had A Gee! Spot!"], for TA DA! finally finding her G-spot! She won a lunchbox full of tidbits, including a wet/dry vibrator. We have had some private correspondence and I've been instructing her on a few things. Happily, she wrote me saying:

"Remembering that, feeling-like-I-had-to-pee, spot...I found it all on my own with that little friend you sent me, on my tummy with a pillow under me to prop me up, and FOUND THAT LITTLE SPOT. Oh my god...you didn't tell me it was THAT incredible. I don't remember ever having an orgasm that lasted that long, actually as I'm typing; I'm still throbbing inside. I love you, I love you, I love you. Thank you so much Goddess."

I had a few blind dates this week and even more lined up for next. It's all so exhausting. Actually there is no such thing anymore as a blind date, not with the magic of the Internet. I like to demurely (cough-cough) demand a photo first. I mean, who really has time to have freakin' coffee with all the possible suitors? It's just easier to weed out a wasted afternoon that way. To be stuck staring at an unshaven hose-head while he drones on about the play of the day in a football game or the wonders of some newly released computer game can only lead to possible homicide. While asking for a photo seems vaguely superficial, we all have to admit that personal appearance is the first thing we notice. So, after a few e-mails to weed out the illiterate and a phone call or two to rule out the sensually ignorant, a photo can really just narrow it right down. I have to admit I give women a bit of a break. Somehow they don't seem to have to prove their worth to me as much. Not yet at least, but let's be fair and give it more time.

Good Advice from a Very Bad Girl

Dear Mz. Conduct,

My girlfriend and I have a great relationship and I love her very much, but when it comes to sex, she is, to put it mildly, a very conservative lover. She has never had an orgasm in her life, not even manually. She's 30 years old and from the Czech Republic, which I realize may have something to do with the way things are. She won't have anything to do with my cum and when I ask her to try new things she just freezes up and won't talk about it. I try to show her what I want and she just pushes me away. Don't suggest a vibrator because she won't even hear of it.

I know she'll be hurt if I talk seriously with her about this and I don't want that, but I feel like that if things don't change I may not want to stay in this relationship. What advice can you offer me?

Stuck in San Jose

> Dear SISJ,
>
> Look, you can start by telling her how much she means to you, and that you understand being from another country has its effects, but—bottom line—she's in America now and she's going to need to get some help, for her own sake. Explain that you want her to be happier, plus you need more from her too. There are professionals that could help her, but if she doesn't want to discuss her personal life with a stranger (just a guess), then it's your turn, buddy boy.
>
> Obviously she's not comfortable with her own body or self. If she decides that she does want to work on things with you then clink, clink, cheers baby, but ease into it. One evening, light some scented candles around the bedroom, sprinkle rose petals all over the bed and slide in an Enigma CD (la la, my dream is that someone other than myself will do this for me).
>
> Anyway, both of you get naked and lie on the bed together, just let her know that there is no pressure, maybe even have a rule that there be no sex this time. Touch each other, touch yourselves, talk about what it feels like. What are your favorite parts of your own bodies, each other's bodies? My very first boyfriend (and that's a truckload of boyfriends ago) used to always run his fingers under the back of my knee and say that was his favorite part of me. It didn't necessarily turn me on at first, but later it did. It was the fact that he loved it so much and it is really, really soft there. As I undress, I digress.
>
> So, lay with each other and talk about anything, just relax with yourselves and communicate. That's the most important step. If it goes no further than just lying with one another talking about painting the walls, fine. You'll have to have patience, and my guess is that you already have more than most doctors I know.
>
> The next step is, YOU buy a vibrator and get a porn film, all on your own, lil' Timmy. I recommend a film called *Erotic Obsession* with the lovely and talented Jeanna Fine. It's mild (I promise it won't scare her with ten horse-y men and a chick with her face in the toilet), funny, and Jeanna demonstrates just what good friend a dildo can be when a girl is home alone. Offer the suggestion of watching the film with your girlfriend when the mood is amorous. I'm imagining that she may freak out at this point and call you names that true perverts would be proud of. So, then back off and let her know that you bought those things for the two of you. If she's not comfortable watching with you, then maybe she'd rather peek at them by herself when you're not home. Plant a seed, so to speak.
>
> So, Mister Head-in-a-Hammock, you had better sit down and discuss this seriously with your girlfriend or before you know it you'll be cheating on her with

Mz. Conduct's House of Sin

that sweater snack you saw in the lunchroom. You can tell your girl this fact too. Sure it may be a harsh reality and she'll be hurt no doubt, but it's the only way to grow in a healthy relationship. If she's willing to know the realities and work on fixing them, then it'll strengthen your relationship that much more. If not, either figure on a lifetime of hookers at the Hideaway Hotel or pack her up and off she goes to let some other poor sap deal with it.

Dear Mz. Conduct,

Recently I have started dating again and have found myself involved with a very interesting man. He is extremely experienced in the bedroom, and makes me feel better than I have ever felt sexually. He has the knowledge of when to touch softly, when to be firmer, and asks questions as he is going along. He isn't afraid to ask me to show him. Usually that would make me feel really embarrassed, but with him, for some reason, I don't mind at all. As a matter of fact, in any relationship I have ever had, it has always been boring old missionary, get it over with, okay-let's-eat-popcorn-now sex. This guy wants to give me multiple orgasms before he will even consider letting me relieve him. I know, I know, where did I find him and does he have a brother? Hell yeah. He has two! Anyway, I guess I have a couple questions here.

First, I am extremely inexperienced and I am afraid it might turn him off. He just smiles at me when I say…"UMMMM huh? What is that? You wanna do what?" Is he thinking I'm retarded or is he thinking he will get to show me something new and watch me for the first time?

Now my main question is: we have talked about tying each other up. I haven't ever done that, and that's one thing he hasn't ever done. I think it would be fun, and for some reason I trust him, even though I haven't been seeing him very long. He said the rules would be, "We can't do anything to the other that we wouldn't want done to us," and that sounds fair to me. But then I don't know half of what he does! I don't have a headboard and neither does he. How do we tie each other up so we can't move? What do we use to tie with? I would think rope would kind of hurt if you got all excited and wiggled a lot. Soooooooooo, all knowing Goddess of Pleasure, what do you suggest?

Sincerely, and with lots of freakin' luv

U wanna WHAT??

Oh and one more thing…is there anything NATURAL for enhancing sexual pleasure? An aphrodisiac or something? Herbal? I don't know. I'm new at this stuff. But hopefully not for long, heh. He doesn't have a problem getting me all hot, I just wanted to try it sometime.

> **Dear UWW,**
>
> Okay, to answer your first question, and this is only partially based on your inexperience: whether he thinks you're naive and a dumbass when it comes to sex—and let's face it you are, but such is life, right?—or if he's swinging his heat seeking missile around at the sports bars, bragging about what a stud he is for showing some little filly the big boy corral, you'll have to get to know him better. Oh and please send me both spare brothers, if they can muster up the courage.
>
> On to question number two. Same answer basically. You should get to know this guy better before you go tying each other up. Any sort of bondage requires a great deal of trust between consenting people. You said you didn't even know what things he has done or wouldn't do or whatever. Find these things out before you go roping yourself into an unpleasant situation. If you want to play around with the idea, most sex shops carry novelty type hand-

cuffs and fuzzy wrist restraints, that sort of thing. That way you are never at a loss for control. If and when you get to the point where you want more, nylon stockings are not only sexy, but are workable too. If and when you want even more, Jesus with jumper cables, then I suggest you read some recommended books on the subject. There is a book out called *Consensual Sadomasochism: How To Talk About It And To Do It Safely* and it's written by William H. Henkin Ph.D. and Sybil Holiday. Midori, who is a bondage expert and a writer on SM, fetish and human sexuality—sadly I didn't get to meet her when she was in town recently—has commented on this book. She calls it "Practical, insightful, full of information and gentle wisdom. An essential reference that I keep close at hand as an educator. For the novice to the experienced, offering something on every level." Midori herself has several books out. One that's just been recently published called *The Seduction Art Of Japanese Bondage*.

As for aphrodisiacs, I'll say it again and then I must grab that tight-assed waiter with the stiff one, cocktail that is: talk about all of these things with your man. Most of the time just talking about your sexual desires, imagining them together, is in itself a great stimulating source. It's entirely subjective. Find out what he likes to eat (aside from you) and what scents he likes, what textures turn him on and so on. Explore these things and you will know in time. It really is an individual thing. For instance, just thinking about those, supposedly sensual, fruit flavored oils make me want to toss up my Thai noodles right on the spot. They've been selling them as long as I can remember so somebody sure likes them. My point being that everybody has different preferences. I can't stand perfumes myself, but I do wear pheromone oil that drives my own self into a slick little frenzy. Seems to work on my playmates too. It's hard to find those and they're expensive, but they are nicely arousing to say the least.

Now get to yakking, girl. Who said talk is cheap?

Mz. Conduct's House of Sin

"I shot my mouth off and you showed me what that hole was for!"
–Chrissie Hynde

Mz. Conduct's Top Ten List: Music For Fanning the Holiday Flames

1) "The Reprise Years, the Best of Frank Sinatra" Frank Sinatra (when you're hazily swaying, sampling the rum cake and the scantily clad boy shakes his little leather ass...and the martinis)

2) "To Bring You My Love" PJ Harvey (for those come-on-in-honey, hang-up your-coat-and-slam-me-against- the-hatrack entrances)

2) "Haunted" Poe (for those take-the wreath-off-that-thang-and-grab-me-by-the-hair festivities)

3) "The Singles" Annie Lennox (for those immediate yule log greetings, those hold-me-by-the-hips and bend-me over-in-the-doorway plunges)

4) "The Very Best of Elvis Costello" specifically the gut-wrenching song, "I Want You" (when the emotions are intensely and nauseatingly overwhelming)

5) "Big Red Rocket Of Love" Reverend Horton Heat (for those apron lifting get-ya-from-behind-while-basting-the-turkey times)

6) "Isle of View" The Pretenders (when you're caught up with the moans of romance and the sloshing of gin and loiter under the omnipresent mistletoe)

7) "Until the End of the World" Soundtrack from the movie (for those pluck-the-olives-out-of-my-one-too-many-martini interludes)

8) "The Cross of Changes" Enigma (when the guests are gone and the eggnog is slathered on your thighs)

Good Advice from a Very Bad Girl

9) "Boys and Girls" Bryan Ferry (when you're sitting by the fire, blazing with desire and don't care that your panties have been sling-shotted onto the chandelier)

10) "Al Green-Greatest Hits" Al Green (when the glow in your eyes and the ache in your heart knows the party is over and a whole damn new year is approaching not fast enough)

Others that should've made the list: Billie Holiday, Sinead O'Connor, Marvin Gaye, Talk Talk, Tom Jones, oh and the eclectic list goes on, longer than ol' Santa's scrotum.

> Dear Mz. Conduct,
> How do you get liquid latex out of those crevices and tight places?
> Gooey Girl
>
>> **Dear GG,**
>>
>> Mz. Conduct has never used liquid latex, but the day isn't over yet. I did call my friend who owns a sex shop and she said most kits come with instruction booklets. The Fantasy Company makes a nice little kit that actually comes with accessories to clean. There is also a product called Body Clean that is also helpful for those nooks and crannies. However if yours was a streetscore or a hand-me-down batch then there are a few things to do. If you wash with soap and water and just rub lightly, it will come off. You can also use a little vegetable oil and rub gently with your fingers. That can be especially nice to do when you've got leftover latex in those secluded areas. Whoa, we're going again girl! If you need to get it out of your hair, soak your noggin in warm water with a tad of vegetable oil and you should emerge latex free and maybe with a halo. Well, in my case all halos have been revoked, but you might have a shot.

> Dear Mz. Conduct,
> Why do women like to shop so much?
> phoenixprime69
>
>> **Dear pp69,**
>>
>> Wanton weenies in cocktail sauce, it's a substitute for sex, you dolt. Men bury themselves in television shows and video games and women shop. It's genetic. At least that's my interpretation. Personally I am not a shopper and hate the very thought of it, but there have been those rare times when I have money to spend and just go on a royal spree. It's a sort of high, a lift, a void filled and like coffee and sugar, it can also be a colossal let down when you've exhausted your feet and/or bank account. That's why women get addicted I think. When the high is over, there's that frenzied appeal to head out for another fix. One can be left with a heap of consumer crap piled high on the bed, sale tags dangling, reminiscent of bargains scored, and realize that the purple, fuzzy doohickey that you swore was screaming your name was really calling

Mz. Conduct's House of Sin

"Yoo hoo, dazed and confused sucker" instead. We refuse to answer to that name again and are compelled to have immediate cocktails...until the next sale that is.

So, if you men are up to snuff and make sure that we're too busy in the boudoir to even think about those boots that are half price only this week, then you can shut your pie-hole. Otherwise, mister too tired to pump, fork out the credit card and again, shut your-pie hole.

Dear Mz. Conduct,

My girlfriend wants me to fist her and has been bringing it up each time we're together sexually. I tell her I will, but we never get to it. Actually I think I'm avoiding it because it scares me a little (I don't know how to go about it) and it doesn't really turn me on. What should I do? I want to please my girl.

Fist Fighter

Dear FF,

You're not alone, a lot of people get turned off my this. On the other hand, no pun intended, there are an awful lot of people that feel just the opposite. You may change the way you feel in time. As a matter of fact I'm willing to bet my hatbox full of sex toys on it. It does take time to work up to though. Testicles on a tuna, you don't want to just jam your hand up her delicate flower. When a woman has a baby, the whole vaginal region is slowly stretched over time. Of course you don't have to work up to a nine month mark unless your hand is the size of a newborn. And by the way, childbirth is not a prerequisite to enjoy fisting.

There is a great book I recommend called *A Hand in the Bush: The Fine Art of Vaginal Fisting* written by Deborah Addington. She also wrote an excellent book called *The Ultimate Guide to Anal Sex for Women*. Here is a review of her book on fisting; "Penetrating insights by a longtime fisting aficionado. Vaginal fisting—the intimate, potent sexual act of gradually inserting the entire hand into the vagina—is an increasingly popular form of sexplay among lesbians, bisexuals and heterosexuals alike. Now, for the first time, an experienced practitioner explains in detail how to fist with the greatest possible safety and pleasure. Extensively illustrated, this long-awaited guide has been approved by three fisting-positive physicians. A must-have "handbook" for the sexually explorative!

It can be an amazingly intense and thrilling experience for you both. So, I suggest you work more fingers in each time you're with your girl and read the aforementioned material. Go get 'em Rocky! And leave Bullwinkle at home.

Good Advice from a Very Bad Girl

"The only people for me are the mad ones, the ones who are mad to talk, mad to live, mad to be saved, desirous of everything at the same time, the ones who never yawn or say a commonplace thing, but burn, burn, burn like fabulous yellow roman candles."
–Jack Kerouac

As the holidays approach—who am I kidding? Rather, as the holidays have leapt on our backs and chewed our brainstems into a bloody pulp of pulsating cheer, I think the only way to get through this is to pour those alcoholic spirits "down the hatch"—as my dad used to say—like there's no tomorrow. Hey, there's always the new year for those promises to join the health club, get a nicotine patch and sign up for AA. It beats mowing down those perky holiday shoppers and landing your ass in the hoosegow.

So, needing an evening of amusement, I went to the comedy club with my son and his friends. The first comedy act was just downright obnoxious. It was a woman, a district attorney by day—honey, don't quit that day job—and a spokesperson for repressed, vanilla-wafer women by night. Granted, the club seems to bring out the mullet-headed, giant-wheeled truck owning men with their perfume marinated, gum chomping, big haired women in tow. A big night out in the city.

Anyway, this comedian woman gets up on stage to start her set. She first complains about her lousy dates and such and then asks the crowd, "How many women get stuck on a date where they're expected to give head?" Well, the hands are clapping away and she continues to complain and say, "Unless there's a diamond on my finger and a Lexus in the driveway, that's just not going to happen, am I right ladies?" I waved over the waitress, as I could plainly see that this act would require a double martini. I didn't clap or hoot like the room full of agreeable hyena-like women. I drank my martini. Then she asked the cackling women in the room to raise their hands if they like anal sex. My hand, and one other woman's, shot up in proud honesty. Now, my son wrote a paper in first grade about "his wild mama" so he's less appalled at me as life goes on. The wannabe comedic wench was all over that like flies on a ham sandwich. She belted out that we—us two anally uninhibited trollops—make it that much rougher for the rest of the ladies because butt sex is just not going to happen. I held back the impulse to bend her over right there and shove my strap-on all the way to China. Nuns in a Knapsack, what was she telling these people, women especially? That we should all just shop and gossip and consume and give our man the bare necessities when we feel he deserves them? We should keep repressing our own sexuality and other's as well, until we finally snap and do something completely insane? Doing something perhaps like getting up on a stage and grinding some women's fantasies and prospective sensual pleasure into a pile of degrading and misunderstood fodder? So, I was feeling the smoke seep out my ears at this point.

She went on like this for awhile and thankfully the gin was numbing my brain. She ended her set by talking about "this shaving thing" and asked if any women shave every body hair they have. Again, my hand and one other girl's flew up in glorious self-respect. Again, she tries to take that self-respect and make it a hand-slapping, go-to-your-room diatribe. I was glad to be sitting at the back of the room because the gin hadn't numbed my tongue and lord only knows the feedback I would have given. The girl, sitting in front, got it instead. The D.A.-By-Day launched into a speech about how her boyfriend only likes to have sex with her because she looks like a six-year old. "He's a pedophile!" she screeches and points to her man. This only got a smattering of applause at best. All I could think of was somehow mouthing off, breaking some law and ending up with her face on the other side of my cell. Not a pretty picture. I behaved and remembered the first amendment. She must've realized she had done all the damage she could and introduced the next act quicker than you could refill your RadGirl razor.

The Lil' Princess took me out for cocktails to celebrate a personal conquest of mine where we had a drunken, philosophical party with two engagingly pierced, rock-n-roll boys. What Mz. Conduct has in store for one of them is beyond telling. My face hurt from laughing so hard and Moses on a matzoh

Good Advice from a Very Bad Girl

ball, it's been awhile. Well, since putting on a show at a nearby porn theatre I guess. Ah, the memories, ah the mammaries.

It's monsoon weather and my little house of sin is rattling and banging and getting wet in places I never knew existed. At four in the morning my mail slot starts banging, my windows rattle and an ice bucket full of storm water comes racing through the rotted window frame. Lovely. I run around, cussing like a sailor and stuff towels everywhere and try to hammer the uncooperative windows shut. The dogs are hovering on the bed, shaking in their cowardly skin. They bark at the mail slot once in awhile and I guess that comforts me some. Mz. Conduct apparently needs a handyman. Hmmm...a boy with Popeye arms and a tool belt sure sounds good. Well, when doesn't he, though?

Mz. Conduct needs to go find that big, ol' jolly Santa and sit on his accommodating lap. I got all beside myself to hear that the *Vagina Monologues* will be in this city soon. Oh Santa (or any of my beloved readers), please, oh please give me tickets for Christmas!

> Dear Mz. Conduct,
> Tell me something please. Why is it that when one of my buddies has a girlfriend he turns into a totally different person when she's around? My boys and I will all be just hanging out, having a good time, everything's cool and then the girlfriend shows up and my buddy acts completely different. It's like I don't even know him. This is really pissing me off.
> Irate in Idaho
>
>> Dear III,
>> You unhinged little spud, you. I'll give it to you in one lovely word: pussy. The bottom line is that boys—until they become men, which sadly sometimes never occurs—will do and say anything to get and keep the pussy they're getting. It's a damn shame and there's nothing you can do about it short of telling him what you think. It's your right, but don't expect it to change.
>> Hopefully the time will come when your buddy will realize that any woman worth a swizzle stick would never want him to be anyone but his own true self. When she can be part of his life without you witnessing the Jekyll and Hyde routine, that's when you can give him a little more respect. Until then, put up with it or take him into the alley and tell him how you want to grind him into meatloaf when he turns into Captain Dumbass.
>
> Mz. Conduct,
> Why is it that the other guys in my band—who are assholes, actually—always get the girls? They don't care about the girls they meet and aren't even nice to them

Mz. Conduct's House of Sin

most times. I consider myself a decent guy and have been told I'm very sweet. Some girls say they like that about me, but why am I not a babe magnet like my rude and tasteless friends?

Drummer in a Bummer

>Dear DIAB,
>
>Bad boys aren't boring. That's my first instinct. For instance, you meet a girl that's really sweet, always there for you, calling you frequently, and willing to do whatever you want just to make you happy. Sounds like a bathtub full of naked, oily fun doesn't it? Truth be told, it gets boring after awhile and you know it. Women like that are usually insecure and can't stand up for what they want or don't want. It's downright annoying when someone doesn't express their own opinions about things for fear of not being 'nice.' They can't be a bitch because, oh no, you might get mad. Ugh...bitch slap time in my book.
>
>Anyway, my point is that it goes both ways. I'm not saying that you are any of these things, but I'd bet a fifth of Beefeater on most of it. The key is, both men and women want to spend time with people who are confident, have stuff going on and have opinions to express. No one likes a doormat. That's where the so-called 'assholes' gain points.
>
>Assholes or jerks usually exude a certain amount of confidence and independence, which is really freakin' attractive. Gaad, I remember having a boyfriend that was as hunky as anything I'd ever laid eyes on. He was overly generous with his wallet and his time and everything else, but when it came to having any sort of accelerated conversation, I might as well have dated Mister Coffee. Instead, I pined after the cocky musician with no interest whatsoever in me. In the long run, I dumped the nice guy and got the cocky musician of course, but that's beside the point.
>
>So just remember; it's independence and confidence—not bad treatment—that attracts women to these men. Also, passive guys attract user women. If you act like a doormat and a victim, you will undoubtedly attract those women that are unscrupulous users. Try not being so passive and don't forget to express what you think even if it contradicts the girl you're with.
>
>Women—and also plenty of men—of this type search out easy targets: insecure people who are willing to give anything for a relationship. The result could be a destructive relationship, which may only further your low feelings of self-worth. So watch it mister rockstar.

Good Advice from a Very Bad Girl

"How could I become a destitute woman when I have all these treasures locked in my heart?"
–Blanche DuBois from A Streetcar Named Desire

Cuff me up and call me Candy. Candy Cane that is. All this holiday hoopla is getting on my nerves. I know I'm being a Bah Humbug girl this year, but I can't help it. Let me offer a tidbit of reason: So I'm clutching my ten dollar bill from a poem I just sold, standing in a God awful line at the hideously decorated grocery checkout. I had tampons, toilet paper and wine—all the necessities of a destitute woman—when this superfluous perky woman in front of me is bouncing around like she's got crack in her nasal spray and humming holiday jingles in a nails-on-a-chalkboard voice. UGH! She's flipping around her freshly coiffed head and wiggling her Gucci butt around, which by the way is about the size of my left thigh. Double UGH! I look at her in utter disgust only to notice she's wearing the black boots that I've wanted...well, forever. I despised the joyful air she breathed and secretly wished her ill. When I go to hell on a headboard, oh and I will, I doubt if PMS to the tenth degree can be used as an excuse.

So anyway, at this store there are 'door greeters' which are women as old as Methuselah who say things like "How are you today?" all sunny and sweet. I feel sorry for them because most people ignore them Then again they do have a job and probably make more than I do. These old birds must either have loads of self-esteem or are on the verge of Alzheimer's. I can just see me working that job, running after people, kicking them in their fat asses and asking if they heard my happy greeting or what. I know I'd feel compelled to lecture about common courtesy and blah blah blah. This coming from the biggest bitch around. Hey, I was raised by psychotic nuns, my behavior speaks for itself.

I'm still standing in the checkout line. I'm reading the headlines in the Enquirer squealing that Hilary Clinton is having a secret affair with an alien and not from behind a border, but from another planet. So, I'm still behind little

Mz. Conduct's House of Sin

Miss Too-Happy-To-Live, in the boots I should be wearing, and this tobacco chewing, squalid looking guy walks in with his woman about three steps behind him. He looked like he down shifted a tractor to the store with one hand and scratched his scrotum with the other. Well the old lady greeter does her thing and asks "How are you folks today?". Mister Scruff E'Nuff blows right by her, leaving his woman in his dust, passes my ear with his nasty breath and says "I'd be doing better with something like you". Now this is when I can see the use for a handgun. I'm instantly repulsed and refraining from up-chucking into an empty baskcart. Instead, I clandestinely slid my foot out in the aisle, sending him sailing into the stacked bags of fertilizer where he truly belonged anyway. He started swearing and looking around. I know I felt better already.

Meanwhile the sloth-like cashier is ringing up my tampons, toilet paper and Bordeaux and I looked at the thirty-eight cents she handed back to me. As I walked out through the parking lot, I started planning just how to spread thirty-eight cents out for two days. Just then a metallic green Impala pulled up next to me. A 400 pound, black man turned down his radio and asked me how I was doing. I knew he didn't really want to hear so I just said "I am good, thanks." He started whistling across the parking lot and yelling "You sure are looking good baby!" Okay, I thought, there has to be a way to make more money. Hmmm...but could I? Dare I? Why not?

So, now I've decided to research the psychological aspects of having sex for money. I'll let you know when it pans out. It's a whole new year ahead and I, for one, am going to make the most of it.

Ruby Liscious aka the Transient Trollop, which is what I'm back to calling her, just called from somewhere in the southwest. She had just won a buttload of moolah playing the lottery at the Blue Jeans Lounge. An all but swanky hole-in-the-wall that fired her the previous week. She was explaining to a drunken and dense patron, that tipping was not a city in China and things got out of hand. The big win was perfect timing, as she was down to her last two bucks, the dog is pregnant, the hotel bill is due and blah and blah and then her phone card went dead. I love her madly, what can I say?

I figure that if I ever win the lottery, and before I flew off to Paris to stroke those beautiful baguettes, I'd open some sort of philanthropic place. Something to the effect of "Mz. Conduct's Homeless Shelter for Wayward Wenches and Their Unruly Offspring". I can see the marquee now, with red light bulbs and flashing stars. Big fluffy beds and velvet couches, books by the scores, and maybe free classes. Okay, I'm getting carried away. In any case, it would be dreamy.

Mister Bo Dangles gets Mz. Conduct's Big Fat Jingle Balls award this month. I'm personally handing it over, as I've caved beyond compare. He has demonstrated a strength of character which is hard to find in a sensitive man. We're all tempted by our weaknesses—i.e. those loves of our lives who can't decide what they truly want in this world—when we watch The Sound of Music or in his case, a Sandra Bullock movie. But a definite big YAY as I postulate a power potent pioneer—say that three times fast—in the game of life for him, in this new year ahead.

> Mz. Conduct,
>
> In lustful desperation I signed up with one of those online dating services. Aside from the fact that the listings seem replete with woefully imperfect humans seeking (nay demanding) utterly perfect ones, there is a particular Sexual Interest category that the ladies are allowed to choose, and quite a few of them do. The interest they express is "Sex with no intercourse." Now I guess I understand "Online sex." You chat dirty, work the mouse and keyboard with one hand, and get off under the desk with the other, or something to that effect. But why would you want to meet someone online, go on a date, and have "Sex with no intercourse"? Does it have anything to do with the Bill Clinton number?
>
> Desparate
>
>> **Dear Desparate**
>>
>> That was a puzzler question and I conferred with Mister Bo Dangles who is a hyper intelligent sort and gave me some of his manly and insightful thoughts. Here is what we think: Women who have placed those ads have thought it through. They want the control, the power, and maybe some oral pleasure, but aren't willing to have a one night stand with someone they really don't know. For some reason, some people feel more intimate having intercourse than just cuddling and stroking and licking. Mutual masturbation can be quite nice as

well. You don't have to worry about STD's so much and you haven't given up the nectar of your flower, which can be quite sacred for some women.

I think it's a safe starting point that some women find comforting. It's like they want to let you know that they are not opposed to sex and in fact really enjoy it, but are not willing to actually insert your car in the garage just yet. The driveway seems safer for an easier getaway. It is a strange venue in a dating service, but not totally uncalled for. I wouldn't give up. If you run into the right woman then things will work themselves out. If you just want to get laid—and most men do—then try a different service. Maybe something like "Poly Anna and her Put-Out-Princesses" where you can rest assured you'll drive your meatcar right in the roomy garage, gun the engine and blow the carbs right through the roof. Watch out for Santa who may be up there. I don't want him injured, as he hopefully will be delivering my Nutcracker Barbie. I picture her in leathers and cap, single-tail whip in her hand and ball harness in the other. Oh I hope that's what she's like! And Clinton's wife is dating ET, what do you expect?

Dear Mz. Conduct,

I'm having an affair with a married man and I know all the usual repercussions, but this disturbs me to no end; After we have sex, each and every time, he immediately goes into the bathroom and washes his penis off. Sometimes he'll even spit too. It leaves me feeling cheap and dirty and I hate it. I have told him the way it makes me feel and asked him why he has to do that. He just says he has to because his wife is at home and he can't take any chances. What do you suggest?

Ms. Washrag

Dear MW,

Do you have a blunt instrument? If you're not of the violent type then I suggest you reiterate to this subhuman swine licker that this is not acceptable. I'd want to chop the damn thing off and toss it down the toilet myself. Say, "let's see how clean that gets it!" and then call his wife to come get his bloody carcass off your floor.

Seriously, I would dump his inconsiderate ass, being that you've already spoken to him about how this makes you feel. What a dolt and so are you if you let this go on. If he is so worried that his wife will pounce on his arrival and sniff his crotch like a bitch in heat, then he could get a box of those handy dandy weenie-wipes for his car. Drive and wipe buddy, it's not like you haven't done that before. He could stop at a freakin' gas station bathroom for all that matters, anything but at your damn house. Even if he cleans up elsewhere, you'll know he's doing that and UGH! do you really want a rude sonofabitch like that? I know one thing: he's not that good honey and you're worth receiving much more respect. Santa on a swizzle stick, have enough respect for yourself!

Good Advice from a Very Bad Girl

So this guy walks into a bar. He looks around and sees no one. He sits at the bar and orders a drink. All of a sudden he hears a voice say "You're sure a good looking guy!" He turns around, but still sees no one. Puzzled, he sips his drink and again a voice says "You are such a sexy man!" This time he asks the bartender what the deal is, he's hearing voices yet no one is in the place. The bartender points to the bowl of peanuts on the bar and says "It's the peanuts". The guys says "What the hell are you talking about?" and the bartender says "They're complementary".

It's a new year, a full moon, an eclipse even, and time for life changes, but that's (i.e. the bowl of peanuts) about as verbally generous as Mz. Conduct's going to get this year.

So, my derriere has beautiful, purple circles covering it. I thought I'd have to explain them to my massage therapist, but he knows me all too well. He greased me up like a holiday ham and said "It looks like Mz. Conduct got a new paddle?" He was right on target. I just saw it and immediately wrote a bad check. To hatch my holiday spirit, I had a wee, wild party. The electricity slut a.k.a. Greedgirl attended, as did Not Your Average Joe, Wild Bill and his Amazing Appendage, Mister Bo Dangles and moi, the hostess Twinkie with the mostess. The next day, after everyone left, my nostrils flared at the aromas in the house. It smelled like gin, cat food and ass. But in a good way!

The Lil' Princess dragged my ample ass down to meet her latest pootie licker. We met him at his local hootenanny club hangout and Christ on a crab cake, she told me he was old, but I wasn't prepared to meet Moses himself. He was a decent guy and I'm glad she likes him. I'd just be more impressed if he could get an erection. She has the worst weenie luck imaginable and may want to consider a penis embargo this year. When they jaunt off to the beach for New Year's eve, I hope she remembers to bring the beautiful glass dildo I bought her for Christmas.

> Dear Mz. Conduct,
> I was just wondering—why do guys become alcoholic womanizers? And why are we, as women, attracted to them even though they're mostly blithering idiots?

Mz. Conduct's House of Sin

Thought you might have some insight on this subject with your breadth and depth of experience. Thanks.

Just Wondering

> Dear JW,
>
> For the love of labia rings, guys become alcoholic womanizers because after a few drinks even those shy boys start swinging their weenies and thinking they're going to score with us. Then there are just the alcoholics who smell like beer at eleven in the morning. They have their own set of problems. And then there are just the womanizers who feel no need for any brewed enhancement, thinking we goddesses will just drop dead at the sight of their bulging Dockers. Need I say more about them? Ugh. So what do we have left? Yeah, I know it's depressing, but that's why we take them home and then wonder why the next day, or worse yet, two years later. To be fair, I suppose there are exceptions, but I've yet to find them. The Lil' Princess and I are designing our wedding dresses (with no men in mind) for the Old Lesbians Club that we will have in full swing by the time we're eighty. You're welcome to join.

Mz. Conduct,

First off, LOVE your show. I always look forward to the next issue's words of wisdom. So wise in fact, I now find myself seeking an answer or two. Here goes—I'm a 41 yr. old man, widowed and a single parent. I've always been perpetually horny. It was common for me to masturbate at least two or three times every day (with or w/o partner). I've played on both sides of the sexual fence and consider myself bisexual with a slight preference towards women. After my wife passed away three years ago I've only had a short fling with one woman. Lately my perpetual horniness has been waning. A lot. To the point where I'm only masturbating maybe once a week (sometimes not for two!). I'm thinking less & less about women and men. Just don't look at 'em THAT WAY anymore and I'm starting to think that something is real wrong somewhere! I feel like some sort of eunuch who is so numb below the waist I might as well be dead. What's wrong Mz. Conduct? Did I use up my lifetime allowance of sperm? Do you start thinking about retirement more than sex after 40? Is this normal? Can you please suggest something to help me get my libido back—I'm real serious and I really miss it?

Signed,

No Desire & No Fire

> Dear ND&NF,
>
> Wow, I'm thinking you may need a lengthy visit from the Transient Trollop and Mz. Conduct herself. The three of us, strap-ons, thigh high boots, dry martinis. It's your lifelong fantasy and you know it. We'd tip the scale on the old peter-meter baby. So, did it move yet?
>
> I would say that yes, it is normal to have these down periods in one's life and no you did not use up all of your sperm. This down time seems to have gone on long enough however. You have a lot on your plate. Raising a child at whatever age can put a damper on the ol' dipper. Something to consider is that some medications such as antidepressants, blood pressure medicine, and anti-anxiety agents can have a negative effect most definitely. I am a firm believer in vitamins and especially vitamin B for the energy levels and sex drive. As I always say, the biggest sex organ is in the brain, and if you are not getting brain boners then you may have a hitch. Without the true desire to be sexually active, you aren't going to get excited or have orgasms at all. And in order to maintain sexual health, you need to feel desire and feel desired, and to have your body and mind in synch.

Generally as people get older—men, in their mid forties to mid fifties—can experience a decline in sexual arousal as well. Diet, exercise and good mental health are all very important factors though. I've been told I have been an excellent remedy for this though, so you can send me a plane ticket. We can discuss this further mister meat puppet. I'll sit on your lap and we can talk about the first thing that pops up.

Mz. Conduct's House of Sin

"What is most beautiful in virile men is something feminine; what is most beautiful in feminine women is something masculine."
–Susan Sontag, Against Interpretation, 1966

My landlord is here, puttering around aimlessly, for the third time this week. He keeps telling me he's forgotten some tool or something and has to come back yet again. Yeah, right. Meanwhile back at the ranch, when turned on, my kitchen faucet (like my landlord) spurts in all directions. So today instead of walking around in my boxer shorts—with cartoons depicting domestic violence on them—and my wife-beater, as a hopeful deterrent, I decided to scuff around the house in my torn, chenille, bathrobe, my green, dog-chewed slippers and leave my bed-head hair looking just like Rod Stewart's. Never mind lipstick or even brushing my teeth. Now let's see how fast the dolt gets the repairs done.

I attended a fabulously informative class the other night called Sex Toys 101. It was held at "It's My Pleasure", a salaciously, saucy, store that caters mainly to women. We covered everything from lubricants and female Viagra to dildos and harnesses. Of course I own half of everything shown, but now have my eye on a deliciously wicked, two-headed, dildo. It's made of 100% silicone and comes in a lovely marbly black and white pattern. They're hand made by a one-woman company called "Vixen", thus the eighty-five buck price tag. Silicone is by far the longest lasting and most durable. By the way, silicone is also best at not harboring bacteria and easily washable with hot water and soap. Oh I just must have that thang!

Mister Wild Bill and his Amazing Appendage took me to see an amusing play by a performance troupe called The House of Cunt. As the playbill describes "experience a roller coaster of raw emotion" and that's barely stating it. It was six people entrenched in multi-media extremes that made me almost pee my panties, if indeed I had been wearing any. I developed a crush almost immediately on one girl in the cast. She was brilliant in all her skits. Not only did she play the guitar, singing a sweetly sensual song she wrote, as two naked cast members crawled slowly out on the floor, making naughty gestures with their fingers, but she also portrayed a little girl who was supposed to be eating her sugarless cereal. She found it boring and played with her twat instead. That's the sugar I like too!

Oh and big balls o' joy, I found a righteous remedy for my crooked tailbone affliction …oh yes darlings, I've found that anal sex has even more booty benefits. Once upon a time, when I was in the sixth grade, some bean-headed, lice-haired, boy pulled a tall chair out from under me and I landed—a prelude to my non lady-like behavior—on the cold, hard, linoleum with my dress over my head and tears streaming down my bespectacled, little face. So, now on some occasions when I launch into some sort of acrobatic amusement—or wear my new, six inch, Mary Jane shoes for two days straight—my tailbone goes painfully out of whack. I have to hobble like a hunched over snail directly to the chiropractor for adjustment. The only way the good doctor can adjust my pushed in coccyx is to go in vaginally or rectally, pushing the bone back out gently. And voila! I turn into a new woman. Just to think, now I can wear any of my tall shoes whenever I damn well please. I may have no more need of my chiropractor now that I have my sure-cure-waltzing-wonder-weenie. So much more pleasurable at that. Hell, I can even swing from the chandeliers again wearing nothing but my tiara and lipstick, what a concept!

Dear Mz. Conduct,

I've been married for thirteen years to an asexual amoeba. I love my wife, but she has no sex drive whatsoever. She isn't taking any medications and as far as I can tell and there seems to be no physical reason for her to be this lustfully limp. She wants nothing to do with me when I try to touch her and I'm seriously considering cheating on her just to fill my needs as a man, but hate the thought of hurting her. What advice could you offer me?

Itching in Ithaca

> Dear lil,
>
> Holy dish rags and enema bags, I figure there is one of two things going on. One may be you're a man who hasn't looked in the mirror for about a decade. No physical reason, HA! You're a dumpy, unshaven, crotch-scratchin', loser or a reasonable facsimile to what your wife may see. Not a turn on, big boy. Not to her, not to anyone.
>
> Then again there are some people that are just asexual. However I doubt that you didn't see this before you married the woman. I tend to think it's some-

thing gone awry after the fact. You don't give me much information on this though, so I'm left to believe that maybe your wife is living a financially comfortable life—with you footin' the bill—and that your little amoeba may be doing some deep sea diving of her own. Perhaps with another lipstick wearing plankton.

Here's a thought, Homer, you could sit down and ask her what this is all about. Tell her you want and need to have sex in your marriage, because duh, it's healthier that way. And tell her that if she's not willing to work with you on the matter then you'll be launching your heat seeking missile elsewhere. The countdown begins. And try not to land in the amoeba-filled ocean.

Dear Mz. Conduct,

I'm a college student, a good looking guy with very high standards in girls. There are a lot of pretty girls on campus and I'm not shy about approaching them when the time is right. It seems that the girls that do meet my standards turn out to be total bitches. Here's my problem, there is a girl that I keep running into over and over. We've never spoken, but she gives me this sultry sort of look each time. She's incredibly gorgeous and I'm nervous about actually trying to approach her. I'm afraid she'll be like all the rest of the high maintenance, snotty, and self-absorbed girls that I seem to have a history with. It's driving me crazy because I really want to talk to her, but don't want the fantasy to end up in the trash. What should I do?

Campus Puss

Dear CP,

From the beginning of time, beautiful women have intimidated men. First you should understand that being a gorgeous creature has it's drawbacks. Every Tom, Dick and Harry (and all his hairy cousins) continuously hit on you wherever you go. People awe at you and paw at you and eventually those girls build up a bitch-shell. However when the right guy comes along, those same bitches can become putty. So, how do you know if you're the right guy unless you try? I understand your jaded attitude in your efforts to keep at it, but life goes on. If you're so nervous about this one girl then take your time. Tube-steaks in a textbook, the school year just started! Give it time and enjoy the fantasy. The next time she flaps those lusty lashes at you, just smile back and leave it at that. There is something extremely seductive about an unattainable man. Keep in mind that there is nothing stopping her from coming over and talking to you either. Play it out baby.

Now, shut your blow-hole and get your "high standard" ass to class.

Good Advice from a Very Bad Girl

"Take what you can use and let the rest go by."
–Ken Kesey

As I drove through my lively Latino neighborhood, past the "Car Stereo Alarms/Joyeria Burrito Mart"—which always just cracks me up for some reason—I realized that some things in life can be so gaaddamn joyfully rewarding. Things wickedly wonderful and karmic, such as always wondering what your body building ex lover —and one of the best lovers in your life—is doing these days. Always thinking that maybe it was a mistake to let him go. Well here comes the kick: one night I get a phone call and although it's been over a decade since I heard that voice, I knew it right off the goddamn bat. Lo and behold it was the aforementioned, muscle-head from Molalla. I'm still not clear on how he finagled my number. So we start yakking about old times, new times. He said he's now completed his nine years of school (yeah, he was never the sharpest scalpel on the tray), and to my udder amazement, is now a full-fledged chiropractor. We kept blathering away and right in the middle of my sentence he says to me, "What would Jesus do?" Thinking he was joking, I came back with, "I bet Jesus would jump on a crack whore, bind her limbs with rosary beads and ride her for all she's worth." Doctor muscle-head was aghast and said he couldn't believe I just said that. Instead of apologizing, I told him flat out that if he had gone all-religious, that was fine and dandy, but I didn't want to hear about it. I changed the subject and asked about his relationships. He launches into a long-ass diatribe of how he'd been married, but was accused of raping the former Mrs. and she took him for twenty grand. And how ironic it was that now an ex girlfriend was accusing him of the same thing. They were bitches of course, he said. Of course they all just wanted his money. I kept pretty quiet on this note and then he continued, saying he'd done a huge amount of 'blow' last week and needed to get to church to repent. After all, he had patients to see later. I was listening to this meshed mass of muscle-headed utterance when he then, completely nonchalantly, asks me out to dinner. Oh happy freakin' horseshit, I thought to myself, yeah that's what I want to do, go to dinner with this accused rapist, coke-headed, born again Christian! Well, I was born okay the first time and I told him "Hell isn't handing out Popsicles yet, honey, but thanks so much for asking". I hung up feeling an immense sense of relief and downright sympathy for anyone he ever comes in contact with. Thank the Goddess of Good Riddance, I would never be one of them. I stirred up a batch of stiff martinis and re-applied my lipstick.

The Lil' Princess has been frolicking in those Taboo booths again with a big-weenied boy toy. The boy has his drawbacks, but hell, with her magnetic charm for the penile dysfunction set, she's taking the good with the bad with this one. However, after a rough bout in the booth 'o lust, she immerged with alarm, noticing her glasses were missing an all-important rhinestone. "I'm missing a Diamelle! Oh gaaad, the Princess cannot possibly go around with a missing Diamelle!" Mz. Conduct is donating one to her in the name of royal roustabouts.

The Transient Trollop called from a city bus somewhere on the East Coast. She had a job interview at a nightspot that went rather well. All I caught before the line went dead was something about an old queen who said he wasn't hiring, but then they had cocktails, and are now fast friends.

I have more dates than a California palm tree this week, and needless to say, each should provide a story in itself. And of course, darling readers, I will disclose any juicy details fit for your ears.

> Dear Mz. Conduct,
> Is it really true that is I masturbate before a date that I'll last longer when having sex? And won't it cut down on the amount of cum? I know that when I masturbate a lot, after about the fifth time, there's not much more than a drop of cum left, if that. I want to give my date a full load and am concerned that I won't if I jack off beforehand.
> Straight Shooter
>> Dear SS,
>> Jesus in Jheri-curls, what's your intention, drowning the poor girl with a tankfull of wanker juice? And isn't this a bit presumptuous of you to plan all this facial fun with each 'date' you go on? Some girls may just want to see a movie and go home afterwards. Ever thought about that? No I think not, you're too busy whacking yourself into a frenzy. You probably need to be bitch-slapped and butt fucked, but that's beside the point. This is a loaded question (pun in-

tended) and I must flag down that buxom bar maid first. Oh, since I'm here by myself, I guess that would be me <giggle> and I mustn't forget my miniature penis cocktail stirrer, not for this question, oh no!

Okay, mister stroke machine, there really isn't any advantage to ejaculating a larger amount of semen, unless of course you're working on a full, eight-ounce protein shake for your partner. And by the way, even porn stars have a rough time with that. Yes, if you masturbate before you have sex it will make you last longer. The amount of the ejaculate varies in each man, as does the consistency and the color. And just so you know, the amount of ejaculate has nothing to do with the amount of sperm contained in that fluid either. The average volume of ejaculate in men is about 1.5 ml. The volume depends on the glands that secrete the seminal fluid, hormone levels, amount of sexual stimulation and, as you asked about, period of abstinence prior to ejaculation. If you have an enlarged prostate it will however limit your fluid amount and then you'd want to hip-hop down to the weenie doctor's shop.

Basically, to answer your question, yes, masturbating before a sexual encounter is good to prolong your pumping but it will cut down the amount of seminal fluid. It takes a day or two to build it back up to the same amount. By the way, zinc is an excellent mineral for men to take if they want to maintain a healthy prostate and seminal flow. A man's body continually manufactures semen so perhaps you shouldn't concern yourself so much about showering your date with weenie juice. Instead, focus on the rest of the time 'spent' with her.

Dear Mz. Conduct,

How do you know when a guy is just feeding you a line?

Suspicious Girl

> Dear SG,
>
> Mz. Conduct has heard them all but even still, I'll bet my titty-clamps that sporadic blurts of buffoonery are yet to enter my future. What I have learned is that what people say—and this goes for all folks—and what people do are entirely different things sometimes. Words are just that. Words are immediate ways to get a reaction. Behavior, on the other hand, takes time and requires more effort. You don't get to know someone by what they say, you know someone by their behavior.
>
> I see girls all the time falling over themselves for flowery spews of flattery and it just makes me sick. Bitch-slap and butt-fuck time again, honey. Sure, a bit of flattery is nice to hear but you have to think enough of yourself in the first place to already know whatever it is these guys are telling you is true. You know when a guy is feeding you a line; his behavior doesn't back it up, bottomline. Figure out what you want first when you meet someone. If it's a relationship you want or a partner then take your time and learn his behavior patterns. Take his words with grains of salt and go from there. Then again, if you just want to straddle his trouser trout, then take his hook, line and sinker, reel in the flattery, the tackle box and bait, and rock that boat 'til the gulls come home.

Mz. Conduct's House of Sin

"The older I grow, the less important the comma becomes. Let the reader catch his own breath."
–Elizabeth Clarkson Zwart

Tease my titties and call me Tank Girl. I threw a wee, little birthday bash for a dear friend and woke up the next morning to snow, a raging hangover—on eighty-dollar Spanish wine, no less—a house full of paella-caked dishes and the phone ringing incessantly. I crawled out of bed, slapped my Judy Garland CD on, ignored the phone and smoked a ciggie. Then I went outside with the dogs to play in the snow where I promptly stepped in a snow-disguised pile of soggy dog crap. Oh yeah, I made rude gestures to the dogs, swore like a sailor and Judy's "Clang Clang Clang went the trolley" came ripping off the CD player. I decided to start over and bee-lined my ample ass right back to bed.

I had a suitor with promise this week, Sir Have-Weenie-Will-Travel. He had mucho potential that is until he came over with a bottle of...get this...screw-top wine. Jesus in a Jell-O bath, do I seem like a girl that would drink screw-top wine? I think not! I opened it, took a whiff and decided it would come in handy to strip some furniture with. Needless to say, the furniture was the only thing that was thought about getting stripped that night. On his behalf, it was very late and...ohmagaad, you know what? To hell with the 'on his behalf' crap, there are no excuses. Yeeesh, I sometimes have to bitch-slap myself. And why is it that men feel compelled to whip out there schlongs thinking we girls will just faint at the mere sight of it? Okay, so it's true to a point, but damn it all to hell, why can't they just leave their magic meat on the coffee table and get the hell out?

Having sex for money was a new ambition of mine to report on. So, yay, I can do that now. A relentless pursuer and visitor to the House Of Sin got farther than the welcome mat this week. The guy was decent enough and I invited him in this time along with the two crisp bills in his hand. While the conversation was appallingly boring and his cologne strangled my nostrils, I focused on the lovely loot he laid on my dresser. So we got to it as I remained focused on the green stuff. That loot would buy the little, black dress (pump pump) that I had been ogling, food for the (pump pump) mutts and a few other (pump pump) necessities. I decided it was totally worth it and for an hour out of my night—and as long as I wasn't missing *Sex in the City*—I rocked this guy's boat (safely in a latex weenie raincoat). As a matter of fact, I rocked and rolled his dinghy so far out into the wicked waters of oblivion that I thought I might have to bury his depleted ass at sea. It felt naughty and slutty and oh so right and I'd do it again damnit...when need be.

Mz. Lula la Paintbrush had a good point the other day. She said "You really know that it's time to move on in a relationship when you notice that lump-line down the middle of your bed." You know, the big ridge that grows between each other, the one that's too mountainous for either person to roll over. And so there you lay in your little trench of mattress. If the relationship is worth it, instead of shopping for a new partner, there's always the option of getting a new mattress I suppose. Mz. Lula is a lascivious, little she-devil and she phoned her Catholic priest/lover last night. She gave him a tad of naughty talk while he was in the abbey. I picture his fingers frantically kneading the strand of rosary beads draped around his wrist and under his starched, black cassock, an enormous boner pointing the way right to the confessional. Oh Lord love us bad girls.

I've got parties to throw, bashes to attend and exotic dancers to interview. Oh how I need my hot bubble baths accompanied by my 'Wash Those Sins Away' soap and one large, dirty martini, three olives of please.

Dear Mz. Conduct,

I've been seeing a married man for about six months and I know you're going to rake me over the coals for this, but I really think this is a different situation. He and his wife haven't slept together for years. She has severe health problems and not interested in sex at all. We sneak off and have amazing sex and I feel so great afterwards. He makes me feel like a queen. He says I make him feel just as good. But then it's sometimes weeks before I hear from him. I haven't put my life on hold however, and date other men in the meantime. It's just that none of the other guys make me feel as good as when I'm with him. So, here's my question: should I sever it before I totally fall in love with this married guy or just enjoy my time with him and hope someday he'll leave his wife and be with me as he says he wants to do?

Mz. Conduct's House of Sin

The Other Woman

> Dear OT,
>
> Good God in a Good 'N Plenty box, to paraphrase Dr. Phil, could you be more stupid if you lopped off your freakin' head? First of all, this is no different than any other 'I hope he'll leave his wife' stories. Whether it be the ball and chain's lack of libido, the insane head case wife, the 'we have nothing in common' situation or any other of the million and a half reasons that men slip their slimy salamis into 'the other woman'. Get it through your thick skull that if a man is going to make changes in his life, he won't talk about it forever and a day, he'll just freakin' do it. That's what real men do anyway.
>
> This guy's wife has health problems and that makes it all the less likely that he'll ever leave. What he will do is keep wrapping you around his weenie until you won't wrap anymore and then he'll replace you with another brainless bimbo.
>
> At least you are seeing other guys and I give you two points for that. The reason this married, spineless, cheatin' on his disabled wife, wart-weenied, son-abitch makes you feel good is because there's a dangerous aspect in it all. Danger is almost always a big thrill. Plus the fact that you know his wife can't please him as you do, duh…ego boost. So, put it together. Rather let me do it for you. Okay, you have: danger + ego boost = power tripping, delusional, duncette. Oh, that's you by the way!
>
> Things will most likely never change. Weigh it out, if a few hours of blinded bliss is worth three weeks of being ignored then have at it. If you decide it is worth it and you indeed keep pole vaulting with his weenie and you do fall in love, then be sure to write me back so I can point and laugh and say "I told you so!"

Dear Mz. Conduct,

I met this beautiful woman a few weeks ago. I got brave enough to finally ask her out and to my surprise she accepted. We went to a cafe, had a nice afternoon and we talked about getting together again. Things were going really great until I walked her to her car and she kissed me. I know you're thinking I'm crazy at this point but the thing is, her kiss was horrible. Maybe this is shallow of me, but I could feel her teeth cutting through my lips and it was awful. The thing is that I truly like this woman. I'm wondering if I should ignore this faux pas and see if she's any better next time. Obviously I don't need to worry about her being interested, but I am worried about losing my lips in the process. What would you do? What should I do?

Bitten By Vampira

> Hooters in a hatbox mister, I know I've been here before. I bet we all have. For me personally, if the individual in question doesn't soak me to the ankles on the first kiss, they're getting nowhere fast from there.
>
> I think the way a person kisses tells so much. It's a window to the way they will make love to your body. I know a few times when I really liked someone—but had too many weenies on the stick already and didn't want to muck it up any further—I've wished with all my might that they be a horrifying smoocher. That would cement the deal right there…friends and only friends. Sometimes when the kiss happens it's yuck, ptui, and then it's easy, no incurred problems. But then once in a blue moon, oh fuck me running, you get the fourth of July and New Year's Eve all rolled up into one big tongue tangling, throb-a-thon. Somebody slap me…my mind is drifting and my panties are dampening with just that dash of memory.

I would say that since you like this woman so much and she apparently likes you (and your skin for a snack), it wouldn't hurt (or maybe it will) to give her another try. The next time you find yourself in a locking stare and you feel her coming in for the kill, take control of the kiss and see what happens. May the force be with you.

Mz. Conduct's House of Sin

"Did you ever feel like the world was a tuxedo and you were a pair of brown shoes?"
–George Gobel

Last summer I picked up a little paperback book at a garage sale for a quarter, no less. All the Grand Dames of advice are my motivational goddesses and I had to have this one for sure. It was Amy Vanderbilt's *Answers to Everyday Etiquette*, published in 1957, the glorious year Mz. Conduct was born screaming into this oh-so-deserving world. The back cover describes the handbook as "a down-to-earth guide to gracious modern living; carefully arranged and ready for use." It's a hoot to say the least and full of chuckles such as this one:

"Dear Amy,
In my work I travel quite a lot on trains. Is it ever correct for me to permit a man to buy me a drink, either alcoholic or non-alcoholic, on these trips?
Miss W.P."

Here is Ms. Vanderbilt's answer:

"Dear W.P.,
No, never permit strangers, especially men, to buy drinks for you on a train or in a terminal. And do not accept any invitations from such strangers for entertainment at the end of the journey, unless you arrange for friends or business acquaintances to join you. This rule applies even to older women traveling for business or social purposes."

Well, tawdry trollops in a bar car, my advice would be a tad different of course. I say if a man wants to buy you a cocktail, you let him girl! And my rule applies especially to us older woman. Unless he's drooling pools of saliva on his pocket pencil protector and has a problem forming a sentence, I would graciously swill gin until the end of the line. And if he invites you to a wild bash in the hills, Beverly that is—swimming pools, movie stars—Sushi on a swizzle stick, woman, you go! Have fun, meet people. Life is shorter than my last date's dick.

A box full of sex books I ordered just came in the mail and I am a damn happy hoyden. It's snowing monster flakes, the fire is blazing and my martini waits. I can't think of a better way to spend an evening than reading about the clitoris, the illicit behavior in the 16th century King's quarters and the challenges of masturbation. Actually, I can think of a better evening but there seems to be a moratorium on penises tonight. And there's nothing like checking one of your email accounts and having big blue letters come up to remind you "your box is empty". Thanks so much. Well, as Winnie the Pooh would say (and I'm pretty sure he was without a penis as well) "Ho Hum".

> Dear Mz. Conduct,
>
> I am 34 and my husband is 45. We have been married for seven years. He works constantly and I rarely see him at all. When he has time off, he wants to either be alone or just watch sports. I have asked him to spend more time with me and he will for awhile but then it always goes back to the same old thing. I am getting so frustrated, what should I do short of killing him dead?
>
> Losing the Love in Rome
>
> > **Dear LtLiL,**
> >
> > Yeah, you don't want to kill him at this point. You most likely haven't checked his will or insurance policies lately and besides, it's messy and exhausting and dragging the body around will just throw your back out.
> >
> > You need to sit him down without any interruptions taking place and tell him seriously that you must have some more of his attentions, bottom line. Ask him if he really wants to be with you because it's not what his behavior is telling you. Ask if he's willing to try some counseling with you. When you're in a partnership with someone, there has to be communication going on at all times. In a partnership each person must listen to the other's needs and then make certain compromises based on those needs. When one person refuses or procrastinates and doesn't fulfill their end of the partnership, then it's up to the unhappiest one (you) to make some changes. We can't depend on someone else to make us happy, it has to come from within first. Basically, ask yourself this: is it worth it to you to remain in this relationship and stress yourself into a murderous frenzy? If it isn't then suck or get off the cock. If you decide it's worth it to be ignored and disrespected then live with it and quit whining. But honey, at least grab that pretty, young man at the shoe store, and on a regular basis, have him stuff that size nine into your empty, little Roman box.
>
> Dear Mz. Conduct,
>
> I'm a 43-year-old man in a twelve-year marriage. My wife and I have been using the chat lines and ICQ to bring some fantasy into our sex life. It has been fun, but lately my wife gets extremely jealous when I'm on the computer so much and it's not

Mz. Conduct's House of Sin

working so well anymore. Now I want a real threesome but I don't know how to go about it. Can you help?

Asking in Aussie Land

> Dear AiAL,
>
> Kangaroos on a keypad, why would you try and coax your wife into a threesome when she's already made it clear that she's become insecure with the cheap thrills of a chat room? I can only assume that you want your wife and another woman concluding this threesome. How would you feel about another man with you and your wife? Whatever the menagerie, hold off for now.
>
> Listen to what your wife is telling you when she says she's jealous. Jealousy is an unnecessary emotion, mind you, but nevertheless if it's what she's feeling then it's coming from somewhere and there's an insecurity behind it. Why not put the ICQ on "out to lunch" for a while and concentrate on the just the two of you.
>
> A bit of role-playing may be just the ticket. Act out your fantasies with each other even if you feel silly at first. Maybe she needs more attention. I wouldn't know anything about that, mind you (cough cough). Maybe too much of your time is spent on the Internet instead of focusing on one another. Thus, your wife isn't getting your time, some acne scarred, four hundred pound "blonde, blue-eyed, model type" is. You don't need as much of the Internet as you need your imagination.
>
> Sexual Role-Playing can be very bonding. Acting out your fantasies is an extremely healthy way to explore your sexual life. Role playing, taking on the persona of a different person (i.e., French maid, pirate, nurse), is essential to fantasy. By taking on a different role we free ourselves of our so-called 'normal' boundaries and it helps us to discover new things about ourselves.
>
> Just get your head out of computer and put it into your wife. Bring up the threesome idea only after you two have resumed a closeness. Make it a fantasy for now which can be great in itself and see how she reacts. You don't have to put the idea in the trash, but for now, put in in a Hefty bag near the back door. If it starts to stink, figure it's a no go.

Good Advice from a Very Bad Girl

"We were once so close to Heaven/Peter came out and gave us medals/ Declaring us 'The Nicest of the Damned'."
–They Might Be Giants, from their song "Road Movie to Berlin"

Scratch and sniff and get my drift, honey. Every damn Valentine's day is always a huge disappointment for me. We all have our little favorite things and mine happens to be flowers, well and, as we all know, beautiful appendages. I was a florist for eight years and even owned my own flower cart for a few months, until some lunatic burned it down. That's a whole other story. Anyway, I make it abundantly clear to all man/boys that I adore flowers. And every year, no freakin' flowers on the holiest of days and honey, I'm so worth it. I'm full of fire and penis desire. Granted that on the holiday of the chubby little cupid, prices go skyrocketing for flowers of any kind. Hell, at the flower shop we used to cackle at the businessmen who'd almost forgotten their sweeties and raced in before we closed, looking for any crap we had left. At three times the price, they'd snap up some withered Carnations, the ever so lovely 'hearts on a mug' arrangement, or wilted, blown open roses. So, for that day, Valentine's day, I'll accept a gift instead because it really is slightly unattractive to foolishly pay those prices for faded old Forget-Me-Nots. However, and yes there is a however, potted, blooming plants such as orchids are nice, as you can purchase them weeks beforehand to save the holiday price hikes. The rest of the year leaves no room for excuses. Now I'm not talking about yanking a prized azalea out by the roots of some old woman's yard, as one of my exes used to do when he had been drinking all night. He'd stumble home through the neighborhood only to slobber out his late-night excuses and then proceed to try and pee in the closet. That's not the sentiment I'm talking about. It's the little things that matter in any sort of relationship such as: a single lily on your doorstep with a note or a bunch of spring flowers on a gloomy day. A day perhaps when you've thoroughly explained to your sweetie, down to the tiniest detail, which they love hearing of course, what it's actually like when you're bleeding like a stuck pig and feel as bloated as an overcooked shellfish. That's what I mean.

Mz. Conduct's House of Sin

The Lil' Princess has a keeper of a Keeper at the moment. I called to let her know I was safely home from a blind date and her man had strewn rose petals all over her candle lit bedroom and surprised her after her bath. That was before he banged her big, bootiful, booty...sigh. What a man.

Most of my dates lately have been, for the most part, uneventful. Other than being suffiently sodomized by a couple of well endowed boys, my dates usually consist of me graciously gathering my gifts, drinking fifty martinis and blathering my opinion and advice to everyone at the bar. When it comes time to leave I pick the most suitable sycophant to escort me back to the House Of Sin...and sometimes it's even my date.

> Dear Mz. Conduct,
> I'm a 38 year old, attractive women who is married, and feeling love starved and rapacious. I so want to meet somebody, say who feels the same about his situation. He must be a male on a Seattle website that I can hook up with. Is there such a site or must I head out to the bar??!! Please help?
> Ms. D
>
>> **Dear MD**
>> You ravenous little ho! I know for a fact that there are infinite amounts of people in the same boat. As a matter of fact that boat is bigger than twelve of the Titanic...but this one stays afloat through hell or high water, honey.
>>
>> There are lots of things to do in your situation you big wannabe ho. The first thing I suggest is to talk to that lame ass hubby of yours. Crap on a cracker, that's his stinkin' job. Communication is the thang baby. When he ignores you, stares at the computer continuously, or digs in his ass while you talk, THEN I say go to it, woman. This way you've tried, you've warned him and off you go.
>>
>> The personal ads are great. Check the Seattle Weekly or The Stranger. You're bound to find some tidbit in there. I really suggest, and I've said this before, that you place an ad instead of answering one. This way it's free (in most papers) plus you have control (oh sweet control!). You can state just what you're looking for and weed through all the Cro-Magnons that, yes, you will receive. It's all part of the fun though. Be patient and if you can help not going to a seedy bar—although I picked up a nice specimen once at the Nightlight in Seattle—then refrain. It's just better to put what your needs out there discreetly and see what fellatio loving flounder you can reel in. I know the whole thing can be frustrating and sometimes that sparkling dildo just doesn't replace the feel of penis meat skin. Sigh...okay now I'm going on my own fishing expedition. Deep sea baby, deep sea.
>
> Dear Mz. Conduct,
> I haven't had sex in over four years. The craziest thing is that I've been married for seventeen years. My wife and I sleep in the same bed and have a decent relationship but just not sexual. Four years ago I had an affair, my wife found out and confronted

me. I confessed but she wasn't at all upset. I have a suspicion she has been seeing a man for a few years now. I hear them on the phone making lunch plans and things like that but the funny thing is that I don't seem to care. I need to have sex soon but wonder what to do. What can you suggest?

Sexless in Salt Lake

> **Dear SiSL,**
>
> My suggestion is that you go throw your stupid self off the nearest high rise. Lawrence of a labia, do you not know how to talk to this woman you've been married to for nearly two decades? That was rhetorical, obviously you don't and that's your main problem.
>
> You probably have this secure little relationship, dog, house cars, etc. and don't really want to muck it up. You most likely even really love her. Fine. Work with it. Okay, she wasn't upset at you having an affair, you're not upset with her sneaking around, what's the big conundrum? It's simple. You learn how to form a sentence, sit down with her and just tell her that you are not happy sexually. Talk about your past affair, ask her flat out about hers and then see if you can come to some middle ground where the sneaky stuff desists. You may be surprised at what she says. Maybe you can work on an open relationship together. Many people do this successfully, but communication is number one in any type of relationship. So start talking mister and the closer you'll get to dipping your wanton weenie in something wet (other than the carpet cleaner hose, that is).

Mz. Conduct's House of Sin

Amy: *"The hell with it. I shall become a bitter, twisted hag with nothing but rouge and one-liners to disguise the emptiness of my existence, and I shall drown the memory of numerous loveless affairs in a tsunami of vodka."* **Tulip:** *"I think gin's more traditional."*
–Amy Grinderbinder and Tulip O'Hare from the graphic novel The Preacher

I'd like to report that Mz. Conduct was not a happy hoyden for Valentine's day. The previous week, an entire Ella Fitzgerald song was emailed to me through slobberspace, and although the gesture was ultra romantic and totally swept me off my eight inch heels, apparently it was supposed to 'tide me over' through the holiest of holidays. Ha, fat chance. My only phone call was a message from a boytoy's jealous woman (how unfortunate), a psychotic hag who screamed illiterate obscenities into the receiver. No flowers, no nothing, and honey I was livid. The Lil' Princess sent the only gift I was given on my porch and that was stolen, wouldn't you know. The girls came through, as always. Ms. Lula La Paintbrush bought me a book and an overflowing ashtray magnet. Okay, I did get a mushy card from the Lion King and a couple of sweet e-mails, but I've decided, from this day on, that my Valentine's day will consist of giving my man/boys a proper education. I'd like to perform Mz. Conduct's home vasectomies on all of them, and when needed, Mz. Conduct's home circumcision. Needless to say, there will be no anesthetic in the vicinity, except for mine, of course.

So, I'm out on the most boring date in the world, a blind date at that. I'm hornier than a locked up bitch in heat and stock market expectations and George Dubya's blunders are not my idea of stimulating topics of conversation. The guy is monotone, bony and above all, unshaven, albeit trim and neat. I'm about to talk to my soup I'm so uninterested. Just when I think all is doomed for the evening, the waiter (a young coffee-skinned lad) succeeded in slipping me a small piece of paper. Intrigued, I thought...hmmm! My date never even skipped a beat in his diatribe of economical downfalls. I opened the piece of notepaper in my lap and read the words "you look like you could use a rendezvous. Go to the ladies room now". Well, my stomach got butterflies and my pulse raced. We were just finishing our entree and I politely excused myself to go to the bathroom. When I got to the door, this beautiful boy intercepted me and grabbed my hand. I thought, what the hell, I'm impulsive trollop, and followed him to a supply closet. He locked the door and immediately slammed me up against a giant rack of paper products. His hot breath was on my mouth in seconds and I returned the heat inside him. We banged ourselves into oblivion and he quickly muffled my screams with a pack of towelettes. I composed my disheveled self in the real ladies room this time and walked back to my table. I know I had that freshly laid glow about me and at this point, when my dolt of a date said "Should we get dessert?" I thought, sure what the hell. He would sit and blather away and I would bask in that firm eight inches that was just thrust upon me. I am not dating that guy anymore but will be back to the restaurant on any other blind dates I end up on. A girl's gotta eat, doesn't she?

The Lil' Princess and I went to a sex writer's reading at a bookstore last week. It was to promote the *Best Bisexual Erotica* book that was just published recently by Black Books. The first speaker asked, jokingly, that they see our hands at all times. Carol Queen was absolutely fabulous and M. Christian was his usual twisted mo fo, Darklady read a poignant piece, Bill Brent (Black Books publisher) delivered a story from one of his other books, Margaret Weller read a hysterical story in her tie-dyed gown. Charles Anders, cross-dressing expert, read some tidbits-bits of advice to those wanting to solidify their 'look'. I was bummed that my friend, Jamie Joy Gatto (mindcaviar.com) wasn't there, but as she explained it's Mardi Gras in her hometown and she wasn't about to go anywhere.

I had the utmost—oh geez that's my mother's word, and may she rest in peace, as she's probably teaching aerobics in hell—embarrassing incident in the elevator at the bookstore. Against my better judgment, I am telling this to you. I guess I figure that if you can't laugh at yourself, then who can you laugh at, right? So, the Lil' Princess and I waiting for the elevator and this cute little dyke walks up, wearing a stunning leopard hat. I love leopard and had to tell her that her hat was fab. We started a conversation about proper attire with

Mz. Conduct's House of Sin

leopard and such. The elevator comes and we get in, along with several others going to the reading. I was wearing tall Mary Jane shoes, black lace tights and a black, lace, retro dress. The cute, little dyke turns to me in the semi-crowded elevator and says "Oh my God, I just realized that you're lace from head to toe". Well, Mz. Conduct was confused and heard "Oh my God, you're just LEGS from head to toe", which was such a flattering remark to me being that I am not that tall. So I beamed back "Oh that's sooo nice of you, no one has ever said that to me before...I think I love you!" At this point everyone in the elevator looks at me like I'm nuts, and rightly so. We get off, go to the reading and after all of that, we're walking out and I again go on about what a nice comment that was (as I was still all flattered like a dork), from that cute little dyke. The Lil' Princess asked me what I thought she said, I told her, she laughed so hard I thought I smelled urine and right away, cleared up the misunderstanding. I wanted to die. Yeah sure, some cute girl is really going to rave about my long, more like sausage legs...when hell serves Dove bars.

Mz Conduct,
What is "queening"? I saw it in a magazine, but with no explanation.
Curious George

> **Dear CG,**
> The term "queening" used to be sort of a derogatory term for a gay man, although it's not such a big deal anymore. I think though that maybe you may have had your head (both of them) in a deviant sort of magazine, and why not? If I had a choice between *Ladies Home Journal* and *Watersports and Whips*, I'd read the latter of course.
>
> But the sort of "queening" you are most likely referring to is when a woman straddles another person's face and forces her vulva into their mouth and nose.
>
> It could be a form of simple mound munching or it could be a type of breath control. Breath control is autoerotic asphyxiation. It's a game involving control or restriction of air and/or the supply of oxygen to the brain. These games are dangerous to play alone and even with a partner, unless of course they're annoying the hell out of you.

Dear Mz. Conduct,
I've dated this guy a few times and I really like him. The trouble is that I don't know how he feels about me. He's hard to read and I don't think he's very good with emotional expressions. When we're out together, all I think about is that I hope he likes me as much as I like him and I worry that I'm not acting too stupid and I look okay. He never says anything and it's driving me crazy. How can I know?
Worried Girl

Good Advice from a Very Bad Girl

Dear WG,

Bourbon and backwash girl, I'll save you the big mystery. Yes, you are acting stupid and shallow and self-absorbed and shall I go on? Let me tell you something very important: The best thing you can ever do, when attracted to a man as much as you are, is make him feel good about himself. Ditch the dizzy-ass fretting over yourself because I'll have to personally come and bitch-slap you. And that'll just work up a crazy thirst in me and God knows I've had everyone's share of martinis this week. So, obviously he likes you well enough, being that you've gone out more than once. Now it's time to pay attention to him. Believe me, guys don't notice your smudged mascara if you're busy listening to their stories, complimenting them on how sexy, smart and interesting they are. That's the absolute best thing you can do for any guy. Most of them need a big 'ol ego-hoister, at least in some respect, as much as we all do. Don't overdo it though, just lose your vanity and concentrate on his. Don't get me wrong, we girls do need to feel like princesses (and in my case a Queen), but in time you should be able to find a royal balance. It's up to you to find the places he needs emotionally filled and then fill 'em, cupcake. In return you'll probably get your snatch filled as well.

Mz. Conduct's House of Sin

When Good Things Happen to Bad Girls

"It's the way you love me down. Every time we kiss you bring out the woman in me. Every time you holler out my name you set me free. I am a sex-o-matic venus freak when I'm with you."
–Macy Gray

My week has consisted of nursing a bruised uvula from my ex shoving his enormous, Cuban missile down my throat while I was trying to pee, fending off a darting tongue from an old, hippie, ex boss who bragged about his love for Viagra, and canoodling with horny boys who have no apparent employment and promise me the freakin' moon. Well, I'm a sunshine girl, boys, just so you know. Little Miss Sunny Delight, that's me, all smiles and rainbows and all that happy horseshit. Now where are my ciggies and coffee?

Not Your Average Joe called me from the lovely Jefferson Theatre the other night. This is a porn theatre that specializes in audience participation and performance art, let's just say. I have been there once with the Lion King and loved the standing ovation I received when my fishnet-covered ass was hiked in the air while I drained his member. I'm an exhibitionist I admit, and feel quite comfortable with it, thank you. So, Not Your Average Joe calls me from inside this wild theatre and since I wasn't home he left a message. He was like a twisted version of Howard Cosell or something as he commentated on his swarthy surroundings. "Mz. Conduct you should come down here. There are two couples getting it on in one section and another woman getting her wrists wrapped with electrical tape. Now, over on the other side, it looks like we have several guys spanking their monkeys." He then went on to say he bought a great piece of art at a gallery earlier that evening and blah and blah. I had a mental picture of him in this darkened theatre, his cell phone in one hand, his ample appendage in the other. His moniker was acquired for a reason.

Ms. Lula la Paintbrush and I went downtown to put some of her gorgeous artwork in a salon. It was one of those swanky places, one of those 'massage, nails, and hair' salons with perfectly coiffed snoots running around fiddling with everyone's 'do. Well, they took one look at my 'hair-don't' and offered an emergency, (mere) sixty-eight dollar conditioning treatment. Thinking of all the martinis that could buy, plus a new pair of black-seamed stockings, I declined...and not so politely. After all, I could have shot back with "Ms. Fancy Pants, it looks as if you haven't had a good orgasm in years, let me help you out with that immediately, and for just sixty-eight bucks." After that fiasco, Ms. Lula and I decided to go to Leonard's tobacco store and browse. We automatically turned into Lucy and Ethel and made his poor life a living hell for the good part of an hour. We know he loved it. Ms. Lula and I looked at cigarette cases and lighters and pipe tobacco and smutty magazines and purple candy. Then it hit us, we just had to have some sort of elegant cigarette holder. Not too long, but just long enough (my particular weenie motto at that). This was something I always felt I should have anyway and today was the day. We picked out lovely amber and silver holders and then spent the entire afternoon walking around with them like we were some sort of movie stars from the thirties. I stopped on the way home to rent the video—for the umpteenth time—the classic Sunset Boulevard. Oh swoon and smoke baby, I absolutely adore that film.

It looks like I may soon be writing for a new fangled dating magazine. One which is featured on some new, daytime television talk show. I will also be doing the quarterly booze and bitch column on Mind Caviar called Bottoms Up. My edible editor friend says I'll be going on Oprah any day now. Now that would be a hoot and a half. Me and Oprah just yakking it up, that is, until she brings out Dr. Phil to hack my gin soaked advice to shreds. Ha, let him try! I'd love to make him cry, honey!

Well daahlings, I must go. I have a lunch date at the Labia Lounge and my libations await within the walls of a luscious red head.

> Dear Mz. Conduct,
> I am a loyal, faithful reader of yours and get a gigantic monstrosity of a kick out of your writing. Now I'm wondering if you will answer a question of mine?

Mz. Conduct's House of Sin

I am in what I would consider to be my 'middle' years. In 1987 I was diagnosed with Multiple Sclerosis following a traumatic loss in my life.

My problem is as follows; In the more recent past, I broached the subject of Cannabis as a form of relief for persons suffering from diseases like cancer and M.S. I told my neurologist that when I treat myself with Marijuana it really helps. He sort of hemmed and hawed about the whole thing, explaining to me that he thought I was doing "just fine" handling my M.S. and that I don't need to smoke anything that can be "a potentially dangerous drug".

At night it sometimes causes me to feel so relaxed that I'm able to achieve an orgasm of extremely high quality with my husband and/or by myself. I usually experience up to four orgasms during one sexual encounter, because of Marijuana and my own insatiable needs. Why can't the damn plant be more readily available without me and my household having to fork out sometimes up to $300.00 per month? Is this something you can help me with?

Fondly, and anxiously awaiting your wise response,

"Turned on by an ILLEGAL SUBSTANCE"

> Dear TobalS,
>
> My advice to you, since you do have MS, is to see another doctor. While your neurologist may be someone you're comfortable with, he doesn't seem to be listening to you with an open mind. He sounds like a misdirected, uptight old coot, actually. Plus, if he can't just keep you on all the pharmaceuticals, he won't be able to buy that new boat he has his eye on. This guy thinks you're "handling it fine," well, hootie and a blowjob, you just explained how it could be handled better. Furthermore, his crack about marijuana being "potentially dangerous" is a bunch of theoretical toe-jam. What can be "potentially dangerous" is his ignorance. Oh, honey, don't get me started. Too late! Yeah, let's call marijuana a potential danger to a woman who has a chronic illness and then we'll prescribe huge amounts of unnecessary drugs to everyone we know, pop a couple over-the-counter "legal" drugs with lunch, have a few legal cocktails after work and then drive home where the wife—on her antidepressants—will hand you a 'muscle relaxer' and a scotch. Sure, that makes sense and that's America.
>
> There are doctors that are more liberally minded when it comes to medicinal marijuana use and you should find one. You'll have to establish a good doctor/patient relationship first and not just go in on the first visit and ask him/her to sign a form. After you've established this relationship then see if/how they can help you get what you need. You can get a card showing legal rights to carry marijuana and use it. Depending on where you live in some cases, if you can't find a place to buy it, you can grow it yourself. There are a few good web sites you may also want to check out. One web site is www.cannabis.com/medical/. Another good site is TheCompassionClub.org (instead of .com).
>
> I agree with you wholeheartedly that marijuana should be more available for medicinal purposes. I think it's fab that it helps to transpose you into an orgasmic goddess. It does have different effects on individuals though. I knew a guy that said he could never even drive without smoking a joint first. On the other hand, if I did that I would be putting at about three miles an hour, sweating profusely and glancing into my rearview mirror every third second, thinking every car behind me was a copper. I'm happy it works well for you and good luck. Take two bong hits and call me in the morning.

Dear Mz. Conduct,

Good Advice from a Very Bad Girl

Could you tell me why this woman I've been seeing for weeks now refuses to kiss me? I really enjoy spending time with her when we go out. She's made it clear that she's attracted to me since we've dry humped and rolled around for hours on end. When I want to go farther, she puts a stop to it and says she has to go home. I asked her why she's playing me like this and she says she doesn't want to get emotionally attached. What's going on in this woman's head? Please help!

Blue Balls in Baltimore

> Dear BB,
>
> I know what's not going on in your head, the release of yum yum juice and that's just a damn shame. Granted, I did this sort of thing when I was a teenager, but I assume your woman is as grown up as the pulsating bulge in your slacks. Send her to me a.s.a.p. and I will promptly bitch-slap and butt fuck her.
>
> Seriously, I think this floozy has issues, as a lot of women seem to. If she really likes you, then she should be kissing you, and often, and by someone who knows how—Gaad I love that line when Rhett Butler says that to Scarlett O'Hara. It's true, though. When you really like someone you crave their kisses like melting sugar cubes in honey, like butterfly wings and soul surging suction. Okay, I'm drifting into a bit of a moist reverie here.
>
> Chastity belts and paddle welts, I don't have time for such nonsense myself. If you want to have sex with someone then you should. Take a risk of loving and celebrate the connection in the meantime. If she won't kiss you (what is she a prank-call girl?), she may be right about the fear of attachment, but then why the hell does she roll around with you for hours and not give up the pooty? She's a lunar case sweetie, that's why. If she really wants your steamin' stem o' flesh then maybe she's worried that she's not experienced enough or perhaps she's groped your monster meat and is wondering how to fully take it on (hey, someone should try to make you feel good). Or maybe she's just an immature, teasing little ho and you should tell her just that …but in a nice way. Simply say that you enjoy going out with her, but if she's really not going to have sex with you, that it'd be best to not to allow yourselves to get into the dry humping-horizontal-hoopla again. If she persists on being a whack-job then suggest she play elsewhere. On her way out the door, slap a sign on her stingy ass that says "Does not play well with others" (you know, just to warn other undeserving men). Moooove on mister, find another girl that isn't a Pandora's box of penis-punishing-puzzlement and bang her 'til the cows come home.

Mz. Conduct's House of Sin

Wet Between the Rabbit Ears

"Cunt" is not slang, dialect, or any marginal form, but a true language word, and of the oldest stock. It is a derivative of the Oriental Great Goddess known as Cunti, or Kunda, the Yoni of the Universe.
—Barbara Walker

Tweak my titty and call me Kung Pao Kitty, I remember when I was a young spring chicken, the word cunt used to make me cringe with rigid disgust. The media has always held complex controversy with this word especially, (even in this publication I am careful not to actually spell it out). As I got older I realized how much I verbally caress and actually enjoy the intricate use of the word. I love to pooch out my cock sucking (I love that word too) lips to deliver the word. Roll out my bottom lip and say it with emphasis, with total meaning, embracing the succulent syllable for all it's worth. Cunt...mmmm. And with it's own raspy-voiced inference, it seems to envelop all that I am as a woman.

My wise, ol' Yippie* mentor Stew Albert and I were discussing this topic just the other day when he reflected into his amazing past, as he so often does. Stew told me that he was the first person to ever say the word cunt on national television. Wow, I thought, and grabbed my pen and pad. This is his story and a bit of the etymology of the word itself:

It was 1970. Stew and Jerry Rubin, two of the founding members of the Yippie organization, were invited to the London version of the David Frost show. The show was a live discussion forum and the crowd was full of radical, left wing, hippies and Yippies. The anti-war movement was at hand and the discussion became quite colorful. David Frost was interviewing the two when he described one in the group, Jerry Rubin, as "a reasonable man". Stew shouted back, jokingly, "He's not a reasonable man, he's the most unreasonable cunt I've ever known in my life!" The atmosphere turned to pandemonium and a riot ensued. Marijuana cigarettes were being passed through the audience and general upheaval persisted. David Frost then called the British police and Stew and Jerry had to flee into the London subway system. A week later they were

Good Advice from a Very Bad Girl

deported. Stew has yet to set foot on London ground, other than a quick plane transfer. The Yippies have been described as media terrorists who demonstrated an uncanny ability to manipulate the media and consistently tried to be offensive. Oh Stewy, my hero!

After this first use of the word cunt on television, the world's first cinematic outing came the following year in the film *Carnal Knowledge*. Jack Nicholson called Ann-Margaret a "ball-bustin' son-of-a-cunt bitch". Oh Jack, do you kiss your mama with that mouth? In 1972 there was a double-bill of cunt use at the cinema, John Waters' (hail, hail the great!) *Pink Flamingos* and *L'Ultimo Tango A Paragi* (the French and yummy Last Tango in Paris). In *Pink Flamingos*, the Sandy Sanderstone character says of another, "You're a real cunt, you know that? A real fucking cunt!" In an out-take from the same film, another character spouts, "A lot of people like cunt…but your eyes are like cunt to me. Them cunt-eyes". Then in *L' Ultimo Tango A Paragi*, Marlon Brando sits by the deathbed of his wife and addresses her in a long, emotional monologue: "Smile, you cunt! You pig-fucker. You God damn fucking pig-fucking liar". Oh, Marlon, you twisted genius, no one could have played that part as you did. What a memorable film.

Then Lisa Kuhne titled her 1993 lesbian porn film *Cunt Dykula*, though other uses of cunt in films titles have been limited to the fictional *My Cunt Needs Shafts* and *Girls Who Crave Cunt*, and the heterosexual porn, such as: *Mondo Cunt*; *Cunt-Eating Frenzy*; *Cunt Hunt*; and of course, *Cunt Hunt II*. I have a sudden hankering for popcorn and a stiff martini and gee…a cunt?

Thankfully, these days the word is used much more liberally and acceptance seems to be building. Just this year the *Vagina Monologues* played in town and I attended a play by a performance troupe known as The House of Cunt. It was fabulous! By the way, if any of you readers have any objections to me overusing the word cunt…well then, lick mine!

Mz. Conduct's House of Sin

Stew Albert's biography is now available at independent bookstores everywhere and through his website at http://stewalbert.com.

*Yippie = highly theatrical hippies that mixed their performance art with their political activism, calling themselves the Youth International Party.

Some information used is from a PhD thesis from the University of Coventry in England.

The Catch O' the Day is Trouser Trout

"Is sex dirty? Only if it's done right."
–Woody Allen

My ex told me the other day that I'm every man's best dream and worst nightmare all rolled into one. I polled my boys and they all agree. Hmmm…such is life I suppose.

I should have known it would be one of those days. I woke to a phone call at an obscene hour, a wrong number at that, then heard the recycling truck screech up like an intergalactic battleship. I heard each bottle being thrown into the truck separately and what seemed like an hour-long process. I just knew it was a deliberate act on the recycler boy's part. I mean, they saw two big bags of empty liquor bottles and they assumed I was hung over and were going to really piss me off. I bet they thought that if they had to get up at the butt-crack of dawn then why shouldn't the party girls? Maybe they couldn't get laid and they were somehow trying to take it out on me, I don't know. They won. I dragged myself out of bed, waited for coffee and went in the other room to slip in a Parliament CD. Hey, if I was awake, I was going for all the way. As soon as I pushed in the CD tray, my phallic shaped cactus that sits atop the CD stand, all at once came toppling down on my chicken-haired, head. True, I had been neglecting it, but hookers on a hymnbook, it's a freakin' cactus. So, after a few colorful expletives that sent the dogs running for cover, I carefully picked up the eight-inch stem of prickly plant and carried it outside. I tossed it on the cement and stomped the holy hell out of it. Reminding myself that I was, for the most part, sane and almost completely in possession of my faculties, I went in to have my glamour girl coffee and ciggie and start the day over.

Later same day, I was out on my porch, shaking out a hairy dog blanket when I see my old, green and silver toothed neighbor, Jackson, come cruising up the sidewalk carrying a white bag with grease oozing from its pores. Since he saw me last summer in my backyard (lurking lustily from his apartment window),

Mz. Conduct's House of Sin

mowing the lawn and gardening butt-naked as I always do, he's never let go of his lurid, little fantasies. He's asked me to go have a drink several times and each time I tell him, unless they hold the Ice Capades in hell, it's never going to happen. I also told him that he blew it by telling me that he spied on me in my backyard because he'll never see me in the buff again. He shakes his head saying, "Oh damn now". Not a mental giant, poor Jackson. So on this day he asks politely if he could come up on my lawn, as he wants to ask me something. I give him the okay, and he sticks out of his greasy bag he's clutching and offers me some sort of stanky fish. "No thanks" I say "I don't really eat fish." "Oh that's right, you're one of those veganarians. I be needin' a woman like you to make me healthier," he says. I told him I bet he could do that all by himself, thinking to myself, inevitably like everything else. Knowing that wasn't what he really wanted to ask me, he hem-haws around a bit and I'm still shaking the blanket, beating the dog hairs into canine oblivion. I tell him to spit it out because I have to prepare for a shindig I'm throwing that evening. After begging me not to get upset, he finally says—with his soft spoken, yet jive talking self and his greasy fish hands going up and down his body for effect—"I be waking up evvvery mornin' just thinkin' 'bout you, girl." I said that I'm sure he did and asked, was that all? He continues with his Ebonic plague and says under his breath "I was just wonderin', uh, if I could come up wit a hunded fitty dollars, could I please have some sex with you?" Well, I, for some reason wasn't offended and just told him "Ol' Jackson, that's just never going to happen, not even wit your hunded fitty bucks, but hey, you go enjoy this beautiful day and your bag o' fish." He walked away shaking his head and groaning like the day was going to be extra long. I shuddered, thinking about those greasy fish hands stroking that old man weenie meat and went inside to make a martini before my guests arrived, a damn stiff martini at that, stiffer than a greasy ol' Jackson weenie.

Dear Mz. Conduct,
I am a medical doctor, but I'm at a loss for this and thought maybe you could help. I had a patient come in and while I was giving him a physical I noticed he had a peculiar piercing. I see many a pierced body parts these days, but this was in the rim under the head of his penis. I didn't ask him like I wanted to so I'm asking you. Also I wondered if it's a pleasure thrill for him or more for the woman?

Good Advice from a Very Bad Girl

Dr. Dumbo

Dear DD,

First of all, how presumptuous to assume that the pleasure could only be for himself or a woman. He could very well be a gay boy with a lover that gets a bang (pun intended) out of the sensation. Consider yourself bitch-slapped.

You weren't terribly specific so I will tell you what comes to mind. Penis, mmm, penis head, rim mmm…okay I'm there and honey, it doesn't take much. Well, let's see, you have your Prince Albert which is probably the most common in male genitalia piercing. It's usually a ring that enters through the urethra and then immediately behind the glans, or the head of the penis. Nipple rings on a Nazi, what am I telling you this for, you're a doctor. Anyway, for some people, the piercing is purely aesthetic, but for others, it is highly sensual. I should add that some women find the piercing uncomfortable. Want to know a bit of the history you say? Well, a lot has been written about the history of this piercing, but very little of it is true. The most common story is that it was a "dressing ring" used to pull the penis into tight fitting fashions, and that Prince Albert himself had one. Other people have suggested than he wore it to keep his foreskin retracted and "fresh smelling" so as not to offend his Queen. Others have suggested that it was worn by divers to hold on a urine trap as an alternative to a catheter. There is no conclusive evidence that any of these is particularly true.

You also have the ampallang, which is a male genital piercing passing horizontally through the body of the glans, whether through the urethra or above it. Initial jewelry is almost always a straight barbell. Historically this piercing was performed in various Polynesian cultures, specifically the Dayak people of Borneo, who wore this to emulate the rhino, which has a similarly equipped penis courtesy of nature.

There is also the frenum piercing which goes through the little piece of skin on the underside of the head. Not all men have these slips of skin to do that sort of piercing with though. You can even have implanted tiny balls around the head of the penis. The majority of those implants are inserted using a pseudo-surgical method. Obviously there are several kinds of piercing for male genitalia so perhaps I've touched on whatever it was you saw. Basically there are contradicting explanations of male/female stimulation and it really depends on your partner. Personally I would have inspected it closely, tried out the sensation, smooched it just a bit, you know because I must, and been promptly reported to the authorities. I suppose it's good I do what I do, eh?

Now take two weenie rings and yank them in the morning.

Mz. Conduct's House of Sin

"Life is a banquet and most poor suckers are starving to death."
–Rosalind Russell in Auntie Mame

Gaad, I love that movie! Auntie Mame is hung over and as she exclaims, "Honey I'm hung," and pulls up her satin sleep mask to answer the elaborately decorated telephone. When the crotchety, old coot from the bank says he's on his way over to check out the status of her newly adopted nephew, Auntie Mame panics and asks "You're coming…now? Repeating what she hears, she says with disgust, "Spitting distance?" Moaning under her breath she drawls, "Howwww vivid".

I feel like Auntie Mame today. Flog my flanks and call me Fortunate Fanny. It's a good time to write. It's 3:47 in the morning and I am doomed to insomnia tonight. I fell right to sleep in front of a blazing fire, all cozy and warm, only to be woken by a knock on the door at midnight. Well, I don't answer my door at that hour, so I peeked out from the curtain. It was Yolanda, a homeless woman I give my beer bottles to from time to time. Too bad Yolanda, you may be homeless, but you can find a clock. I crawl back to bed, determined to drift away into a sea of sexy dreamland, only to hear the wind banging the hell out of the bamboo shade on my porch. At least something is getting banged. Try as I might to ignore it, no such luck. After wrestling and tying it down, back to bed I go. Almost to sleep, the sheep's baas are fading and then Bing, Bing, Bing goes the gaaadaaam oven timer, which has always possessed—key word here—a mind of it's own. Three times I shut it off and knock on wood (where's a firm penis when you need one?), it seems to have finally stopped. Once again, insert body in bed. Well now I realize that I just can't sleep so on goes the television. I have a choice of two infomercials, the not-the-least-bit amusing and resurrected—for this time of night only—*Charles in Charge*, and the crap I chose in the end. It's one of those creepy, road movies with Mark Hamill as a psycho who just yanked some morbidly obese woman's fake eye right out of her head. Horrified, I watch for awhile, but after he slices up some innocent young girl with a switchblade, I come in to write. Luke Skywalker, what's happened to you? Perhaps that's what too much butt banging will do to you.

Good Advice from a Very Bad Girl

So I attended an S&M 101 class last week and for three hours watched about twenty people blush and hang their mouths open in amazement. There was quite a motley crew in attendance: four-hundred pound dykes; timid, little, mousy girls; what looked to be a homeless man with matted hair and filthy pants; and even a yuppie couple that looked as if they had mistakenly entered the place thinking it was a Starbucks. For me the stuff taught in class was mostly old news. I did learn a few things, however. I learned that, unless you're a pro Dom, handcuffs are not recommended for play. They can cut off circulation and cause permanent nerve damage to the wrist area. If you've ever been in police custody, you know the impact they can have, and they're not playing consensually. The two instructors were serious eye candy by the way and I was a bit worked up just watching their interactions and vivid explanations of things. They both agreed that since they actually like handcuffs, they do use them. But they recommend if you do use handcuffs, you should attach restraints (either leather or the washable sort) to the wrists and then attach the handcuffs to the restraints, then to the bedposts or eyebolts or whatever you're hooking the person to. That way you have the aesthetics as well as the clink clinking sound. Makes sense to me. They passed around at least twelve different flogging devices and when I had passed the last one around (my favorite, the horsetail), I was as moist as a damn snack cake.

A quick check back to the movie and Mark Hamill is running amuck with a surgical saw, covered in blood and laughing manically. Vulvas and villains, then Robert Mitchum, of all people, appears as the seemingly self-medicated psychiatrist. What next, Martha Stewart in a French maid's uniform, using a scalpel on some pathetic craft project?

The Transient Trollop called and has been parading around with her gay boy. Hey, they can be fun in the sack too! They went to a drag queen cabaret, which turned out to be a pants-peeing hilarity. Poor girl hasn't been laid in months and if I were there, we'd be smoochin', strappin' on and pouring good champagne, that's for sure.

Mz. Conduct's House of Sin

Dear Mz. Conduct,

I'm nineteen and a Catholic altar boy and have been feeling guilty because I can't stop looking at porn lately. My girlfriend doesn't know and I'm ashamed when I see the things I see. Some of the things that I look at are extreme, like some S&M and really dirty things. How can I stop this and save myself?

Bad Altar Boy

> Dear BAB,
>
> Oh geez how I love altar boys, all pristine and proper and sprouting young wood under those ironed, linen robes. Oh I'm supposed to be helping you, aren't I? Perhaps I'm taking the place of the confessional or maybe you just feel the desire taking hold and need the bad girl extraordinaire advice. Either way, dear boy, listen up.
>
> There is nothing wrong with porn. I'm a dirty girl (and have the soap and wash cloth saying just that) and damn proud of it. There's really no real health or pleasure without your own freedom to enjoy sex. Looking at gigantic men's appendages thrusting into some tight little hole turns you on because, well, you're human. Plus the fact that you're freakin' nineteen means your hormones are raging, honey. By the way, I certainly don't consider SM to be dirty. Sure you do because you're Catholic, home of the hypocritical movement, pedophile priests, unchanging viewpoints and sexually repressed men and women. So okay, I'm biased; I was raised by psychotic Catholic nuns and have a slight attitude. You're in the House Of Sin now though and you may find even a fetish that appeals to you. It's okay sweetmeat. If you sit there all damn day and night wanking away and ignoring your girl, then I would say you may have a problem. Just like computer games and gambling, it, like anything can become an addiction, so watch it. Otherwise lose that Catholic guilt, maybe try and share your view of vixens with your girl if you think she can handle it. If not look into finding an experienced Dominatrix to teach you the ropes (pun intended), and enjoy yourself. Remember, shame is a worthless emotion. It's up to you if you share that with the confessional priest though, he'd most likely give you six thousand Hail Marys and flog himself.

Dear Mz. Conduct,

I needed a spot of information and I wondered if you could help me. I want to give my husband a nice massage, but don't know which massage oil to use. The one time I gave him a massage, I'd used Johnson's baby oil, as nothing else was available at home at that time. In spite of the oil, he enjoyed it so much that I want to give him one with a proper good massage oil. Can you please tell me what sort of oil would be good? And also can you tell me if I need any other accessories other than oil for giving a massage?

Oil of Oh Lay

> Dear OoOL,
>
> Massage...oh lord, what a slathering of good oil and some magical hands can do to uplift (pun intended) a person. The last visit to my masseur, he got a tad carried away and greased me up like a holiday ham, gave me an erotic massage to cum for and by golly I did just that. I can be such a bad, bad girl, but sensuality is the essence of who we are and very important in the longevity of life.
>
> Okay, back to you. Good oil is crucial. Baby oil is mineral oil, it may feel nice on the skin, but it can clog your pores. I like using olive oil myself. The skin ab-

sorbs it well and it's completely natural. I called one of the highest rated spas in Portland, the Finlandia Spa, and the masseuse there agreed with me. She's been in the business for over a decade and feels it is the healthiest by far. I also talked to a masseuse at the Dosha spa and they prefer to use jojoba oil, which is also a natural oil and absorbed easily through the skin. She likes to use jojoba because it isn't quite as thick as olive oil, which makes it easier to spread than Mz. Conduct's legs, and it also has a neutral scent. If you want to add a scent, be sure it's only an essential oil in whatever oil you decide to use. A lot of men really like the scent of vanilla, but you can ask your husband what he likes. Give him a snoot of some little testers such as cinnamon, vanilla, etc.

As far as other accessories, candles are always a thumbs up and be sure to pick a nice relaxing music to soothe the mood. Enigma and oil…okay I'm drifting again. Make sure you put the oil in your hands first so it warms to your touch and then slather up that man of yours. And you know what? Ask for one yourself sometime, girl!

Mz. Conduct's House of Sin

Time Flies and So Do Queen Bees

"Maybe some women aren't meant to be tamed. Maybe they need to run free, until they find someone just as wild to run with."
–Carrie from Sex in the City

Maybe it's because of a big digit birthday on my doorstep (damn that welcome mat), or maybe it's a reflection of past experiences, past penises and the fact that having a queen bee complex simply complicates everything.

Queen bees love attention; our honey is by far the sweetest and we dare to have deviant double standards. Then we can't understand why people don't get us. We are not jealous or possessive until we find ourselves in a love thang, which we fight like hell to avoid. Sometimes it just creeps up and bites us on our beautiful, round asses. Because we get turned on even more by the pain of the bite, we feel as if we've lost control. We will always gather back control, that's not the issue. It's the abruptness of the sting and the vacancy in the hive.

What is it that we queen bees want? Why is it that we need everyone to love us more than anyone else? We want brains, romance, nurturing and undying love, but we also want a man who is strong enough to put us in our place when need be. Personally I want to be banged in the library bathroom. I want strange adventure and uninhibited lust, anywhere and anyplace I so desire. I want flowers and surprises and to be told I'm a raging bitch when I am. I want to be slammed up against the wall and told how much I'm wanted. I want tenderness and humor and nasty exchanges all day long. I want sex in the morning and in the middle of the night and every chance in between. I want to be held when I'm crying and my hair stroked when I'm a blathering, drunken mess. Is that too much to ask? I don't think so. But maybe that's why no man can handle me and stay sane or physically intact for long. Men see me as a challenge and then fizzle out somewhere down the line. I wonder if any one person can alter your spirit within, or finally put a muzzle on the little green monster that shadows us from time to time. Is enough ever enough, and will I live long enough to know?

Good Advice from a Very Bad Girl

I thought back to third grade when David Madrigal was my boyfriend. He was sweet and very cute and hid lots of gifts for me in the big oak tree down the street. I loved it but wanted something more. Danny Fisher was popular and with his little overbite, I decided that I wanted him too. Eventually, and as the years went by, I roped him and then juggled the two pre-pubescent punks until I dumped them both for Eddie H. Eddie H. was a bad boy. Trouble with the law and the works and we were only in middle school. He threw rocks at me and was mean, but I knew he liked me because when he wasn't with his friends, he would call me at home and talk nasty. I thought, this was the boy for me. Well, until another one caught my eye, at least. He already had a girlfriend, but that was beside the point in my should-have-been-banned book, and when I finally got his undivided attention, I dumped him like a bag of week old trash. There is something about the unattainable to us all that remains so tempting and alluring. I just want everyone's love, damnit. Hey, it's not like I don't make it a point to spread it around myself.

Anyway, my life has always been this way and I wonder why it is that we queen bees need more than simple girls seem to. The uncomplicated and simple girls that men end up marrying...and then inevitably cheat on with us. Maybe because we're wild, spirited and on fire in the sack, and can never be tamed.

So, the transient trollop called me, peeing her panties in laughter. She had called her voice mailbox and heard a panting sort of breathy sound but no message. Well, after getting all worked up and listening to it four times she realized it was her own damn voice. She had called and hit the wrong button an hour before and left herself the unknowingly titillating message. Too freakin' funny. Since I was feeling unloved and rejected, she informed me, "Hey, at least I don't have anyone to reject me where as you and your whining self allows yourself a pasture full of boys to reject your demanding queen bee self." I guess she has a point. She said if I complained further, she'd kick my ass so hard that I'd be wearing a colostomy bag. Then I could shop for shitty shoes to go with it. Point taken.

Mz. Conduct's House of Sin

Dear Mz. Conduct,

I know this is an odd question, but would you consider stepping/walking on a man? Would you choose to wear shoes and if so what type? Is this a strange thing to ask?

Footing the Bill

> **Dear FtB,**
>
> Oh, it's not an odd question and in the mood I'm in, you betcha! Yes I would wear shoes, my shiny, black, stiletto heels and I'd start marching away at your groin, honey, like I was putting out a fire. Don't take it personally though, you're just a man.
>
> It's not that strange, as you have a foot fetish of sorts. You like to be demeaned by the opposite sex and have a definite submissive side to you. In actuality this activity would have to be planned a bit and discussed ahead of time with the woman who would do this. You may want to start with her bare feet and work your way up to heels of any sort. Afterwards, a nice massage and some intimacy are a must. You can always hire a professional dominatrix to do this too. She will know what she's doing and inadvertently show you what to do with a non-professional for next time. Not a new fetish, and nothing to fret over. When I was a little girl I remember Nancy Sinatra's sex ridden voice on the radio as she sang "These boots are made for walking, and that's just what they'll do. One of these days these boots are gonna walk all over you." I used to get chicken skin just thinking how cool that would be. Of course it was a metaphorical verse in her case, but I always preferred the literal interpretation. If the shoe fits, wear it and walk on a man who loves it.

Dear Mz. Conduct,

Recently a woman told me I have an abnormal penis. She said it was too short, too fat and the head curves too far under. I have only been with a hand-full of women in my life and never really compared my erect penis with another man's so never thought anything was wrong with my little friend. I respect her opinion and wondered if you could help?

Deviant Dick

> **Dear DD,**
>
> Panty liners for post-it notes, at least this woman was brutally honest with you, I commend her for that alone. From what you tell me, it sounds like you may Peyronies (pronounced pay-row-knees) disease. I found out about this when the Lil' Princess had a man with such a penis. Sometimes a penis with Peyronies is very short, abnormally so, say about three inches when erect. It also can be very thick and the head is severely curved up or down or to the side. It can make it difficult to penetrate a woman and can also be painful at times. There are surgical procedures that can help, but they are painful and sometimes shorten the penis even more. There are exercises you can do though, and if consistent, may also help and certainly be less painful without losing anymore length. It sounds like surgery would not be a bright idea for you, stubby.
>
> If any of these things sound familiar then there is a site you can check out at www.peyronies.org which may answer some further questions. If not, then maybe you just have a mutant little stub of manhood and should go find a submissive little woman who will love you first for who you are then happily take whatever hangs between your legs.

Good Advice from a Very Bad Girl

"My God, I haven't been fucked like that since grade school."
–Marla Singer in Fight Club

I got birthday money from my papa...hooray, hooray! I immediately ran out and bought the video *Bend Over Boyfriend*, which I've been wanting for awhile now. It's a bit more tutorial than I had hoped, for me at least (because I'm little Miss Know-It-All), but I highly recommend it for women wanting to explore anal play with their man. Next on the list: boots and dildos. What else does a girl need?

I've been a very bad girl this week and perhaps need a swat on my sassy, plump ass. I made a naughty, little movie with a longtime, artist friend. Initially, I trotted on over to his purple, Victorian house so that he could draw out the tattoo I've been planning. I wanted vines, he insisted on flowers. This went on for a bit. Then he showed me footage, on his digital camera, of flowers that he photographed when vacationing in Central America. The next thing I know, we were shooting yours truly, and honey, you know I'm a ham for the cam. I was having a blast and my black, lace, bell-bottom pants were an aesthetic addition to each scene. We made cocktails and played my movie back on the big screen. Christ on a crutch, it was smoking. Suddenly I heard the song blare in my head, "You Oughta Be in Pictures." I'm not a narcissistic, exhibitionist, gutter slut. Really, I'm not!

Sir Have-Weenie-Will-Travel came swinging it by the other night and handed me a box of British tea like it was a big gift or something. When I asked what it was for, he pompously told me it was for "when he comes over." Well, he drinks gin at night and tea in the morning, so that meant one presumptuous thing. He was planning on spending the night. Now I never let anyone spend the night, for the simple fact that I don't especially want to wake up and look at them in the morning. My usual line is "Leave your penis on the coffee table and get out." Hell, it'd been a very long time since I caved, and his damn accent was making me as wet as my cheeks at a French film festival. Was it worth it?

Mz. Conduct's House of Sin

Well, the morning after, I vowed to resume my original plan of booting out the booty before I hit the hay. It's never been worth it, so far anyway.

The Little Princess and I share the same royal birthdays and have been celebrating all week. Basically, I've been hung over for eight days straight. We had a cathartic little week, though (a necessary thing when approaching big birthdays). We danced, we sang horrible seventies tunes, we picked at our French fries, we blubbered into Bloody Marys, we smooched in the bathroom, we shopped for shoes, we admired each other's titties, we drank too many cocktails, and we degraded—in an honest manner of course—all men in every way possible. That's our job, isn't it?

> Dear Mz. Conduct,
> I'm happily married and have been for nine years. My wife is a wonderful woman, but isn't interested in sex anymore. This is my question; what would you tell me if I were to have sex with another woman? There's a woman I have been with only once, but I want to continue seeing her. We can both be discreet, which is very important to me, as I know my wife would divorce me if she ever found out. I don't want to lose my wife and son, but my manhood is wasting away. Please help?
> Sneaky Pete
>
> **Dear SP,**
> Men, they have only a handful of hormones while we women have an entire slew to deal with. I'd like to tie you to a lamppost on your little yuppie street and butt fuck you until you fall into a coma. But then you'd probably like it. It's not just up to your wife to spice things up, you know. What have you done lately to make things more fun? She may be so jaded at seeing you whip out your weanus and expecting her to faint at the mere sight of it. So this is my diatribe for you, mister: you need to talk to your wife about this problem first. Why do men have such a hard time with freakin' communication? Is it because you're afraid of the confrontation, the truth, and the conflict? And would you rather just slip back into your slimy holes of cheatin' darkness and not have to deal with your woman freaking out? Well okay, granted, some women do freak out over the slightest things and also have communication trouble. We can make things way more complicated that need be, thus sending men off to cheat like a pool hustler under a full moon.
>
> You do need to talk to your wife though, and see if you can work towards some sexual satisfaction together. If she's unwilling and still uninterested only then would I tell her flat out that you might look elsewhere for your sexual gratification. See what she thinks of that. If she's unable to understand, then at least you gave it a shot. Just remember a few things when having a fling: you set yourself open to falling in love with someone else or vice versa; you will lose some of the sacredness you have with your wife; she may find out and leave you. Also think about the tables being turned. How would you feel and what would you do if she were cheating on you? If you're willing to take all of these

Good Advice from a Very Bad Girl

risks after talking with you wife then *via con Mz. Conduct*, and off you go into the wild humping yonder.

Dear Mz. Conduct,

Can you masturbate too much? I'm a guy that sometimes feels I have road rash from too much masturbation.

Sam and his Sore Snake

> **Dear SahSS,**
>
> Vulveeta and cheese, if that was the case I'd be in the Hall of Fame. I only think it's a problem if you feel compelled to massage your crotch in the dill pickle aisle of the supermarket.
>
> In the late 19th century and early 20th century western doctors blamed masturbation for every illness known to man, from tuberculosis to loose morality. We are lucky now to have fabulous resources to tell us differently. One of the best sex toys shops in the states is Toys in Babeland (www.babeland.com). They have a store in Seattle and one in New York and hold workshops on just this topic. In May they, along with Good Vibrations, are hosting a Masturbate-A-Thon that perhaps you could look into. If I were a judge, I'd be there wearing raingear and a smile. You sound like you're a competent candidate. Like Woody Allen said, "What's wrong with masturbation? It's sex with someone you love." I agree. It exercises your fantasies and it's safe sex.
>
> I know men who masturbate all day long, whenever they can and others who wank the wiener only on occasion. It depends on your drive and no matter what yours is, it's healthy and perfectly okay. If someone says they don't masturbate, they are lying, honey. If your meat whistle gets sore or dry then grease that baby up with some olive oil. Vroom, vroom, now off you go.

Mz. Conduct's House of Sin

"Happiness lies neither in vice nor in virtue; but in the manner we appreciate the one and the other, and the choice we make pursuant to our individual organization."
–Marquis de Sade

So, what did I get for my birthday? Tickets to see "Dirty Blonde," the story of Mae West? No. Elvis Costello tickets? No. The wonderful glass dildo? No. Toss a feather down my panties and call me twitchy, bitchy and a year older, what I got was a big dash to the ER, only to discover I had a kidney infection. I suppose that was my gift from my ex-husband: to drive me and wait with me in a white trash filled emergency room for five hours. As he so eloquently stated, as I lay in the ER waiting room, throbbing in pain in a fetal position, "We've just spent a whole six hours together, you know." Yes, I knew.

Ms. Lula la Paintbrush swung by later and offered me her kidney and presented me with a painting she did. My son gave me a lecture on how I need to stop making such a big deal about my birthday because I'm always disappointed. He may have a point, but my papa is the one that would spend hours constructing a beautiful and ornate crown for me on each of my birthdays. It was always decorated with bright gold paper and my name written in glitter across the front. It's a hard thing to let go of, but it's not his fault. After all, he is a man and had no freakin' idea what he'd inevitably started.

Okay, I can stop bitching now because I did get a gorgeous arrangement of my absolute favorite flower, freesia, from Mister New York, who will be jetting to the West Coast to see me soon. It's one of those online meets and I will divulge all the juicy details as they unfold. I was also surprised, in the wee hours, by mister Have-Weenie-Will-Travel. He was standing on my doorstep looking like the cat that ate the canary (instead of me), and holding a dozen pink roses. I received a glorious bouquet (and the best booty banging ever) from the Lion King as well. The Royal Diva sent me a huge, colorful bouquet of spring flowers and the Lil' Princess and her man came by with lilies so I have a house full of beautiful blooms and that makes me one happy hoyden. I was given wine,

Good Advice from a Very Bad Girl

candy necklaces, chocolate, and delightful French postcards. Tickets to Cirque du Soleil came from Ned Flanders, my brother sent me a book signed by an author (a now shopping-cart-pushing recluse), and a box o' treasures from my country-fried girlfriend. Wild Bill and his Amazing Appendage promises that when I'm feeling better, dinner, cocktails and the wrath of the amazing appendage. My Yippie mentor wrote me a poem that downright tickles my fancy, and my fancy is damn hard to locate sometimes. My son took me to dinner and a French movie and told me "Mom, you're a handful, but I wouldn't change you for the world." Now that's a birthday I deserve.

On a previous note, a kidney infection is not fun, it is not painless (even for those of us that have very high thresholds), it takes too long to recover from and it's just downright annoying. Big tip: when you've had several pitchers of bone-dry martinis and only three Triscuits, and you're having a wild night screaming "Bang me baby and bang me in every hole and do it now," be sure someone is sober enough to remember how important it is to hose off the magic wand before it enters another orifice of your body. Common sense is lost even on Mz. Conduct sometimes. Since I already got a butt fucking, I'll just bitch slap myself and move on.

So off to another year of canoodling and cocktailing and searching for a wildly spirited Sir Prancelot and all his merry men.

Dear Mz. Conduct,

I have a rather embarrassing confession: I can't seem to get off with a blowjob. With or without a condom. It just doesn't seem to do the trick. Frankly, it's a little disturbing, especially when a lover wants to show me her kindness by giving me what most men are dying for, a little lollipop pop. Usually, what happens is that she goes down on me expecting to blow my mind, and then I have to resort to some other method to gain my satisfaction.

Not that that is all that bad for her since it usually takes me a good long while before I discharge my manhood. I've never been the quick-like-a-bunny type.

Is it possible I haven't had the right experience with an experienced fellatio artist? In the end, I don't want to disappoint my lover, because, after all, she wants it too. I just don't want to keep her down there for an hour before anything happens.

Your advice is most appreciated. Thank you.

DJ BJ

Mz. Conduct's House of Sin

Dear DJ BJ,

Hmmmm, I recall a recent thirty-eight minute (yeah, honey I timed it) sausage sucking episode with nobody coming but me. Some men just have a difficult time having an orgasm with oral sex, that's just a fact. My ex husband never could and I used to think that if I can't do the trick then nobody could. Then again, I have been told by the man of the hour, that he's never been able to cum with a blow job so I shouldn't expect it, but all of a sudden…thar she blows.

Sometimes the inability to orgasm may be age related. Men as they age will at some point become less reliable in their ability to ejaculate. It can be a let down for your partner, but it's the way it goes (or doesn't). I know, for me, it's like sucking on a Tootsie Pop without ever reaching the center. But this shouldn't be the big concern. People are just different, in so many areas. Sexual compatibility is just like any other aspect of human nature. Your partner should accept this if they love you and if they can't, then they need to move on and search for what they truly desire sexually.

Speaking of which, desire is a package in and of itself. Keep these five things in mind:

1) Desire Phase: Without the desire to be sexually active, men are not going to get excited or have orgasms.

2) Excitement: Manifesting by penile erection in men and vaginal lubrication in women

3) Plateau: Full sexual excitement during intercourse.

4) Orgasm: A highly pleasurable sensation occurring at the peak of sexual excitement. It is associated with ejaculation in men and rhythmic contraction of pelvic floor muscles in women.

5) Resolution: Relief of sexual excitement and a feeling of relaxation after orgasm.

I found this tidbit on a men's sexual health site and you can give it some thought:

The inability to reach orgasm and ejaculation during any kind of sexual activity, in spite of normal erections and night emissions, is known as 'primary absolute anorgasmia.' If a patient was able to reach orgasm in the past, the term to describe his condition is 'secondary anorgasmia.' Several factors might interfere with reaching full sexual excitement and thus failure to reach orgasm. Suggested psychological factors include obsessive-compulsive personality, interpersonal factors and various fears. However, in many cases there is no clear-cut cause, and anorgasmia may puzzle both the patient and physician. Patients might fall into a performance anxiety trap. Instead of relaxing and enjoying the sexual experience they might focus on their performance and on reaching orgasm. Performance anxiety would thus inhibit sexual excitement and orgasm.

My advice to you is that if you're going to get together with your partner and you want to give it another go at filling her throat up, then hold off from masturbating for a few days beforehand. Also, you could read some erotica together and masturbate while doing so. When you feel yourself about to release then ask her to take you in her mouth and see if that works. Aside from that, I wouldn't worry about it so much…just relax and be creative.

Dear Mz. Conduct,

Good Advice from a Very Bad Girl

I've been married to the same man for almost twenty years. He's never liked me to initiate sex in any way. I could be completely sex starved and if I acted on it, it turns him off and he gets irate. Lately when I go swim at the pool, there's been a man who I talk with. He's very intense and has made it clear that he wants to be with me sexually. He's so different than my husband and I can't help but fantasize about being with him. If my husband ever found out I'm afraid he would become abusive, and I don't want that to happen. Should I have this fling I can't stop myself from thinking about or just put it away and be a good wife?

Wendy In The Woods

> Lord love a lapdance, you should spend a weekend at Mz. Conduct's Retreat for Stupid Bimbos. First of all, your husband is already abusive. There is no possible way that you can be happy with a husband like that. If you are afraid of physical abuse then you need to run (or swim) like the wind, honey. This man has brainwashed you into behaving a certain way to fit his egotistical and self-serving needs. I'd like to strap him to a garbage truck grill and use a cattle prod on him while his friends drink beer and scratch their pathetic crotches, but that's beside the point.
>
> I think you should sit down and tell your husband that this is not what you want out of a relationship. You want to be the aggressor from time to time and if he can't handle that then you may be forced to have to look elsewhere for your needs. I say, after twenty years of his sinker, go for mister swim master and have a wild time, you certainly deserve it. It may even help you rethink your marriage and realize that you may desire your freedom now, or at least a weekend at my retreat.

Mz. Conduct's House of Sin

"The truth can't hurt you/it's just like the dark/It scares you witless/but in time you see things clear and stark."
–Elvis Costello from the song "I Want You"

Why do we sometimes refuse to see the things that are there in front of us, in dire hope that they will someday turn into or fall into the places we desire and need? It makes me think of a lost quote that says "It takes one relationship to define another relationship" or something to that effect. I know that people are placed in our lives for a purpose, but maybe they aren't always for the purpose that we thought or that they are intended to be. Let's open our eyes and hearts to what we sincerely want in life, c'mon we can do it!

I had to let the Lion King go. He is feeling compelled to hunt and gather and rightly so. He needs to be running in the wild for now and I must ditch my double standard ass in the dirt. And moi, well, I'm stronger than even I know and I must thrust my heart out into the world again, ready for stomping and risk-taking and maybe, just maybe, to discover a wild beast in heat, jungle-bungle fevering and one who can truly love a wacky lioness like myself.

So on an effort to slip back into a non-monogamous headspace, I call up the pizza delivery boy (have I been watching too many porn flicks or what?). I ask for this one boy specifically and he knocks on the door thirty minutes later. Wearing my tall Mary Janes, a short, plaid schoolgirl outfit and crotchless fishnets, I ask him to come in while I get my wallet. He's a surfer boy with bleached blonde locks, tall and thin with blue-eyed lust, what my ex-husband would call a "faggy boy" or a "Mz. Conduct special." When he closes the door and sets the pizza on the coffee table, I look him in the eyes and say, "Your shift is over baby." I can tell that I've taken him by surprise and he doesn't know what to do, but that's okay, I do. I grabbed his face and kissed him like I was having an orgasm right there. That night, I wrapped my fishnets around every part of that boy and made him scream (Gaad, I love it when boys scream almost as loud as I do) like the naughty schoolgirl I was trying to be. Four hours later, he plans an unlikely story to tell his boss, and asks me if he could come back the next night. "Is it your night off?" I ask, and he says "it is now." Oh there are definite possibilities with this one. Large salami, lots of sauce and hold the dough and cheese, please. I'm such a bad girl, but damn, I'm so good at it.

I was deep into a compelling, S&M thriller, (*A Tangled Web* which you can buy on Amazon.com) written by my friend, Gregory Lions, when I get a call from Mister New York. Well, *A Tangled Web* is about a cyber affair with both parties interested in the S&M lifestyle. They finally meet and psycho madness unravels. I put the book down and answer the phone. So, it's Mister New York and he's telling me he already bought a ticket to come to the West Coast to see me. My stomach did flip-flops and Christ on a crouton, it had me a tad nervous. It will be a few months until he flies out, but I will keep you posted. If I end up dismembered in a ditch with a serrated bread knife on Highway 46 then you know the column will be a deader too. After three martinis and a shot of something clear, I decided to look at this as and adventure of the heart and loins, one of those risky yet thrilling affairs that just may sweep meaning into one's life. Stay tuned, film at eleven.

Cinderella Cyber Twat has been on a bit of a libidinous rampage lately. She's been loyally following her Mz. Conduct strategies down the rabbit hole of lust. She was a bad little bitch and straddled a boy, in a public place, giving him the thrill of his meek little life. With her short, leather skirt hiked up to China, she made him hotter than Georgia asphalt and they took it to his van in the parking lot. You go girl!

The Transient Trollop was once again down to her last dollar and once again she hit it big on the lottery. The rent was paid, the dog was fed, and then, of course, cocktail swilling ensued, thus leaving her broke and inebriated as always. Or until the next swoosh of blessed luck, if there is such a thing. Baby, everything happens for a reason.

Dear Mz. Conduct,

Mz. Conduct's House of Sin

Is it true that having a circumcised penis increases stamina? This is a rumor in Europe and I wondered if it was true.

Belgium Boy

> Dear BB,
>
> Holy peters in a pie pan, I think this is one of those man-type rumors that really has no substantiated answer. I asked my friend, Darklady (www.darklady.com), who is a wise woman indeed, and this is what she had to say: "I've never heard anything about this. My guess is that there's probably some reassuring male legend that associates the foreskin with potency and that any change to the penises natural, uncut status will somehow make said man "less" of a man. Never been my experience.
>
> "What a circumcised man will experience is less sensitivity. Frankly, if anything, that would be more likely to increase how long it takes a man to achieve ejaculation since it may take him more time to experience the same amount of sensations as an uncut man. But stamina? That's got to do with testosterone and overall good health, not whether or not a guy has a sheath of skin he can pull over the head of his dick. It's *faintly* possible this has some sort of roots in racism somewhere in the dim past, too, since it was primarily Jews who were circumcised until it became all the rage."
>
> So, keep in mind that nothing will improve stamina better than a good diet, a healthy mindset and the knowledge of your own body. No get out of my face and go eat a waffle.

Dear Mz. Conduct,

Why is it that I can't get completely hard lately? I find myself excited and wanting to be hard, but when push comes to shove, the old schlong just doesn't want to go there?

Limpy

> Dear L,
>
> There are several reasons that can cause a limp dick. What medications are you on, is the first thing that pops up (not that you've been there lately). Seriously, they can have a large effect on impotence.
>
> Normal erections require a healthy psychological response to the arousing stimuli, along with a relaxed state of mind. You could have performance anxiety. If you relax, get to know your partner—and if she's any kind of a real woman she'll stick around and understand—and don't stress about performing like a porn star. The most likely and most common causes for erectile failure or dysfunction are psychological. There are other reasons for sure, but here is my info:
>
> *Psychological*
>
> Psychological causes of erectile failure are often mistaken for physiological disorders. By far, the most likely causes of erectile failure are related to mental or emotional problems. The most common of these is performance anxiety. When a man feels pressured to achieve an erection (often spurred by occasional difficulty), he will commonly become anxious and nervous when in a sexually demanding situation. Anxiety conflicts with the ability to achieve an erection, and then failure results, perpetuating further anxiety. If you still find it impossible to break free of this cycle, it is strongly recommended you find a sex therapist to help you and your partner learn how to overcome this reversible problem.

Key word is reversible!

Neurological

Any neurological disorder which interrupts the nerve supply to the erectile tissues will generally cause an erectile failure. There is little known about the nerves which cause erection and therefore it is difficult to predict how damage to certain nerves will affect erectile capacity.

Blood Flow

If the blood flow to the genitals is halted or impeded, then erectile failure may occur. Vascular disease can cause the blockage or constriction of the arteries in the pelvis and/or penis. The blood that normally rushes to the penis is partially stopped. Vascular disease may also be the cause of leaks in the arteries or veins; this too can cause an erectile problem.

This little list holds some of the main causes, however there are other reasons this may be happening to you. You were quite vague in your question and I don't want to scare you limp (oh sorry you're already there) with diseases and such. All I have to say (that'll be the day) is God bless Viagra and God bless the cock ring. Those might be an option as well.

Mz. Conduct's House of Sin

"I took a deep breath and listened to the old brag of my heart. I am, I am, I am."
—Sylvia Plath

I am shamefully smitten with the Blue Sky Boy. That's a good thing, for what it's worth, but I must be careful, as for once in my life I'm concerned about being the dumpee rather than the dumper. This whole re-thinking of the Queen Bee thang can be tough on a tootsie-pop girl. God in a gunnysack, I don't want to be tossed like a salad, like cookies, like a dwarf, or a horseshoe. So, I'm simply a happy hoyden for now. It seems that just when you think your day is rained out and the game is cancelled, a beautiful blue sky comes rolling 'round and suddenly the game is on and all the bases are loaded. And no one holds a bat like I do, honey.

So, I dragged the ex hubby out to the Bang Me club, one of the oldest strip clubs in town. I bought him their famous four-dollar steak and sidled up to the bar to watch a tantalizing girl make the Neanderthal dolts jealous as she showed me all she had. How guys eat their sloppy ass burgers up there while the girls are trying to dance in their faces, I'll never understand. It seems so rude, but then again, some men haven't evolved much.

The Transient Trollop called from a state not far enough south to explain this annoying and puzzling habit of the indigenous folks: everyone, and she means everyone, uses the non-word 'conversate' in nearly every clumsy sentence they spew. "That bar is so loud that I just can't conversate with anyone, Gad!" or "I conversated this morning with the barber over my would-be comb-over." It's got her and her gay boyfriend in an absolute tizzy and forced them to have cheap whiskey in the morning. Hey, I understand completely. Just hearing that made me need to whip a bone-dry martini.

May is masturbation month (yeah I know, we've all got a jump on that) and a friend is holding a Masturbate-A-Thon shindig at a dungeon in town. At first I hesitated about going for fear of seeing a bunch of fat, hairy oafs sitting around

Good Advice from a Very Bad Girl

in a circle jerk. I could live my whole life without viewing that, but she's having celebrities such as Ron Jeremy (I know, the ultimate fat, hairy oaf) and maybe Dr. Carol Queen, who I love and admire to death, and a decent band to play as well. So, Mister Bo Dangles and I will go and check it out. Don't fret, I will report back with anything juicy. I may drag the Blue Sky Boy along as well, but I almost know for a fact that as soon as he steps in the room, the fountains will blow. I may need to carry a splatter shield just in case.

I just roped in a job as a phone sex operator and start yakking filth as of next week. Oh the joy of gushing girths while I do my nails, dishes and perhaps even myself. Men in need, that's my niche I suppose. Amusing stories are sure to be discovered and I will report to my readers with promptness.

And so it goes, 'round and 'round and up and down, my bucket is full to paint the town!

> Dear Mz. Conduct,
>
> I need some advice. I have a friend in San Francisco, a girl that I used to have a crush on. When I moved to another city last year we started emailing and have developed a good correspondence that has made us good friends.
>
> I mentioned that I had this same old crush and thought she was pretty darn lovely. Usually, I hear from her within a couple of days, but she hasn't written back in a week. It is very unlike her. I wrote and apologized, told her I valued our relationship, told her I trusted her and that I imagined us being friends until we were wrinkled and gray. I also made an indication that if I was being cavalier about flirting and caused any confusion I was sorry for this as well. Why won't my friend write? It is giving me heartbreak and grief.
>
> How long should I sit on my hands? There goes my heart being a fucker.
>
> Waiting in Wonder
>
> > **Oh just settle down, big boy. Put on *Miles Davis Live* and listen to him play Cyndi Lauper's "Time after Time." Have a Mz. Conduct martini and close your eyes. It will bring new meaning to your drab little, obsessive life. Stop jumping to conclusions about your girl. I'll bet a new pair of boots that she went on a vacation or her computer crashed or something like that. You opened yourself up and you feel vulnerable, it's okay baby, really. You should never feel bad about giving your love to someone. Perhaps she wasn't expecting that, but that's her problem, not yours. People should accept all the love that is given to them and it didn't sound as if you attached any strings. Leave it alone from here. Get off your hands and give her a call. And yes, honey, the heart is a throbbing hunk of a mo fo, but without it we would not feel what life is all about. Now quit whining before I feel compelled to bitch-slap and butt-fuck you mister!**

Mz. Conduct's House of Sin

Dear Mz. Conduct,

I've been chasing this girl for three years and now that I have her it's great. I fell in love with her and she fell in love with me. We've had our share of problems. She says I've changed, but I don't know how. I just want to make her feel safe, even though she says she's fine. I know that there's something bothering her, but she won't tell me. She says that I'm not the guy she fell in love with. She said at the start we talked about anything and everything, and now we mostly talk about sex. I find that it's hard to stop, but we decided to take it slow. So, the question is…How can I get back to that person I was? We've been going out for 8 months. I love her so much and want to be the best for her. Can you help please?

Losing Her Quickly

> Dear LHQ,
>
> Trollops with titty clamps, we all change and hopefully grow as the years go by. At least we should be evolving as individuals, this is a necessary thing. Every relationship has plateau stages where the initial interests seem to have worn off.
>
> You need to have a discussion with your girl about this. If she can't pinpoint what it is exactly that's 'changed' about you, be sure to make her know how important it is to figure this out and stay together. There might even be things about her that she feels have changed. Some people project their own life conundrums on to their partner instead of facing it themselves. Just a thought. It's good to self-evaluate the relationship from time to time. Relationships are work and both parties have to get involved, bottom line. In this case, she says the problem is the pressure of sex. She may be feeling as if all the focus is on a sexual relationship, and not a romantic one. There needs to be an equal balance, and women in particular need to know they are wanted for more than just a means to an end. My advice would be to take some extra measures to woo her. Go out on date, without dipping your boner in her honey trough, make out, dry hump like you used to. And don't forget the damn flowers you dolt! We absolutely love them, and the thought of you picking out a bunch of pretty posies just for us really rocks our world, believe me. Communicate to her through your actions that you want this to work. Just writing the words dry humping has got me all a-tither. Now where is that boy with the boner that I seem to be addicted to, damnit!

Good Advice from a Very Bad Girl

"Cherish forever what makes you unique, cuz you're really a yawn if it goes."
–Bette Midler

Why do we sometimes refuse to see the things that are there in front of us, in dire hope that they will someday turn into or fall into the places we desire and need? It makes me think of a lost quote that says "It takes one relationship to define another relationship," or something to that effect. I know that people are placed in our lives for a purpose, but maybe they aren't always for the purpose that we thought or that they are intended to be.

That said, I ventured out on yet another blind date. We met at the Tiki Lounge and since I was early, wanting to get the show on the road, I swilled two martinis by the time the girl walked in. Yes, honey pies, I finally hook up with a girlie girl and there she was…sauntering in the dark room, looking soothing yet smoldering, like a nun with a past. Tall and curvy, she wore her black boots and short leather skirt like she knew what she had. We sat for hours, drinking, smoking and laughing uncontrollably until we almost peed our panties, if we had any on. We decided to go to the bathroom together and then call it a night. We split the bill and I left a generous tip for the impeccable, gay boy waiter who had to deal with us all evening. Through the plastic palm trees and totem poles, we made our way to the flamingo-covered women's room. We took out turns and when I heard her trickle come to a stop, I opened the door and said, "let me wipe you baby." She sat there with those big green eyes and smiled. I wiped her beautiful little snatch and flushed for her. Still she sat there, and as I was on my knees in front of her, she pulled me towards her. Our gin soaked mouths met in a ferocious force of feminine energy and our hands searched for one another's scared spaces. Her chestnut hair in my face, the smell of cherry bark, sage and vaginal heat, I banged her right there on the toilet seat with a million faded, pink flamingos watching. Her muffled screams soared down my throat and settled somewhere inside me. We kissed until our lips felt invisible and then with our blushed cheeks, we laughed and slinked out of the Tiki Lounge swirling in our skirts and drunken delight. I guess I would call that a hot date for sure. That night, I gave her myself and my tele-

Mz. Conduct's House of Sin

phone number. Why am I reminded of the badge the Transient Trollop once gave me that said, "I gave myself to Jesus and now he never calls"? Well, she wasn't Jesus and she will call.

I was at the Vortex Room the other day with the ex hubby and my son—who incidentally informs me on a regular basis that I've traumatized him for life—and who should walk in, but Ann Drogenous and her new girlfriend who I'd been hankering to meet. Those girls are absolute dolls and I had to take them both on myself, but I swallowed my offer along with my cocktail and just yakked and had fun. Girls just want to have fun, ya know!

On that note, and hotter than Satan's stovetop, I may have to call up a boytoy to complete my day's fun. I sympathize with him for the simple fact that when I unleash my pent up passion, he will be writing his own epitaph for sure. Here lies Mz. Conduct's boytoy, firmly delivered into the next world. May he finally rest in pieces.

> Dear Mz. Conduct,
> We are a couple in search of bi-females in the Puget Sound area for fun and more, but all we seem to find are other couples looking to swing. This would not be so bad but the only man I really want to be with is the one I already have. Where are the single females I always hear are looking for couples?
> Tethered Two
>> Dear TT,
>> Well little Miss Unswingable, I for one, don't hear about single females looking for couples. Perhaps when you do hear of them you could confront these solitary she babes with a casual offer of drinks or a movie.
>> Women are different then men in that area—along with about a zillion others—and don't just look for a couple to bang in their boredom. Women tend to like to get to know a couple first and then maybe ease into a ménage à trois. Or maybe they're friends with the other women and love her and love to lick her and...oops, having a mind slip about the Electricity Slut. Anyway, back to you, my suggestion would be to join a group of polyamorous people, even if they are swingers. You may meet some juicy Lucy to join in your fantasy.
>> Another suggestion is to put an ad in the personals and be explicit as allowed. It may take awhile but you may get lucky. It'll help if your man is a hunka hunka burnin' love so spruce up the mister and good luck sister.
> Dear Mz. Conduct,
> I have a feeling my girlfriend is going to dump me, but nothing has been said yet. I guess it's just a vibe I've been getting lately. My question is: should I dump her first

so I don't get hurt so much or hold my breath and hope that I'm wrong and it'll just blow over?

Chicken Boy

> **Dear CB,**
>
> Yeah, why don't you hold your breath. Hold it until there's world peace, okay? Roosters on a rampage, if she is going to dump you I wouldn't blame her. No one wants a guy who can't communicate his feelings, at least to some extent. You're feeling 'a vibe' so that's a sign to talk to your girl and see what's going on. Who knows, maybe her period is late or her favorite shoes just went off sale. My point is that you don't know things about people until you ask. Don't second-guess her, dumbass. You seem more worried about saving face than what may be really going on between the two of you. Maybe, deep-down, you want to break up with her and are reeling this whole thing out of proportion just to give you an excuse. Maybe she's banging the soccer team and is simply annoyed with trying to make time for you, or maybe it's nothing at all and you're a paranoid pissant who deserves to be dumped his whole sorry life. If you care, then talk to her. If you don't, then come over to my house and do my sink full of stinkin' dishes, paint my nails, mow my lawn and then get the hell out.

Mz. Conduct's House of Sin

"Time wounds all heels."
–Jane Ace

The Transient Trollop was fired from her job, where she held the title "Waitress from Hell" and right before her freakin' birthday. She had planned to quit at some inopportune time, during the lunch rush or when the table of thirty lawyers were asking for more water, but sometimes things don't work out the way you want. As she so eloquently put it, "Getting fired from a job you hate is like being dumped by a mercy fuck."

I was at Spa Phoo-Phoo having my eyebrows waxed when I noticed how cute the girlie was that was ripping the wax off my brows. At first, I confess that I had deviant thoughts, but then realized she was much too young and seemingly innocent, so decided to hook her up with my studly son. She was totally into meeting him after I whipped out my wallet photo of him. I'm such a 'mom' sometimes, but he never doubts my judgment, as Mz. Conduct does have a knack for the love thang.

Sometimes my loved ones don't want to hear my blunt blurbs of advice, but then it dawns on them that I just may have a point. My ex-hubby hung up the phone on me after I gave him a few pointers before his blind date. All I said was "be sure and clip your loose cruisin' nose hairs and for the love of labia, when you play pool, don't put on your stinkin' gloves and look like an idiot. " The phone went *click*. Such is life, eh?

The Masturbate-a-Thon was a gas and a half. I was supposed to be working the coat room, but there were plenty of volunteers so I got off scott-free. Okay, even though I did get off, I'm not entirely sure there wasn't somebody named Scott involved. It was held at a local dungeon and I attended the bash in garter and stockings, scantily clad schoolgirl attire and very tall shoes. I was escorted by the Boytoy Bitch and Not-Your-Average-Joe, both looking edible and ready for anything. Greedgirl showed up later and the fun began. One of the main attractions was the Orgazmatron, a huge, motorized, dental chair-like device with a penis installed underneath. The boys were teasing me that if got on it I'd break it and ruin the party, which I thought may actually be the case, so I withheld from straddling the alluring concoction. However, Greedgirl slipped off her thong and put it around my neck, jumped on and went for a ride. I snapped some lovely shots of her pleasure ridden self and she got lots of justified applause afterwards. There were a couple of good bands in the main room, and a huge room full of apparatuses that tickled the fancies of many: leather slings and hydraulic benches hanging from chains, a cage, O-ring suspensions, several other rooms for different purposes, a cozier room that later turned into a bath of splooge and suffering, all directed at one individual, with yours truly as the fluffer. I just provided stimulation for the masses, that's all. Let's just say that the mouth can be a wicked and wonderful body part and between Greedgirl's and mine, the scene was definitely worth a celebration. Since I was supposed to be working there, I only felt it my duty. I danced with a very sexy boy, made use of the gynecological table, drank some sort of unidentified alcoholic beverage, and met Corina Curves. She was very sweet and despite the fact that she just had painful dental work done, was making her appearance as planned. Not-Your-Average-Joe snapped a couple of photos with me biting her monstrous mammaries. That's what I call 'big' fun! I met yummy Betty Boop and her cougar wrestling boyfriend from Seattle. They were funny and had lots of energy. All in all, it was an interesting evening. As Boytoy Bitch and I drove home, he calmly says to me "Baby, you'll understand if I don't kiss you right now?" and wanting badly just to get home to gargle and shower, I told him I did understand.

Mz. Conduct's House of Sin

"All really great lovers are articulate, and verbal seduction is the surest road to actual seduction."
–Marya Mannes

Blind date time again. This time a boy who wanted me to fulfill a fantasy of his reeled me in. His fantasy was—extremely sensual—to meet someone for the first time; no phone calls beforehand, no words spoken, just walk into the designated place and kiss. Wow, it sounded pretty hot and any titillating dare like that gets my panties wetter than a seal in heat. In fact it made me wonder why I hadn't thought of it. Of course, revisiting the thoughts of my last two blind dates, I was a bit freaked out about the possibility of the guy looking nothing like his picture again, perhaps resembling a recent parolee or even worse. However, this boy gave me a nice little 'out'. He explained in his email that if for some reason, after seeing him, I didn't want to kiss him, I could simply say "hello" and he would understand. We would continue our date without even a mention of the initial fantasy. Well, yank my thigh highs and call me saturated, this was worth trying.

I arrived at the dimly lit Orbit Room a bit early, my body clad in black lace and oozing with anticipation, so I could swill a quick martini and prepare for anything. I was ready with a boisterous vocal "hello" at any given moment, but throbbing for the opposite. A few men walked in, balding and entirely unappealing, and I was mumbling a silent prayer to the Goddess of Guttersluts. A few more minutes passed and in walks a beautiful, dark haired, hunk of yum yum meat. Beautiful black curls on his head and a butt I could launch my teeth into. He looked at me and smiled and I returned one boldly. He walked across the room to be sure it was actually me. Since I hadn't mentioned what I would be wearing or where I'd be sitting, he walked to the other side of the bar and looked around. All I could notice is those ebony curls, his smooth and boyish face, and the way his butt hugged his cargo pants. When he turned around from across the bar, he pointed at me as if to say "is that you?" and I smiled and nodded as his handsome face broke into a white-toothed grin, just a tad of wickedness on his lips. He strolled confidently towards the booth I was sitting in. What green eyes you have my dear, what gorgeous teeth you have my boy, what nice muscles you have and all the better to eat you with, my homo sapiens sex on a stick. He sat down next to me in the sparkly green booth and our mouths entangled in a gooey union of tongue and heat, making me stick to the vinyl beneath me. Where is a Maxi pad when you need one? We yakked and drank dry, three olive martinis and ended up at my house rolling around from here to eternity. The amazing night that followed consisted of glow-in-the-dark condoms, a freak out over my nipples, worship of his almighty appendage, near lockjaw, and slipping my leopard patterned dildo where no man (or woman) has ever gone before. Mister Yum Yum is in New York now, just for a visit, but when he gets back, I'm all over that like red on a cherry.

So, fellow daters, all you whiners out there (and you know who you are) wallowing in self-pity, it just proves that with a little positive energy and persistence in this wacky dating scene, wishes can come true! But as Mister Bo Dangles, the Ex Hubby, The Lion King (and frankly all the boys I know) remind me, there aren't many girls out there in the world to rock it like me.

My phone sex job has proved to be exhausting. All the screaming and simulated cumming and ass slapping, it can really drain a girl, hour after hour, night after night, especially when there are no tangible men in sight. On any given night, I can become a saucy Nubian princess who's getting her big round ass paddled, a naughty little slut, splayed out on a pool table with six men fondling me, a teacher disciplining a student for masturbating in class, a barely legal girlie, still dressed in her Catholic school girl uniform, a cum hungry whore begging loudly for anal sex, and an older woman informing a young boy on how I would drain his nut sack, ruler in hand. The list goes on and on and on. June Cleaver with a vibrator, it's a damn good thing I have a powerful imagination.

I'm interviewing an enormous breasted porn star and must finish my editing process. You, boy with the lift in your Levis...bring that thang over here.

Mz. Conduct's House of Sin

Dear Mz. Conduct,

I met this woman online several months ago and although we haven't met yet, we have established a good relationship with writing and talking on the phone. I told her I was going out with some friends to a party and she was fine with that, but when I was honest with her and told her that I flirted with some girls and ended up in the middle of a gang bang blow job, she really blew up. She won't even talk to me now. I'm wondering what to do at this point. Can you help?

Pantless in Providence

> **Dear PiP,**
>
> The last time you took your dunce hat off, did you remove your brain with it? Suction in the junction, you were honest with her for crap's sake. By the way, you must have a lovely specimen o' sausage meat to get that treatment, so why are you wasting your time with someone who is jealous over a man she's never even met yet? She has no right to be upset. On the other hand, if you want to pursue something with this woman, then perhaps you may need to omit some details of your personal life. She obviously can't handle some of the information. If she's this way now, without even having met, think of how she may be if you did get together. I'd be running for them thar hills if I were you, but you're a man and will most likely keep pursuing this woman, this unmounted mound of conniption fits. Maybe she's just wishing it was she and not other wenches that were swallowing your schlong, but if you do decide to tell her blurbs of your sex life, maybe throw in a "but I was thinking of you the whole time baby." If she's stupid enough, she'll believe it. Otherwise shut your trap with her and have your fun. You don't owe her anything but the truth and apparently she can't even swallow that.

Dear Mz. Conduct,

So what's the best sex advice you've ever given?

Know-it-Poet

> **Dear KiP,**
>
> Hmmmm…let me shake up a dry martini for this one. Where are my penis shaped ice cubes, damnit? I could have consulted the archives, but I'm going to have to say this: my best general advice to people is to lose their inhibitions and realize that sexual self-expression is the absolute healthiest thing that can occur in one's life. To explore one's sexuality and get to a comfortable place with it can bring an absolute inner peace and release the spirit into untellable realms. Repression is still so prevalent in this society and one will never know true pleasure unless they become all they can as a sexual and free being. It is my personal mission to help people along in this area. If anyone wants to thank me, please send donations so I can finally buy that double-headed dildo I've been hankering for.

Good Advice from a Very Bad Girl

"Do you dream of impossible things?" asked the fairy. "Never" replied the girl, "for I am filled with wonderful dreams of all the things that are possible."
–Mary Pat Corder

Wild Bill and his Amazing Appendage came over for a visit the other day. We were comparing naughty narratives from the past weeks since we'd seen each other. He had banged this girl in California until his wiener almost fell off and I could barely walk from a six-timer romp the night before. We laughed at the gutterslut camaraderie we so fondly share. We yakked about Los Angeles; it's pitiful landscape, movies and movie stars. Then somehow he gets around to telling me that his uncle (one he visits frequently) is an ultra famous movie star. I promised not to disclose the information, but as you can imagine, I'm dying to, you know! All I can say is, wow, I've been banging this famous movie star's nephew for two years now! God, I love the smell of fame in the morning. That was a hint, bozo brains.

The Boytoy Bitch has been showering me with the most fabulous gifts. My favorites being the black light bulb in the shape of a decent sized penis and my chrome and leather martini shaker with a leopard shot glass/cap. He just knew I had to have those, and he's so right. Now we're shopping for black stilettos so I can grind them into his back. He says he needs punishment this weekend, but with all the gifts it's hard to see. Oh baby, I'm sure to find something he hasn't done properly.

I now have a volunteer bodyguard, Big Bald Bouncer, to escort me on my bad girl event nights, in which I will report all the sordid details, of course. He crafts flogging devices and has a doeskin one to die for. His expertise is a black leather-clad, over the knee, hand spanking and honey, you know my flanks are hankering for that, and soon!

I was the only one in attendance at the Female Ejaculation workshop, so the beautiful Ms. Yum Yum, who was going to teach the class, and I made a deal. If she and her lovely lover could go home, start their weekend extra early, and

Mz. Conduct's House of Sin

have tons of yummy girl sex, she'd let me attend the next workshop for free. She also saddled me up—sigh, I wish it were in the literal sense—with a bag full of lube and a box of non-latex condoms. I thought it a pretty sweet deal, all in all. Next month, when the next workshop is scheduled, I hope to have a full report on the subject of the G-spot and female ejaculations, which some of you are in dire need to know.

The Blue Sky Boy and I went to the Tasseled Titty Club and had big fun. I flirted with the gorgeous girls and smooched a doll of a dancer in the bathroom. He loved watching me get all the attention and forked out loot for my tipping pleasure all night long. The Blue Sky Boy is an entertaining entity in and of himself. He's beside himself over his latest acquirement. He has two new pussies to play with and invited me over to romp with them all. Okay, so maybe they're of the feline variety and actually say "meow", but I love playing and smooching frisky critters. I love playing with him too, especially with my strap on. I did avoid the litter box and stuck to the scratching post, and oh my, what a beautiful scratching post it is. Purrrrrr.

A fan from Jordan, yeah the place near Israel, instant messaged me the other night and invited me to come to Jordan along with my sexy feet. Okay, you know what his fetish is. Since I haven't had a freakin' vacation in over a decade, I almost said yes until I was reminded by the ex hubby and Big Bald Bouncer that it was something I definitely do not want to do…for so many reasons. Think about it. So, I simply enthralled him in a cock stroking fantasy with both feet and he seemed satisfied for the moment.

Ms. Lula la Paintbrush is heading over today to borrow some naughty yet classy garment to wear when she flies off to see her Catholic priest this week. I thought an ultra short length nun's habit with garter belt and stockings would be wickedly sacrilegious, but perhaps the fact that she's banging him is enough. Oh, we're all going to hell in a hand basket anyway, get over it.

Now where is that juicy girl with the pigtails, boytoy in tow, and my heart?

Good Advice from a Very Bad Girl

Dear Mz. Conduct,

My girlfriend and I have been purposefully abstaining from sex until we tie the marriage knot. Now don't get me wrong, we've been seeing each other for nearly two years, and for the first year and few months we were fucking like minks. We recently agreed on a mutual decision to abstain until, well, last night. We both were on the brink of going completely nuts and ended up in my bed. We had some of the best sex ever.

I'm not asking any kind of religious or spiritual or ethical question, but do you think it's good to "abstain"—in the sense of purposefully doing so for an extended period, so that we you do reach the breaking point the sex is so much better? I guess it's probably pretty obvious, but I thought I'd at least get your thoughts anyway.

Wally in Waiting

> **Dear WiW,**
>
> Water weenies on lawn boys, I think you answered your own question there, Einstein. I think there are many ways to spruce up a sex life and abstinence is just one of them. Tortuous as it may be, it can bring you back to appreciate all that you had/have with your partner. You can even throw in things, like planning to meet somewhere, pretending it's the first time you saw your other, striking up a conversation, running your hand up her leg, and sneaking away to dry hump in the bathroom of whatever establishment you choose to meet at. Then you go home, not saying a thing about what happened and slide back into the norm of whatever your relationship agreement may be. Another thing that can be kind of hot is to call her up, make believe she's a phone sex operator and blah and blah. You get my drift. It's all about sustaining the passion. A point to remember is, it's fun and sexually nourishing to do these things even after you get hitched. Keep it going, honey and if you're not using your dick then use your imagination. That's what it's all about.

Dear Mz. Conduct:

I have been hanging out with a very attractive lady with whom I share a lot of chemistry. She has a boyfriend with whom she's smitten, but on the East Coast. Officially, we are just friends, but we have flirted a bit. She even showed me her tits the other night when she was drunk. That very same evening at her house, I was dicking around on her computer and pulled up a pornographic picture of a woman. I thought it might be a funny prank if she turned around and saw that girl in all her glory with the vibrator inside her sitting on her monitor. When she did turn around, she was horribly offended and now I think I may have ruined any chance I had with her. She seems to think I'm some kind of damn freak now. I'm guilty of piss-poor judgment and being a testosterone driven sex freak, but I'm not entirely sure I understand why she was so profoundly offended. I care deeply for this woman as a person and her friendship is extremely important to me. How could I have fucked up so bad?

In Love With A Woman Who Is In Love With Another Man And Doesn't Like Porn On Her Computer

> **Dear IL,**
>
> Is this woman a total mixed-up prude, an inebriated titty flasher until she joins the convent? Probably not, but I think this woman has some issues to deal with that are entirely NOT yours to deal with at all. Let's look at the situation, her boyfriend lives far away, she felt comfortable with you, safe if you will, and she's so horny she could take on a Spanish matador head on. She may feel like you didn't understand all this and maybe you didn't. Women sometimes

expect men to read their minds and then give mixed signals. I empathize with men once in awhile for this. Your hormones can never measure up with a woman's, bottom line. Your biological make-up just doesn't allow it. Your penile persona took over understandably because you are a man and can't help it.

I doubt if she was truly offended by your porn pondering, but rather it threw her and her sopping loins into a fiery frenzy of lusty guilt. Apologize to her and then ask her why it is that she was so seemingly offended. You genuinely care about her friendship so try to initiate an intelligent conversation about her re-actionary impulses, porn in general, her faithfulness to this East Coast guy, etc. Sounds like you've opened a door, not closed one!

Good Advice from a Very Bad Girl

"What do I have to rebel against? I don't know, what da ya got?"
–Marlon Brando in The Wild One

I've been wearing my hair in pigtails lately, letting them stick out straight and go where they must, like a twisted punky version of Pippi Longstocking. I'm asked for ID even more than ever, and when I wear my short skirt and over-the-knee stockings, the boys just eat it up (literally for some). Some may say it's a sad reversion back to childhood, but not for me, especially since my childhood sucked big fat donkey weenies. It's just fun. As one of my bumper stickers says, "It's never too late to have a happy childhood." Speaking of bumper stickers, I bought a few new ones for the back of my truck. My favorite being, "Good Girls Go To Heaven, But Bad Girls Go Everywhere." Helen Gurly Brown said that and then started the pathetically self-image disabling *Cosmopolitan* magazine. Poor Helen, she just needed to be bitch-slapped and butt fucked, but then my philosophy is that we all do from time to time...just to keep a proper perspective on life.

Pulling into my driveway, I see my neighbor, ol' Jackson, meandering towards my house. He appeared to be carrying that greasy bag of fish he so loves to munch on. He walks down to the market every other day or so and gazes in my window, trying to catch a glimpse of my bare ass. So, I pull in and get out of my truck and he mumbled a throaty, "Hey Kimi, you sure lookin' good," and I thanked him and talk about the weather as I wrestled with my bag of groceries. "I sure be wantin' to git wit you girl," he drawled and I told him, "I know, Jackson, but I told you before, that will never happen." He got all riled and said, "Why you won't gimme a chance girl?," and I told him flat out, "You're just too old mister." Then he slurred, "Ahhh be showin' you a gooooood time though, I be showin' you what a real man can do," and I reiterated, "Not in your lifetime Jackson, now you go on and have a good day." Then he just walked away, his hand rummaging in his bag of greasy seafood, shaking his head from side to side. I could hear him murmur "Man oh man oh man," like his life was meaningless.

Mz. Conduct's House of Sin

The other night my son and I absorbed the amazing acrobatics of the Cirque du Soleil show. When I remarked, "Ironic! I pulled that same move with a boy the other night," my son reminded me that I had traumatized him for life. He told me, "I'm trying to have a virtuous image of my mother and it's just not happening," and I replied, "Let it go sweetie, it won't ever happen." He laughed and bought me a pretzel. As I looked at the twisted, brown rope of the pretzel, I honestly was reminded of yet another configuration from a recent wild night. My son—reading my dirty little mind—said sharply, "Don't even go there mama!" So instead, I let myself be mesmerized by the flexing muscles and taut French bodies before me...sigh.

Pretty Hippy Boy and I had a lovely vegan lunch at the Labia Lounge. I then lounged on his velvet couch where I sucked down an even yummier protein dessert with Dylan's "Sad-eyed Lady of the Lowlands" playing in the background. Just like a woman, a girl does need her protein and he has a sweet supply, Pretty Hippy Boy that is, not Dylan.

> Dear Mz. Conduct,
>
> Please tell me why a wonderfully mature hotty, like yourself, who is partial to young hairless boys, would pass up an opportunity for momentary bliss with an experienced, ol' hairy dude?
>
> Heartbroken Harry
>
> > **Dear HH,**
> >
> > Let me see, how I can phrase this...maybe because you are HAIRY, OLD and obviously DENSE, and telling you this, well...this is my momentary bliss.
>
> Dear Mz. Conduct,
>
> Here's a question for you: I have a very hot girlfriend who is horny about half the month. I'm talking 'soak a tampon' wet and when she instigates sex, it's incredible! The problem is that the other half of the month she's not into sex at all. If I happen to be the aggressor at these times then she says "I feel like a cheap whore." Since we're not married (in fact her divorce isn't final), is this just a case of morals gone awry? Should I worry that this will linger long after she's blissfully divorced?
>
> Peter Meter Running
>
> > **Dear PMR,**
> >
> > You know, Mister Beavis with a Boner, not all women will constantly faint at the sight of you and your superb schlong sandwich. I would have to say that most definitely her emotions and hormones are kickin' in at those uninterested times. Barbie in bondage, our damn hormones play a big part in things and men have no idea what to make of it. Not your fault, you just aren't built to know. One thing to remember is that women, when they ovulate and when they

stress (for any number of reasons), surely might not be in the mood for a lusty romp. Two whole weeks does seem a bit much for going without sex, at least on a regular basis, so if it remains like this, she may want to get a check-up, there may also be some physical reason why her libido takes an extended vacation each month.

You've got to shake up the mix a little too. Don't expect the same excitement from her all the time. On occasion, when I was married and trying to do seven things at once, feeling bitchy and overwhelmed and hovering over the sink or stove, my ex-hubby used to come up behind me and kiss the back of my neck. Sure it was annoying, and I'd start bitching like a fishwife, but at the same time I was soaking my panties. He'd just yank my dress up and start banging me from behind until I fell to the floor on my shaking knees, giggling with sated breath. There's nothing like a good banging to flip-flop the ol' mood swings.

I do realize that most women aren't like me (are there any?), so perhaps when she's 'not in the mood,' you may want to try a softer approach. To seduce her, try providing a back rub, a foot massage and/or a candlelit bubble bath. All of these things can get the girl purring and when she's feeling less stressed, she'll be more inclined to let your hot dog play with her pussycat. Remember that not every bout o' booty has to be a scene from "Coquette the Cum Whore." Enjoy the variety of passion and whack the weenie meat when you need to.

Mz. Conduct's House of Sin

"You can turn off the charm. I'm immune."
–Pussy Galore in Goldfinger

My bumper sticker hits the nail on the head: "falling in love is hard on the knees." Why is it that man/boys either want to tame me, hoard me, think of me as a challenge, or have babies? Oil me up and call me Olive, toss me in a dry martini and swill, baby, swill…And when I'm in the midst of an obvious hallelujah humpin', the boys are compelled to shush me. There's nothing that gets on my last nerve more (as the Royal Diva always announces). Well, maybe, but I haven't thought of it yet. Ball gags and cute fags, can't they all just shut up and love me?

It was the Boytoy Bitch's birthday so I seduced and reduced him to a sniveling, begging boot licker, his birthday dream come true. Hey, when a wicked wench dresses up in vinyl from head to toe on a sweltering hot day, it means she freakin' cares, honey! We then drove off to the Nipple and Nuts Nudie beach where I flaunted my smooth and savory self under the heat of the afternoon sun, all my metal glistening in the solar rays.

I entered the Blue Sky Boy in a tightie-whities contest. It's an underwear contest judged by the public and we hope to win a fab jaunt to Vegas. He posed all beautiful and hairless, holding a chainsaw, wearing just the snug tightie-whities, and safety goggles. Yumm. I don't know about winning the contest, but when I look at him in all his glory, he sure does win my heart. Or something that throbs anyway. Viva la beefcake boys and Viva Las Vegas! Wait, what's that I hear? Could those be the rotted bones of Elvis singin' to me now?

My sweet, little auntie sent me some loot to pay some bills, bless her ancient heart, but instead of sending the phone mafia money I decided to make myself a happy hoyden. Off I trotted to finally buy myself that double-headed dildo I've been hankering for. I figure, if I get run over by a beer truck tomorrow, I'll be much more thrilled by having experienced that silicone slice of heaven than

Good Advice from a Very Bad Girl

knowing my stinkin' phone bill is paid. The Transient Trollop promises to read that at my eulogy if need be.

So, my horoscope read, the day I decided to try out the double-headed dildo:

"You are probably going to have the urge to show off your abilities to a loved one today, dear Aries. Perhaps you are in the mood to impress them with a bizarre talent of yours that no one else knows about. Feel free to demonstrate your self worth to the people around you. There is no need to hide from the gifts that you have. Other people are apt to find your antics quite witty and entertaining."

I'd say that sums it up quite nicely and may I just say that I worship and adore my new toy. Like they say, two heads are better than one!

> Dear Mz. Conduct,
> I went out with a woman twice and said the inevitable 'I'll call you' afterwards, even though I had really no intention of seeing her again. I didn't call and within two days, she called me. She left a message asking why I didn't call when I said I would and telling me she would call my workplace next. I must say, this worried me enough to call her back, before she could call me at work. I guess I was trying to be a nice guy and made some excuse about being busy. She promptly invited me to the beach, I politely told her no thank you, I was just too busy.
>
> A few days later, I ran into her at a bar and she latched on to me asking me to play pool with her. We played pool and actually had a decent time, but I am just not attracted to her in any way. Now she is calling again and I don't know how to tell her how I feel. Is there a 'nice guy' way to let her down easy?
> Fumbling with Feelings
>
>> **Dear FwF,**
>>
>> Wind-up weenies at Walmart, yeah there's a way to get through to some people. It's your fault for not being a dolt and dishonest with this woman in the first place. Some people have a difficult time paying attention to another's interest or lack thereof and may require brutal honesty. You open your 'nice guy' mouth and tell this indigent, insipid inbred, "Look, I'm not interested in seeing you anymore. I feel no chemistry with you and please don't call me again." If she doesn't understand this, and obviously she's not the sharpest tool in the shed, you may have to further your explanation with something like "If you call me again, then I'll be forced to write your name and number on each and every bathroom wall, in every single seedy truck stop, this side of the border." That should do it. Learn from this blunder and tell people how you feel. Nothing hurts a person more than to be led on, perhaps hoping for rainbows and champagne and finding out all that's there is rain and Cold Duck.
>
> My Dear Mz. Conduct,

Mz. Conduct's House of Sin

I went out with a girl and there was obvious chemistry. We met again and she invited me home. I spent the night in her bed and we kissed and groped, but she wouldn't let me go all the way. I respected that and when I left, she seemed to be interested in getting together again, but then she emailed me saying that she decided she didn't want to have a relationship with me after all. Should I pursue this and ask her why? I thought we really had a connection and am very bummed out.

Sore Loser

> Good God in a gas mask, you are a loser, mister. Okay, so the girl seemed to initially like you. She probably had too many cocktails or was on the rebound or thought she wanted your man meat at first, but then you spent the night and something went awry. Maybe it's not your breath or your lack of smooth moves. It could simply be that what she thought was there between you, just wasn't. Even I've had this happen, or at least I think so. Hell, I don't remember because it's either there or it's not for me, but I do understand the concept of a lost connection.

> Leave it alone. It's a done deal. Move on down the line and quit analyzing the situation. It wasn't a six year relationship, it was a one night thang. Yeah it sucks that you didn't pass Go and you didn't collect the $200. but you aren't in jail so count your freakin' blessings and go mow my damn lawn.

"You cumming is sexy, me going is sexier."
–TM

Tie my tail to a bucket of nails, for I am a bad kitty. Bad, bad kitty! In the last column, "Masturbate-a-Thon", I didn't have the brain function—damn those dry martinis—to mention that the whole Masturbate-a-Thon she-bang was put on by the one, the only, fab beyond belief, goddess of erotica, and creative genius, Darklady! If not for her, I wouldn't have been invited in the first place and I apologize for not even mentioning her. She did a wonderful job throwing the gig together, and we all respect and appreciate her tireless and ongoing efforts…in everything she does. She's in the process of altering a vinyl dress of mine, and with me forgetting to mention her, the dress may come back to me looking like vinyl blinds. But she's a good egg and will forgive me, or one trashy trollop can hope. You can visit her site at www.darklady.com and see for yourselves what a wonder woman really is. Now hopefully she'll invite me to her birthday party and we won't be forced to play Pin the Penis on Mz. Conduct. Hmmm, I don't know, that actually sounds mighty fun.

My snow globe collection is growing faster than a smooched penis. Mister Peanut brought me one from the Netherlands, Ms. Lula la Paintbrush and Pretty Hippy Boy both brought snow globes from New York, each with a different skyline. Most people collect them from places they've visited, but NO, not I. I live vicariously through my traveling troupe of friends, but such is life. Until I'm famous that is. I have four different jobs now, so unless I drop dead in a vat of gin with my dress over my head, as sung on *The Mary Tyler Moore Show*, "I'm going to make it after all!"

As Wild Bill and his Amazing Appendage says, "Mz. Conduct, you are dating at an unfathomable rate of speed!" That tells you something, coming from him. Hey, a girl has to eat, and when a lunch/dinner invitation comes my way, as long as the guy is tolerable, I'll take it. I've met so many interesting man-boys, and have networked among many, in respects to promoting my column. It's all working out.

Mz. Conduct's House of Sin

I've decided to rent my attic space out, as I truly do not want to be pushing a shopping cart filled with my hatbox full of sex toys, my laptop and the dogs, down the main drag of this city. I met a handsome writer, an interesting sort, who was in need of a place to hang his hat, so voila! My attic will be occupied soon. I will never be an existentialist. I believe everything happens for a reason and things are entirely connected in this universe of mad and magical mayhem.

So, last night on the phone sex job was about the most unusual to date. I helped two guys solve their girlfriend problems, which I love and live for, and another guy fulfill a fantasy on a tiki-torched-lit Caribbean beach. That got me so worked up that I soaked through my little leather skirt. But the next guy ruined the whole evening. Except for the fact that being a very lengthy call—good as far as money-makin' goes—he wanted to strangle me and then have me poop in his mouth. Christ on a crumpet, I don't like to judge a person's fetishes, but I'm sorry, that's freakin' disgusting. When I have my own business line, I may have to tell those twisted mo fos a thing or two, "Listen buddy, why don't you eat your own stool sandwich and leave mine where it is, damnit." One of the best calls was from a guy who had a nice conversation with me before he started his pole pounding. He rambled on for a good fifteen minutes and realizing he was in mid-whack mode, I just kept talking filthier and filthier. He obviously finished himself off but apparently forgot to hang up the phone. So, for another twenty minutes, as the line was silent, I read the New Yorker, made easy money and smoked. It was fabulous, daahling!

I've been interviewing strippers again this week, chasing them around to meet up in every strip club in the city. If I weren't flat broke and driving on fumes, it'd almost be worth it. I could stay for awhile after the interview, have cocktails, tip, have a girlie good time, but no such thing is possible, at least not in the near future. What I need is a tall, thin, hairless, 30-year-old, baby-faced, sugar daddy. Ha, when I take over Ann Landers column, that'll happen. In the meantime, bad girl life goes on. For instance, there's a "Find Your Inner Slut" class waiting for me to attend in a few weeks, but honey I've already found it and am polishing it like a genie in a lamp. Let me say, I'm busier than a whore on nickel night.

Mz. Conduct,
What advice would you give to a man with a penis so large that it actually scares women? Seriously, many women I meet are not interested in tackling my organ when they see the girth of it. They don't want to have sex with me and I've never had a woman give me a blowjob. Aside from having it surgically altered, what can I do?
Big Bob

> Dear BB,
>
> Oh boo hoo, mister monster meat. Maybe it's because you're hideous or retarded or stinky and not your greatness of girth after all. Hmmmm, ever thought of that? I'd have to say you're meeting the wrong women. I've known a few women who've complained about the challenge of the oral attack on an extra large appendage, but not one of them hasn't, at the very least, given it a go. You say it 'scares' women, well, think of scary movies. You may be petrified, but you're still compelled to watch it. Sure, I may have watched "Texas Chainsaw Massacre" through my coat sleeve, but I saw it through its entirety and I ended up really liking it. You need to find a girl who likes YOU and then she'll work her mouth around that big schlong of yours with all the gusto one does when one loves. I'm sure you're aware that we women can have the biggest mouths around when we want to. As far as penetration, remember that the vaginal muscles are very flexible and that ten-pound babies actually come through the cervix. Sure, hormones play a part, but it is something to keep in mind. Quit whining, brush your teeth, work on your personality, and go get rich. Make some porn and send it to me when you're finished.

Dear Mz. Conduct,
I work with this great girl, she's 22 and I'm 28, and we sort of flirt a bit here and there, office stuff I guess. The other day, when I gave her the daily report to sign, she took the clipboard and put it on my lap to sign it! She was pressing hard on purpose and I have to admit I got an erection. Then she just smiled coyly and said goodnight. I couldn't stop thinking about this little move of hers, so a few days later when we were at lunch, along with some other co-workers, I walked her back alone and casually asked her out for coffee. To my surprise, she said no. And I asked her two separate times. Now I'm really confused because we obviously are attracted to each other, but I don't know why she sticks to flirting and won't even have coffee with me. Tell me what you think, please?
Confounded Co-Worker

> Dear CCW,
>
> Boys will be boys, won't they? Hard in the Hanes and hay for brains. Not your fault, women have all the power in most situations and this girl knows it. She's too young, too confused, too power hungry for attention and too freakin' catty. She wants you to want her and she's tripping on knowing that you do. Game playing is not a recommended attribute for dating. I suggest you leave it alone. Perhaps she doesn't like dating someone she works with, but let her figure it out first and simply tell you as much. Don't ask her out again, damn you, or I'll be forced to bitch slap you and butt fuck you. She knows you want to ride in

Mz. Conduct's House of Sin

her panty play town and she'll string you on forever…if you let her. Don't you dare woos boy. Just be your charming self and quit flirting with her. If you don't care anymore (try not to show it anyway, honey) then I'll bet you my double-headed dildo—and no one is getting that treasure unless I'm on one end of it—that she may change her tune. At that point you can decide if you really want to date a girl like her. Some women think they have a man wrapped around their little, sparkle-painted pinkie, but suddenly when the guy seems to be completely indifferent, well, that drives them crazier than a loon in heat. Leave it alone in the office and use her for masturbation material at home.

Good Advice from a Very Bad Girl

"With a rebel yell, she cried more, more, more."
–Billy Idol

Blind date time at the Tiki Room again. I got there a bit early and started up a conversation with the bartender. The bartender, a splendid flamer. When I ordered a bone-dry Sapphire martini with three olives, he asked for my identification. The night was starting off on a good foot. "It's the pigtails," I told him. The guy sitting at the bar disagreed and made some not-so-subtle remark about getting my phone number. I gave him my business card instead (no phone number on it, just email). He seemed elated and I planted my leather clad self at a booth, just the other side of the plastic palm grove. A few minutes later, my date walked in. Slightly attractive in a femme sort of way. He was extremely personable and we yakked with the waitress and commented on her fab '60s hair-do. My date drank whiskey with a beer back and the guy at the bar sent over another martini to yours truly. This happened three times and the Tiki Room has the best damn martinis around, honey. Anyway, my date and I got along well and he had interesting stories. The small world syndrome visited us three separate times, as he's friends with one of my oldest friends, has another friend that my friend hangs out with, and has a roommate that used to write a column for a local newspaper. I happen to verbally rake the columnist over the coals before I knew this fact. Oops, open mouth, insert foot, however it didn't change my opinion. Such is life, and where is my martini?

We'd been there swilling for over four hours and closing time was near. I mentioned that I had to pee and he said "let's both go." So he followed me into the women's restroom and when I sat down, he whipped out his weenie and peed right between my legs. After six martinis, I just had to go and this seemed a way to kill two birds with one stone (plus it was sort of hot). We were snickering at our misbehavior as we walked back to finish our last drink. I looked over at him and he had slipped under the booth, disappeared. Where was the boy? Oh my, there he was, there between my thighs, under the lime green booth, lapping away. I caught wind of the waitress headed our way, so I kicked him with my pointed heels, as I didn't want to scream with pleasure right there in the empty Tiki Room. I'm a perpetually, ear-piercing vocalist when it comes to sexual release. Ask my neighbors eight houses down. So, we went back to my house and although I liked the guy and found his spontaneity refreshing, I made him call a taxi…and off he went pointing his way home with a boner compass.

The Blue Sky Boy and I spent an amazing night together, intoxicated with many wonderful things. I spent hours wrapped up in the sheer, crimson, silky material that draped over my bedroom door. I loved the feel of it and danced with it and the wall for hours. Enigma echoing in the background. Blue Sky Boy did the same, his tall, hairless body, his long hair flowing down his back, his movements so sensually rhythmic, oh help me Goddess of Guttersluts. I reached for my camera and started snapping photos. It was a moral imperative, as he was a freakin' vision of perfection. Okay, my vision might have been slightly altered that night, but I feel the same way each time I look at him still. I'll never have him though, not really. This is what saves me, when I know I'm going to see him, I simply yank my heart out (yeah, like self-inflicted heart surgery is ever easy) and lock it in a box, bury it underground. Some place in the yard where the dogs won't dig it up and play tug-o-war until it's shredded like a dying bird in a lawnmower. Shredded tweet. After all, if I wanted to feel that sort of torture, I'd have left it inside my chest.

The Yum Yum Boy, whom I met once, many moons ago, told me he was going to Aussie land for a year. Well, this called for celebration and perhaps a memory of a meaningful romp in another down under. Something for him to take with him over that big old ocean. He drove up to my house looking like heaven on a honey-stick. His long, wavy locks flowed down his back, the jewelry in his face sparkled in the sunset, his tall, taut body strode towards my throbbing skin. My heart pounded, my clit pulsed and up he walked, and his amazing arms grabbed hold of me. Twenty-three hours later, they let go. So much occurred, but when there is a spiritual revelation, sacred remains sacred, and my mouth is zipped, unlike those snug black jeans pants of his. My heart was firmly in place.

Good Advice from a Very Bad Girl

Cinderella Cyber Twat keeps promising to visit me with her matching luggage and pretty snatch. She's up to her ears with bad girl rendezvous and some boys are up to their fists in her. We have big dreams of our meeting and I'm hankering to lickety-split her, seam by seam. Shave your piss flaps and pack those bags girl and c'mon down!

Dear Mz. Conduct,

Present company excepted, of course, what the *fuck* is up with womenfolk? I just received a positively scathing e-mail from a woman who I took out a few times (and with whom I engaged in some heavy kissing, but nothing else). At the end of last night's date, I sensed (correctly as it happens) that she was getting starry-eyed—and that I wasn't. She kind of hinted around and asked me if I wanted to sleep with her. The short answer would have been "yes", but—for once—I thought past my erection and realized that I would probably not want to see her next week and that she would be hurt—more so if we bopped first. So I told her (in carefully chosen and highly diplomatic words) that I felt that I was all kinds of turned on by her but felt that it wouldn't be a great idea. She was okay with that—kind of. But then she went home and called me to ask if I might consider some of the non-exclusive "play" type of sex that she knows I've engaged in—with her. I told her that it's kind of hard to switch to that gear and that I didn't believe it was really her cup of tea (Ahem. Believe me—it's not) Blah, blah, blah. She then sent me a long-ish e-mail regurgitating last night's conversation and I composed what I felt was again—a pretty thoughtful disengagement letter which didn't disallow the notion of our keeping some sort of vibe going. I dated her *twice* mind you. And she went ballistic. Skewered me in a flame-mail. Told me I was a "bait-and-switcher". That I "can't handle the truth". Meanwhile, I've been nothing but truthful and tried to spare her feelings and WHAT THE FUCK IS UP WITH THIS WORLD ANYWAY?

So, can you offer an opinion?

Man in a Mess

> Dear MiaM,
>
> Holy horny cows in a cattle drive, you men! And speaking of which, I could use a stiff one right about now, and an even stiffer martini. Okay, you said that you've been nothing but honest, well obviously SOME people need absolute brutal honesty. Something I cater to daily to avoid just such a thing. Even with absolute brutal honesty, SOME people still feel compelled to surgically attach themselves to us. Is there anything more annoying? Well, maybe a damp thong up the keester on a ninety-degree day, but seriously, you should not feel badly about flat-out saying what you instinctively feel. And yes, leave your penis out of the decision making process. Demand that your penis go get coffee or do some housework for crying in a mutherfuckin' bucket. At the very least, picture grandma in a corset, Aunt Matilda in a string bikini, Janet Reno in drag, whatever works. You are obviously sending out mixed signals, mister buttcheese, so in my opinion, you asked for it! Do not agree to engage in some 'sexplay' if she's already on you like sweat on a boxer's ass. Telling her "it's not a good idea" just isn't graphic enough for SOME. If you need to spell things out, then do so, right off the gawd damn bat! Don't ever go out, call, or merely wave at this woman, even from three blocks away. Leave it alone like a week-old dia-

per. The next time you have a gut instinct, go with it. It may be hurtful to be blunt upfront, but it's a lot less hurtful to the mixed up woman (and less stressful for you) in the end, damnit. The end.

Dear Mz. Conduct,

My boyfriend and I broke up several months ago and granted, it was painful and took a lot out of me emotionally, but I tried my best to move on. The other night he called out of the blue and said he had been thinking about me and missed me. I talked with him for only a few minutes because I was on my way out the door to a meeting. Now I can't stop thinking about his call now and am so mixed up about what's going on. I'm really kind of mad about him doing that, but my heart is pulling me towards calling him back. I was just starting to feel stronger on my own and getting over the relationship and now I don't know what to do. Should I call him back or just let it go?

Pissed Off Patty

Dear PoP,

Good gobs of love juice, you don't tell me anything about how the relationship ended or even was, so I would simply say think about the good, think about the bad, weigh it out and if it's worth giving the relationship another shot, then do it. Your heart is pulling, yet your brain is full of the good and powerful independence you've been working on. Maybe you can use that and have it all honey! If you do, then you get a free pass to the House Of Sin Spa...just for a day!

Good Advice from a Very Bad Girl

"Baby, sometimes you just take me right over that rainbow."
–Lula to Saylor in Wild at Heart

I hope all of you voted for Mz. Conduct's boytoy in Dan Savage's Tighty Whities underwear contest. If not, you deserve to be bitch slapped and butt fucked, and when I show up on your doorstep in head-to-toe leather, you better bend over! There were some chunky bits of manly meat on there, I must admit, but my photo entry was bathed in wicked creativity, and that should count for something, damnit! I've faced the fact however, we're not passing GO and we're not collecting $200. and we're definitely not going to Vegas. Hey, I can still put Elvis on the CD player, make a batch of bone-dry martinis, dress my roommate in a sequined bikini and play make-believe!

Late the other night, as I was on the phone sex job, every Who's Who of mental illness—thank you Blue Sky boy for that great line—seemed to be calling me. One guy was saying my name every two seconds and asked me about ten zillion times to hold on while he went to get a beer. Whatever, dude, I'm thinking as I look at my watch. Drive into town and get another six-pack for all I care. The next guy had me take him into Tijuana to be humiliated. No biggie, I dragged him out in a Mexican public square, naked and collared and on all fours. I had all the local senoritas point and laugh at his genitals. He loved it! Things were going well until he said that this wasn't punishment enough and begged me to take out a giant butcher knife and slice his schlong. Completely repulsed, my facial expression must have been a sight, but my voice didn't show anything other than dominant dignity. I did what he wanted, hacked his manhood up and he promptly shot his load. Stilettos on a stork, what a freakin' nightmare he was. A night full of looneys, out of gin, and I told myself, one more call. Well, this next guy asks me, "Do ya have any rock?" and I play it off and say, "Sure thing, right next to my stash of heroin." This flew right over his head, and whatever contents remained in it, as he begged me to smoke some with him over the phone. I lit a ciggie and mirrored an effect that I saw in some movie once. Whatever, it seemed to work for him and that, my dears, was the night's 'last-call!'

Mz. Conduct's House of Sin

I had another blind date at the Twilight Lounge. This time with a nice looking man who had intriguing stories to tell. But after I swilled four Sapphire martinis, the stories wore thin, and when he insisted on feeling my legs, I ordered him to scoot back to a comfortable distance. I decided to be extra bitchy and bossed him around a bit. He liked it unfortunately. I told him it was time for me to make like a baby and head out.

I'm swooning with the Yum Yum boy right now and can't bear to wrap myself in anyone else's arms. We had a surreal night out last week and it felt like something out of a Gus Van Zant film. We were off to hear his friend's band, and I—being that the Lil' Princess and her man made me three towering vodka frappes just an hour before—was not satisfied with my bland little dress. I ripped off the conformist in me and shimmied into a black, velvet, and low-cut dress with garter hooks on the hem. I slid into my black, spider-webbed stockings and stuffed my tootsies into my tall Mary Janes. I told my baby that I was ready to go and he threw me down on the bed. He put on a Wild at Heart drawl and said, "Gawd damn baby, you shor are purty," kissed me with his hot lips, and off we went into the night. Now, the unhappening town this band was playing in has only been visited on extremely rare occasions by either of us. There's no point, you see. We drove over the river and through the woods and to grandmother's house we did not go. Through the air of the ghost town on a Saturday night, two drugged out kids standing on the main drag gave us spaced-out directions. As we drove off, the Dullsville cop decided he was bored enough to pull us over. The young and buffed blue, jittery and chomping a wad of gum, described himself to us as a "multi-tasked kinda guy" and then had me get me out of the car to explain the problem. My taillight was faded. He chomped his Doublemint and said that my taillight must be red, not pink. His eyes traveled up and down my spider-webbed thighs as I acted like a gave a rusty rim-job. The oh-so-big and multi-tasked guy that he was, he let us go…asswipe. So, we get to the bar and it turns out to be a freakin' mall bar! It was an ever-so-lovely sports bar, lit up like a gawd damn Christmas tree. It was packed with mullet-headed men and mallrat bimbos guzzling down Coors light and hootin' for the band. Christ in a crapshoot, I'm standing at the doorway, dressed for sinning up a gawd damn storm, and staring at the ultra bright lights and brazen boozehounds. Two red necked mo fos, perched on bar stools, made some comment about bending me over and the Yum Yum boy—in his Elvis shades and hat, wearing his black wife-beater which amplifies his cut-with-muscle-meat arms, gave the guys a look that would kill. Not a violent boy, we decided a punch in the face wasn't worth the energy. My hero. Our night consisted of multiple Jello shots, being waited on by my long lost ex-sister in law, me smooching some bi-curious girl, and finally leaving the wacky joint as randy as they come. We bagged our effort of casual copulation in the back of my truck (for comfort sake) and ended up getting lost beyond belief in the wee, alcoholic crazed hours in the town without pity. The Yum Yum boy and I pulled over in an empty lot and passed out until the sun came up. We finally pulled in my driveway the next morning, still half-asleep and half-drunk, wondering if the night had actually happened or was a twisted, twilight dreamscape. We are what dreams are made of.

It's hotter than a whore on nickel night and where is my lizard of unusual size with that Bloody Mary and cigarette?

> Dear Mz. Conduct,
> Oral sex (mutual) is very important to me, but soon after we were married my wife unilaterally decided that we would no longer engage in oral sex on the grounds that it supposedly is unhealthful. I am convinced that she is not correct, scientifically.
>
> I feel like the butt of the old joke: "How do you get a woman to stop enjoying oral sex? Marry her." She knew before we were married what I like, and I THOUGHT I knew what she liked, so I think she should be willing to meet half way at least. But she won't budge an inch. Over the years, my resentment over this has built up substantially, and she still will not even discuss it no matter how tactful or clever I am in trying to bring up the subject in a non-threatening manner. It seems to be no big deal to her, as a matter of sexual satisfaction, because she often becomes completely satisfied before I orgasm. She also often claims to be too sore to continue after she orgasms, at which point the rest is left to me, alone—which, of course, makes it all the more frustrating to me that we do not avail ourselves of the oral sex alternative that not only would prevent soreness, but likely would provide us with more mutual satisfaction.
>
> Thwarted Theo
>
> **Dear TT,**

I'm with you on this one, oh frustrated one, but I wonder why it's taken you years to ask about this. Are you slow on the draw or what? After the first month of this horseshit, I would have asked the little woman to go see a therapist of sorts, along with you of course. This is something that can be done now as well though and what I recommend you do.

You have worded your justified aggravation very well in your question. Your wife seems to have some misconceptions about oral sex. There is nothing unhealthy about it. Unless, of course, you've been sleeping with others and she knows about it, you bastard. I'm inclined to think that she's using her unfounded fears as an excuse not to participate in oral play with you, especially since she was a willing participant before your marriage. Sex should be between the both of you and when one partner leaves you alone to 'finish yourself off,' there grows a gap in the intimacy department and this is the unhealthy part.

There are tantric workshops and sex therapists that should be able to help you two, if indeed your wife is willing. Dr. Carol Queen has a website that perhaps your wife would read with you (www.carolqueen.com). She is my heroine and as wise as they come. Your work is needed here, too, though. Try to let your wife know—in a kind and unthreatening way—that you are not happy in this part of your marriage, and that if she doesn't make an effort to assist you, then there is a big fat chance that your relationship won't survive. There may be medication and/or age factors involved and hormones flying about, but if two people want something bad enough, they can work through it, no matter what. Patience and dedication—and Jesus on a jet ski, you've shown that so far—will get you through. Maybe a round of Mz. Conduct's cocktails and watching someone who has no gag reflex on video would help too.

Dear Mz. Conduct,

How would a very confident, handsome, and well-hung guy go about getting a date with you?

Manly Man

I can definitely tell you how NOT to get a date with me; by describing yourself as all of the above. First of all, confidence can be broken into shards of simple shame in about three point two seconds. Second of all, that's just dandy that you consider yourself 'handsome', but that would be entirely subjective, and I'm not too charitable in that department. If you didn't do yourself in with the two previous adjectives, then you threw in the spewed towel with the last one. Great, wonderful, marvelous…you have a big dick…whoo freakin' hoo! That matters only if I like you…and I don't.

Good Advice from a Very Bad Girl

"I know everybody here wants you. I know everybody here thinks they need you. I'll be waiting right here just to show you how our love will blow it all away."
–Jeff Buckley

The Transient Trollop and her Gay Man with Toolbox are plotting a marriage...to one another! He proposed to her, albeit over large amounts of whiskey, but it looks like it's going to happen anyway. They figure that they don't like anybody else but each other and wearing wedding bands would get them laid more often. The Transient Trollop insists on cheap gold bands from Wal-Mart for the fruitful event. The Transient Trollop is a catch in my book, so is this gay pride or what? Bless the buttplug and get the confetti, I may have to be present for this one!

The Yum Yum boy and I went down to Infinity Tattoo where Paul, the owner of the best tattoo parlor in Portland, crafted a fabulous winged heart right above my butt crack. It took about an hour and a half and turned out painfully pretty. He was just finishing up, and as I straddled the stool, he told me to hang on one more minute, as he had a little mess to clean up back there. I immediately blurted out "Oh I've heard that before," which made the shop chuckle with undue surprise.

The Lion King and I went down to the county courthouse and picked up a set of divorce papers for each of us. We knew our spouse's wouldn't get around to it and we were just trying to get the ball rolling, as it's only been over a freakin' year since I've been single! We laughed at how if it wasn't for either of us and our raunchy rendezvous during our marriages, we wouldn't be in this predicament in the first place. And how funny it is now that if we did get re-married it sure wouldn't be to each other. I still believe that everything happens for a reason, even if it's not the reason you may think at the time. We celebrated by having cocktails of course.

Mz. Conduct's House of Sin

My fab new roommate, the Distinguished Deviant, went on a trek to southern California last week. Upon his return, he brought me the sauciest of sauciest attire. A tiny, red, vinyl skirt that zips naughtily up the front. He told me that when he laid eyes on it, it screamed my name. The Lil' Princess and I wedged my ample ass into it, laying on my bed and laughing so hard we almost peed our panties, if we had had any on. Back to the gym I go starting tomorrow, honey!

The Yum Yum boy whisked me off on a spontaneous sprint to the mountains. Dark and chilly, we found a great, old logging road with not a soul around for miles. We built our campsite by flashlight and a fine fire it was, in more ways than one. We played word games, shared dreams, and bashed our heads together accidentally while freaking out over where we put the vodka. We drank Absolut and cranberry juice until five in the morning. He and I finally keeled over in the cold night air only to waken to the sweltering sun on our naked bodies in the afternoon of the next day. Salacious sex occurred promptly. We decided to continue this evil-slated escapade and headed to the coast. The next night we drove for miles on a gravely, windy road until we found a perfect place to camp next to the roaring Nehalem river. Lust was in our loins once again, but this time there were children down the road. As the Yum Yum boy banged me into oblivion and I screamed my usual Tarzan thrills, no words of discipline said, he simply shoved my head into the sleeping bag and held it down. Now that's my kind of man, baby!

Awkward, embarrassing, oh I don't know, maybe just a typical Mz. Conduct moment that this was; I had gotten some pictures back from one of those disposable cameras I had been carting around for eons. A couple of pictures were on there from last spring, as I had shots of all my fab birthday flowers and such. But when I was showing the Yum Yum boy the ones I took of him there surfaced a shot of a man's wet penis tip through some Calvin Klein's. I told him I didn't remember taking that of him and he calmly reminded me that he doesn't wear that type of underwear and that was not him. Oops. The only thing I could soberly remember is that perhaps it was an old Lion King picture. With

Good Advice from a Very Bad Girl

that in mind, I brought it to him, laughing at my stupidity and telling my silly story. The Lion King looked at me and said that it wasn't him either, as he never had a pair of those underwear in his life. Oops again! I thought I'd better just toss the picture in the trash, as I'd done enough damage already, and leave it be. It must've been the Boytoy Bitch, thinking back, and some things are better left alone.

As I sit here and treasure how good it finally feels to have a beautiful boy adore me and not want to change one thing about who I am, nor I him, I know that Guttersluts may not go to heaven, but I'm almost sure that is about as close as one wicked little wench will ever get.

Dear Mz. Conduct,

I have a friend who I care about very much. This girl is nineteen and engaged to a guy she's never met outside of prison. It was one of those online/prison things and although she's visited him since, I feel protective and uneasy about this. I also have a buddy in the same prison and he told me that this guy she's involved with is a real asshole. He's not due to get out for eight more years and she seems absolutely dedicated to this jerk. She won't date anybody else and she sits at home and writes to him, consumed and obsessed with only him. My question is how can I tell her she's throwing her life away waiting around for this dude?

Prison Blues

> **Dear PB,**
>
> Chill out baby. I realize that you're concerned about your friend, but don't sweat your nutsack off. She's freakin' nineteen years old and I'll bet my thigh high boots (and no way I'm losing those!) that she'll grow up and have a revelation of reality before too long. I'm guessing that if the prisoner in question has eight more years of time to do, he's no knight in shining armor, any way you look at it. The best thing for you to do is to continue being her friend, suggest fun outings and leave it at that. If you try to persuade her that this guy is no good, it'll only make you look like the bad guy in her eyes. Believe me, I was nineteen once and trying to talk me out of something only fueled the fire... hmmm some things never change. Don't worry though, this will.

Dear Mz. Conduct,

How would my wife and I meet other couples that are interested in swinging? We've had some experience with this before but it never seemed that anyone we met was interested in much of a relationship. We'd like to develop a good friendship as well as a sexual one. We are in Oregon and wondered if you had any suggestions.

By the way, we love your column!

More the Merrier

> I would go online and check out some Yahoo groups like the Ace of Hearts Club and Oregon Sex Contact. There are many people in the same lust boat as you two. As a matter of fact, I will be writing for a new branch site of Oregon

Mz. Conduct's House of Sin

Sex Contact coming this September. Also there are some decent polyamory sites as well, such as Portland Polyamory. You can meet online first and find others who are searching for the same particular thing instead of just hooking up with some random swingers. Many of these groups have smaller groups within themselves and have developed very good and real friendships. Go forth and multiply!

Good Advice from a Very Bad Girl

"There's nothing wrong with having bags under your eyes as long as you have shoes to match."
–Steven Tyler

The Royal Diva made a grand visit from Seattle. Over clove ciggies and beer, we had a delightful visit as I cut veggies and cooked lasagna, preparing a big bash for the Yum Yum boy's down under sojourn. She looked fabulous and is working hard on the marriage thang. It's a difficult task to love and commit to a woman hell-bent on stardom, I should know. The Royal Diva is responsible for always keeping me believing in true love we so deserve and the magic that can happen so unexpectedly. I will never give up and neither will she.

The farewell bash was a gas, guests so sincerely sweet, no big spills, no crashes, no jewelry stolen, and best of all, no tears...not even by me. The band, called UNTYD, were friends of the Yum Yum boy's and they rocked the house...or rather my backyard strung with Christmas lights. No neighbors complained and no cops were called. Three old men cruising by in the night yelled a hardy "Turn it up!" and that was it. Amazing. And moi, the hostess with the mostess, surprisingly enough only had four Sapphires on the rocks—which I kept misplacing all evening—and one muscle relaxer. You see, it was important for me to keep in mind that the love of my life was leaving on a trip all his own. It was his dream. Besides, he had his ticket before we met. No blubbering, no uncontrollable sobbing, no weepy woman clinging to his arm. I was bound and determined to give my support and Superwoman strength for the man that had finally captured my heart. Now, as he's flown off to the farthest section of the globe and having the time of his young-ass life—even smooching koalas just for me—I am digging deeply for any ounce of strength left in my soul. I ask myself this; why did I think it a good idea to secretly spray the pillows with his Armani cologne? Wash them I could, but something won't allow me to...not yet. Maybe in a month, when the dog hair has collected and the cologne has faded into a wretched mix of sweat and tear stains, maybe then I'll feel my powers rise again and let Downy take over. I realize that this too shall pass, but until then, it's stomach clutching in my bed with my ciggies and gin. I'll do

Mz. Conduct's House of Sin

what I damn well please...always have, always will, and to hell in a hatbox to anyone who tells me different.

So, okay, in a heroic effort to pry my wild spirit back out of the can, I decided to go to the gym and work out some stagnant endorphins. Strolling in, feeling my oats, I was glad that the place wasn't too crowded. I walked out on the floor full of machinery and Lycra and climbed on the evil Stairmaster, set it for thirty minutes and plugged in my headphones. Listening to Al Green sing about love and happiness, climbing floor after floor, I think how nice it'd be to have an ashtray attached to the stair machine...and hell, maybe even a place for a cocktail. Eighty flights later I dismounted the contraption and reached for my towel and water bottle. When I turned around, a troll of a man with hair on his neck and back, said "Hey sweet one, don't leave now, your ass is giving me motivational skills beyond belief." In no mood, I promptly blurted out "Why don't you get your motivational skills from a good waxing and a class in manners, you wee little man!" and off I trotted to the weight room feeling extra snarky. Ten minutes later the troll man walks in, dripping in hairy perspiration and smiling from ear to ear...at me! Great gobs of gamma rays, I thought, does nothing deter this guy? And of course, now I'm on the thigh machine, up and down and work those loins, and here he comes. "Wow, I need to watch that!" he mumbles and leers with his glandular drippings. Ohmagad, now I'm feeling homicidal and say "What you need to watch is your potty mouth" and he just grins bigger. Okay, I realize he's getting off on my bitchy attitude, but since I'm in a weight room and not a dungeon, and not collecting money from this, I climb off the machine and walk to the front desk. I ask them to please remove the troll man from the floor, as I am bothered. They do, and I continue my workout in peace. Two hours later, after a swim, steam and hot tub, I walk out feeling like a new woman. Not as new as I'd like, since troll man is lurking by the front exit, obviously waiting for me. He apologizes and begs my forgiveness, as I stroll passed him, annoyed and starving, I turn and say "Two hundred an hour—upfront—and next time you can follow me around." He walks to his Lexus and I wait for an answer. He reaches in his visor and hands me four fifty-dollar bills. I take them—not too eagerly—and say "Be here on Thursday. One o'clock." He says he will, smiles and drives off. I think about how I can pay the rest of the rent now and about how I was trying to figure out a way to buy cat food and toilet paper just this morning. Sometimes life seems so hard, but sometimes things can be just that easy.

Dear Mz. Conduct,

I saw this girl from across the room the other evening. We were at an opening, a gallery in a ritzy part of town, and she took my breath away. I'm quite sure that when me made eye contact, she formed a tiny smile. I'm so intrigued by her beauty and wonder how I would go about finding her again. There is an "I Saw U" section in the local paper and thought about putting in an ad. What are your thoughts on that approach?

Breathless in Boise

> **Dear BiB,**
>
> **Next time you go to the gallery, and do this soon, ask the owners if they know who she is. If they don't, let it go. If you don't see her at the next opening—and do I really need to tell you to attend?—then let it go like a cheesy puff in a hot breeze. Those "I Saw U" columns are pretty redundant in my book. We goddesses make eye contact with six dozen people every damn day of our life and a blurb that says something like "saw you at such and such gallery opening on such and such date" with and added "you wearing red backless dress, me in slacks and brown shirt—made eye contact...drinks?" will get you nowhere fast. What lame-ass losers read those things seriously anyway? Oh, you do.**

Dear Mz. Conduct,

I've noticed my girlfriend looking at other women lately. The manner in which she stares isn't just an 'I like her outfit' or a 'cute hair-cut' type of thing, but more of a lusty look. I haven't said anything because I don't know how to ask her what she's thinking. She can be very strong-minded at times and to be truthful, I'm a little scared of her temper. How can I know what she's really thinking?

Threatened Theo

> **She's probably thinking that she'd really like to suck those bouncing breasts and bury her snotty little nose in those warm, scented snatches, that's what. Since you can't seem to find the necessary cojones to come right out and ask your girlfriend (these are important communication/relationship things) then I'd let her go and lick the real pussies and leave you alone.**

Mz. Conduct's House of Sin

"There's nothing to writing, all you do is sit down at a typewriter and open a vein."
–Walter W. Smith

A car wreck started off my day, no, I should say that a whack on the head, a spider bite and a step into fresh dog poop actually started off the day. The car wreck was a little later, once I had gotten my jinxed ass out into the world. A guy in a big, black SUV backed down a steep hill right into my little, apparently invisible truck. He bent my hood and the bumper, and thank the Goddess of Great Workouts, if I hadn't just come from the gym and a long soak in the hot tub, I'd have been bent out of shape too—in more ways than one. I just thought about good karma so, after asking him to smash down the hood and pull out the bumper, I let it go at that. Taking advantage of my good nature, the guy then tries to ask me out. Yeesh! I told him that'll happen when Dubya says something intelligent and off I went.

Greedgirl and I went to the Labia Lounge and swilled one too many cocktails. She was parading around in a skimpy skirt and a good tan and when we smooched good-bye on the street, it turned into a bit more. We suddenly heard hoots and hollers from men with boners, sitting at the cafe across the street. Laughing, we decided to play it up on this balmy night of boob-on-boob bliss, and gave the boys a good show. Wet and wild, we drove our separate ways. We joke at how it's just a shame—sometimes—that we like our boys so much.

I was still missing the Yum Yum Boy so, his buddy—and mine now too—Fret Boy, pried me out to the Tasseled Titty to cheer me up with some flesh for fantasy. It worked to some degree. Only a downpour of pathetic tears every now and again, but it was still too much for a night on the town. After ten thousand gin and tonics, I agreed to accompany him to meet a dancer he had been enamored with at another topless club. I switched to drinking water for the rest of the evening. A good thing. The chickadee he was swept away with was indeed a slice of innocent seduction and new to the dancing thang. Another good thing. She was sweet as candy and she and I established a good rapport right off the bat. I talked him up to her and she listened. For hours, she and Fret Boy yakked about guitars and such and when we finally left, at closing, he had her phone number. In the meantime, I was having a blast with some of the other dancers, sharing Butterfingers and talking trash. I felt like some old Madam, but Mz. Conduct hooks it up, baby!

I went out with my ex, Homer Simpson Junior, and his fab new girlfriend to the Tunnel O' Love Lounge where we ran into some old friends and did a bit of people watching. The room was dark and smoky and eye candy all around. Our waitress was a dish herself, but I felt like behaving, as I had just met the ex's new girlfriend twenty minutes ago and didn't want her running for the streets in screaming mode. Three guys with plaid shirts tucked into their Dockers, were standing near us trying their hardest to look cool. Not happening. As I walked to the restroom, one of them asked if I needed assistance. I turned and sarcastically told him that if he was any slicker he'd be oil down a drain, then added "Oh, you already are!" Still, I gave him my card on my trip back, as Lord love a labia lock, he needs it.

From there, we headed to the Sin Club where a punk band called The Hunches was belting out deviant desires. I left my comrades and sauntered upfront to the stage for awhile. I felt an urge to absorb the tense and troubled boy at the microphone. In his Converse tennis shoes, straight black jeans and tee shirt, through his mop of black, shaggy hair and stop-start crazy crooning, we made big-time eye contact. Damn this celibacy I've chosen. However, it's my choice and parts of me have changed since meeting the Yum Yum Boy. In my exploration of monogamy, I find parts of myself I never knew existed…and it feels good. But he's three thousand miles away now and it's the celibacy thang that has me in a twist and, well, working out at the gym four times a week. It's like this: If you know you're waiting to have a big ol' slab of hot, homemade blueberry pie, you don't want to grab a Quickie-Mart 'blueberry flavored' fruit pie. It may sate you for the moment, but you'll feel like crap-on-a-stick later on. It'll leave a bad taste in your mouth and it just isn't worth it.

Mz. Conduct's House of Sin

Mr. Bo Dangles has finally decided that true love can happen. He just needed to make a real effort and believe. He's happy now with his woman, and a rapturous redhead she is, with a voice like a naughty angel. They're playing music together and working on the love thang. Since I'm the one he whines to when they're not together, I appreciate this union of bliss more than anyone!

I'm off on a date now to the Tipsy Gypsy. He's a fan that "just wants to meet me," and of course buy me dinner and drinks. Most times these fans turn out to be guys that "just want to slide their meat whistle in me," but there are exceptions, and I never know until I know. Besides, I'm hungry and he can gaze all starry-eyed at me as I cram lobster and Cabernet down my throat.

> Dear Mz. Conduct,
>
> I have a great boyfriend and we've been going out a few months now. The only problem is that he never tells me how he feels…about anything. He's the quiet type, but I can't tell what he's thinking about and it's driving me crazy. When I ask him, he just shrugs or never answers. It makes me wonder if he's being faithful, if he loves me, if he hates me or what! How do I get my boyfriend to open up to me?
>
> Girl with Gag Boy
>
>> **Dear GwGB,**
>>
>> There's something to be said for 'the quiet type' and that's this: Sucks donkey dicks! But it's who he is and you can't change that. He's whom you fell for in the first place and you must have liked that shyness in him from the start. Your boyfriend will speak when he's good and ready and if you pester him, it'll make it worse on you both. He's still with you so quit your bitchin' and just leave him be. His behavior will tell you more than his words ever will. Remember that love is a verb, not just a noun.
>
> Dear Mz. Conduct,
>
> Do you think you can have too much sex?
>
> Petered Out
>
>> **Dear PO,**
>>
>> Sure, ask me that question now, you mindless twit! ARGH! My first response would be HELL NO, but then I guess it all depends. I suppose you can have too much sex if you're never being satisfied and you neglect the real reason for your unsated state. And you could have too much sex if you're an unsafe, filthy pig, spreading diseases. You could have too much sex if you're not discriminate in any way, shape or form and/or if you hurt people in the process for your own needs to be fulfilled.
>>
>> If your monkey meat is in high demand and can't keep up the tree swingin' with someone, why don't you just come out and say it? Meanwhile, eat well, take vitamins and quit asking stupid questions. Go wash your hands, you mental giant and make me a martini.

Good Advice from a Very Bad Girl

"Moral indignation is jealousy with a halo."
–H.G. Wells

So, the fans want to meet me, they beg for a lunch or dinner date, no expectations they say. Well, this is one girl who loves dining out (and a good Merlot), so I accept many of the offers in a chance for shameless self-promotion, and to maybe meet a new friend. But why is it that even the tame ones seem hell-bent on wanting to show me their penises? Okay, so I've always expressed my love for the almighty appendage, but not at a random sitting and certainly not after a plate full of crab cakes and prawns. I figure these men are most likely experiencing bothersome bulges and partly just want to release their burdens on me, while staring at my size-able mouth. Some don't even ask, they just whip out their wads in the front seat of their BMW and proudly display their ignorant manhood. That's when I thank them for the evening and diplomatically eject myself for the vehicle, leaving them wilting like a waterless tulip. It doesn't happen all the time, but even once in awhile is really too much. I must admit that when a stiff whopper catches my eye, I can be a bit distracted by its potential beauty, but when the guy is sitting there with a bad tie, bad breath and a pock-marked face with a deviant leer stretched across it, it doesn't much matter what his dick looks like. Face it, I tell myself, men just love to show off their penises, like a bowling trophy or a certificate from some Built-Right Penis School. Let me want it, crave it and find it for myself and we'll all be better off.

My roommate, the Distinguished Deviant, came home with gifts for me the other day, I told you he's fabulous! A blonde wig and a black vinyl jacket with zippers all over it. I look like a waist-less version of Marilyn Monroe in drag, but it could be fun on certain nights, depending on how much is left in the bottle of Sapphire.

I've been trying to get my husband to fill out the damn divorce papers with me before Mercury goes retrograde. The Transient Trollop insisted on this, as she says that all hell will break loose if I don't. I figure there is something to all this because she married her ex husband—the closeted homosexual, Mexican

Mz. Conduct's House of Sin

nightmare—on the same exact day that my husband left me. A year later, to the day, the Yum Yum Boy popped the question to me—albeit over too many cocktails and seven hundred orgasms. The Transient Trollop and I pieced this all together and figure there's something important going on. Something worth our attention in any case. So, I drive over to my soon-to-be ex husband's place, take him to dinner, look over the million-page forms with him in near silence (except for the sound of me guzzling the house red wine). After dinner, we got in my truck and the radio starts playing B.B. King's "The Thrill is Gone", almost as if I had staged it. Wow, this was ironic, and I mentioned it in humorous tones. He didn't catch the humor. When I dropped him off, the song continued and afterwards the station played two more versions of the same song! My entire drive home consisted of a thrill that was gone, but a new thrill had begun and this thrill was more consuming and freeing than anything I'd ever felt before. It's about knowing who I am, what I'm worth, and not capitulating for anyone.

This evening called for cocktails in a bubble bath and thinking about new places to masturbate. Being that the Yum Yum Boy is still down under, and not down under in the places I'd like him to be, I'm straining to behave and just wait patiently (for the first time in my disreputable little life) for the return of the Yum Yum meat. The steam room at the gym is always a little tantalizing, knowing that someone may walk in at any minute. If I could get away with it riding the Lifecycle—sitting in line with eight other breath-stealing contraptions in the middle of the weight room—I would. But I'm a sordid screamer, even with my own fingers, or a bicycle seat, and that may get me booted out of the Christian run YMCA. Either that or they'd put my picture up on the wall, right next to Jesus. I'm not taking the chance.

Dear Mz Conduct,
You are so bitchy and wise and all the things I want in a woman. Could you answer me this: I've been chatting online with this girl for about two months and she's talked to me on the phone too. She's even seen my most recent pictures, but twice now has stood me up on a date. I've been totally honest about myself and would simply like to meet her! Should I just say fuck it or keep after her? It's not like I want her to marry me, just meet me!

Confused, Frustrated, and Crazy!

> Dear CF&C,
>
> First of all, flattery will get you about as far as my cat can fly, so stuff a stiff sock in it, as I'm well aware of my multifarious attributes. On to you now. This girl obviously has some issues to deal with, whether it's that she's introverted and too shy to actually meet someone or that she's just a disgusting flake. Is that the really the type of girl that you want? Think about it mister big brain. Maybe she was repulsed by your picture and can't bring her self to ask you not to call again. She should be upfront and honest, as you have been, but all people are not sane. Leave the tramp alone and move on to a girl that will be considerate enough to, at the very least, keep her word and meet you when she says she will.

Mz. Conduct,

I've had a girl use her strap-on with me many years ago and I liked it…a lot. I haven't done that with anyone since, but lately have been thinking about it again, especially when I masturbate. I'm finding it's a part of what I definitely need in a sexual relationship and I can't let it go. My current girlfriend isn't into it. I've sort of brought up the idea to her once, and she wasn't at all interested. My question is, if I asked another girl I know to do that for me, would that necessarily be cheating on my girlfriend?

Butt Boy

> Dear BB,
>
> Yeah, poke at my weakness (pun intended) in my moments of celibacy, why don't you? Okay, mind off the double-headed dildo that is not in use at the time, damnit all to hell and back. Anyway, YEAH, you insipid sodomite, having another girl fuck you in your tight little pucker would be considered cheating on your girlfriend, even in my little black book! My advice is for you to talk to your girlfriend about this serious need of yours. That's what partners do, try to please each other even if they think they aren't interested in something the other may be hankering for big time. It may be a very intimate experience for you both and when she sees the response she'll get and the power she has—oh good God in a Gucci bag, fan me and pour me a drink—she may be the one bugging you to let her give you a butt banging. By chance, after discussing this with her seriously, she's still not willing, then you could ask her if she minded if you asked another girl because that's how badly you want/need it. See what unfolds from there. It's unfair not to work with a partner in order to get to a place that works for both parties, and if she won't relent, then it's up to you if you cheat or not. Now bend over and grab your ankles, Skippy.

Mz. Conduct's House of Sin

"If you're truly wild at heart then you'll fight for your dreams. Don't turn away from love...don't ever turn away from love."
–The Good Witch to Saylor in Wild at Heart

My comrade in the written word of the wise, Darklady, had her last big bash at the infamous Darklady Estates, before having to move. Her front porch was laden with smokers and a man with a camera that snapped some naughty shots of me draping my scantily clad ass over the railing. There were hundreds of interesting folks in attendance: four-hundred pound drag queens, voluptuous strippers, bikers and leather boys, corseted beauties and Greedgirl and I, of course. It was an immoral imperative that we go to this last party, as we met there, in the love loft, one year ago. We met as Greedgirl was indulging herself in the wand of electricity and I was in full awe of it all. I had to try it out on my bare boobies and instantly became an electricity slut myself. We realized at that point that we shared more than just a love for the purple wand o' sparks and we've been bosom buddies ever since. So, at this last party, we took turns smooching boys and posing for others, swilling numerous amounts of cocktails in between. A lovely vanilla boy that we met at the Masturbate-a-Thon was the focus of our evening. Upstairs in the love loft, he spanked me to orgasm in front of a lust filled audience and that turned me on even more. Greedgirl and he spent the rest of the evening doing much more—because she didn't get her name for nothing! They woke up laughing at jackhammers; the real ones and the good old-fashioned flesh covered ones!

The next night, my roommate, the Distinguished Deviant, did a photo shoot of Greedgirl and I, smoking and drinking, as he's making DVD's to sell. What a night. She and I cracked open the bottle of Absolut just a wee bit early, and before long I was making love to the dining room floor. It turned out to be quite the shot. I later passed out in just my purple tutu and seven inch heels. Fighting the tutu, which was still over my head, I woke up the next morning in bed with Greedgirl. I mumbled something like, "gawd, my breath could knock a buzzard off a shit wagon," and still half asleep, she moaned back, "it's okay sweetie, I can't hear anything." We realized we were still a little drunk, but laughing made our heads hurt. Nothing a couple of Advil and a Bloody Mary wouldn't cure.

The Blue Sky Boy and I went out to the Breasts R Us Bistro and ogled the table dancers, swilled beer and accepted compliments on my pigtails. When we couldn't toss down one more beer or swallow one more compliment, we headed back to his place to swallow other things. I sampled every inch of his skin from head to toe. With the skill of a contortionist, without removing his penis from my mouth, I peeled his socks and shoes off, and soon thereafter, sent him spurting into fire hydrant frenzy. As he would say, "Nice!" He says that so much, I tell him that'll most likely be on his epitaph.

Fret Boy and I ventured out, on an orange colored, harvest moon night, to the comedy club downtown. We were both in need of a few hours of chuckles…and alcoholic beverages of course. Our waitress told me I was 'adorable' and seated us at table number sixty-nine. Perfect. It's always seemed strange to me when a woman half my age calls me affectionate little names. Most likely she had no idea, as I had my pink hair sticking straight up in a Pepples style ponytail and a skimpy little pantsuit on. Other than some poor sap—coiffed and cologned, in a lily-white shirt—puking his guts up outside the place, it was a fab evening.

The last day of summer was a smoldering ninety degrees, so I grabbed my radio, ciggies and water bottle and headed out to the Nipples and Nuts nudie beach. Just as I was bending over to situate my blanket, a man yelled from down the beach, "I'm in love with you." I didn't even turn around to see who the idiotic blurb of jiggling testosterone was. Instead, I ignored him and sat down to turn on my radio. All of a sudden, out of the little red speaker, came an immense voice of a preacher yowling "you're a sinning woman, a sinner! You know you're Satan's slave." I dove for the damn thing before half the pervs on the beach could hear more. Guilt ridden? No, just a tad embarrassed. It must've gotten jumbled around in the car, as the volume was turned up and the station was not my usual one. I quickly turned it to another station and heard Poe's "I'm Not a Virgin Anymore." Ahh, much better!

I was in a mix with the editor of the magazine I write for. It seems that he thought he had paid me for this month. We haggled and bickered, and finally when his damn British accent got on my last nerve, I felt the need to quit right then and there. After a day or two, he called and conceded. He told me I could pick up my check at the office, so I trotted right over, as I hadn't eaten in two days. Thankfully he wasn't there and it was just the two assistants at their desks when I arrived. We all yakked about what a penishead he was and blah and blah. They both reminded me that I get a ton of fan mail and the magazine would certainly suffer without my contribution. Ego-boost. Much needed. Okay, I was feeling better. I spied an ultra-cool martini glass lamp they had sitting on the floor next to the water cooler, unplugged! Well, this lamp is made of metal and stands about fourteen inches high, with a huge green olive on a giant toothpick. The red pimento, in the center of the olive, lights up when turned on, sort of like me. I freaked out over that lamp in my not so demure way and the boys not only decided I deserved it, but insisted I take it. And that I did! I had a smile on my face the size of Manhattan as I carted out the big ol' lamp and my wee little check. The lamp is properly perched in my kitchen now—along with my thirty-eight martini shakers and miniature penis cocktail stirrers. Cheers baby!

Dear Mz. Conduct,

My wife and I have been married for nine years. We have three small children and she stays at home with them. I work ten hours a day and the first thing I see/hear, as I walk through the door, is her complaining about whatever; her day, the kids' troubles, and well, you get the picture. Don't get me wrong, I love my wife dearly, but I don't know what to do about this situation. When I know what's waiting for me each day, it makes it hard to want to come home. We don't get any time to ourselves and I feel guilty when I ask to take off for an hour. She flips out when I ask, so I've stopped. Do you have a suggestion?

Hub with a Headache

> Dear HwaH,
>
> Yeah, I have a suggestion: stand up for yourself, sackpaste! Wait until your kids are in bed and you have some time alone, then explain nicely to your motor-mouth wife how much it matters that you have some time to unwind

when you get home. If she can keep her yap shut and the kids away for even a half hour after you get home, that's a start. When you emerge from your spot, whether it is the garage, den or even the bathroom, then and only then will you hear about your family's day. This is important, as your children will respect you more, the more you respect yourself.

Dear Mz. Conduct,

I've asked my wife to wear wigs while we're having sex, just for the kick of it, the fantasy of her looking like a flight attendant, a hooker, or even a teacher. My wife refuses and tries to tell me that I want to be with other women and that's my reason for the fantasies. Is there a better way to approach this subject because I'm finding myself obsessed with it lately? We both enjoy reading your column, so she will read what you write. Help please?

Wigless Wayne

> **Dear WW,**
>
> I personally don't see her aversion to this. Sounds like fun to me, but that's just me and I'm sick and perverted…but in a good way! She seems to be insecure, maybe you should confront those issues first. You might ask her what some of her fantasies are and be willing to explore those with her. Exchange ideas and talk about them first, then ease into role-playing possibilities as you move forward. Some fantasies are better left as such and it's between the two of you to compromise on the differences. If you want her to make your fantasy come true, then really listen to her, be interested in what she's telling you, and seriously want to make her own fantasies come true. Maybe you'll be the one wearing a wig, lipstick and a uniform, who knows. And if so, you'll do it and you'll like it, you hair hoppin' hump daddy!

Mz. Conduct's House of Sin

"We are going to go to europe, and swill french wine, yell with the greeks, barter with the italians, and lick the sunrise of the east...we will conquer the world, one martini at a time."
–The Yum Yum Boy

Now that I've decided that celibacy is a crock of hooey, butter my buns, I'm on a roll! On my way to workout at the gym, I got stuck on the freeway for an hour and fifteen minutes. I was hornier than a she-devil in heat, it was ninety degrees out (and no I don't have air conditioning), I had no ciggies, and only fumes in my gas tank. All of the cars were stopped on the onramp to the bridge and we all had turned our motors off, waiting impatiently. I sat there awhile, then decided to look around to see if anyone was smoking, so I could go bum a cigarette. An Asian couple —old as Methuselah—to my left, a yuppie woman yakking on her cell phone to my right, some hag of a housewife in a station wagon full of screaming children in front of me. Hmmm...my prospects didn't look good. A glance in the rearview mirror and oh la la, what have we here? A dark haired, handsome gentleman in a white BMW, and, could it be? Yes, he was smoking! I opened my car door and threw my tan legs out to the side, just so he could get a full view of what was coming to him. I sashayed my body over to his shiny, clean car and asked if he could spare a cigarette. He smiled quite nicely and offered me a Benson and Hedges. Okay, so it wasn't my brand, but beggars can't be choosers. He brought out a gold Zippo and lit me up, in more ways than one. We chatted for a few minutes and I complained that I was famished and this whole traffic jam was just elevating my blood sugar to no end. He picked up the hint like a naked hitchhiker and promptly asked me to lunch. We decided to meet at a swanky seafood restaurant downtown in three hours, providing we were out of traffic by then. Our dialogue ended as we noticed cars starting to move forward. I told him I'd see him soon and jumped back in my car. I slammed through my workout at the gym, masturbated in the hot tub, and fluffed myself up for lunch with the handsome stranger.

I arrived fashionably late and there he was, sitting at the bar, smoking and drinking. God bless his vices. I ordered a Sapphire martini, three olives, and no vermouth. His black wavy hair was shiny from some sort of goop, but he smelled good and had healthy skin and great teeth. His shoes were expensive and he had a butt to bounce a quarter off of. I ordered lobster, he had prime rib, and then he surprised the thong off me by ordering a bottle of good champagne. At the end of our meal, he asked me back to his place, but I really wanted to just get home. I also really wanted to see what was behind that bulge in his slacks, so we sat in his BMW and swapped spit to a Sade CD. I decided to go for the goods and hiked my skirt up and straddled this hunk of man. When I pulled out his cock and attempted to slide a condom on, it turned out to resemble a cocktail weenie. Holy handbags full of pennies, was I disappointed! I leaned in and kissed it on the tip and said, "You come and see me when you're all grown up, ok?" With that, I thanked him for dinner and wished him on his way. He looked pissed and as if he was about to yell some obscenity at me as I strutted across the parking lot. He must've thought better of it and realized that a man with a three inch penis shouldn't be yelling anything, except maybe "God help me."

My divorce is final and I feel like dancing behind an electric chair. I will be celebrating forever, the freedom of my true self, the dodging of a bullet, and the lessons learned from falling into a relationship that tried its hardest to control, stagnate, and belittle me. I have won, and thy true self flies into the heat of the wicked night, with the wings of a dirty little dove!

Oh what a night! Greedgirl and I finagled tickets to see, the one and only, Elvis Costello. We purred our kitty selves at the Distinguished Deviant and The Lion King and they fell prey to our soft coats and jeweled collars. Tickets in hand, we paraded like school girls, clutching our handbags, giddy and loud, downtown to the beautiful ballroom where he would play. The crowd was made up of an odd mix of yuppie scum, PTA women with balding husbands in tow, middle aged men dressed in Dockers and too-small polo shirts, folks that looked like they were going to the opera, and wine clutching women that seemed to lack enthusiasm for anything but the latest hair product. We felt like bitches, we knew we were, and we didn't care. We were there to see Elvis and that's all that mattered. When he came on stage the crowd politely clapped without hoisting their lift-n-tucked asses from the seats. Greedgirl and I lifted our naturally rounded ones and kept them up all night. We danced, yelled, sang, screamed and kissed each other, which annoyed the people behind us to no end. Isn't that what a rockin' show is all about, I mean really! At one point the people behind us announced that we were blocking their view. Greedgirl turned around and asked why they weren't just home on their couch listening to the CD, for shit's sake. We thought her remark was funny, but apparently no one else did. Like I said, bitches we were, and we didn't care. We had a blast and Elvis' last song was my all time favorite called "I Want You", which brought tears to my eyes and made me get chicken skin. I thought of the Yum Yum Boy and how he has the same effect on me.

The Transient Trollop was asked to leave the motor vehicles department when applying for her license. It seems, while taking the written test, an old school marm of a wench had seen her pull her water bottle out of her purse. Well, her driver's manual plopped out at the same time and the woman came storming over, accusing her of cheating. She was humiliated enough just to be there—believe me, you want to clear the streets if she's driving—and now in front of a room full of non-English speaking people, she was asked to hand over her test. She's been banned for a week now and is plotting some sort of revenge, I'm sure of it. The Transient Trollop is hell-bent on getting a driver's license so that she and I can take a bad girl road trip on Route 66. We plan to spend the night in Nashville getting drunk, and possibly banging the other Elvis impersonators. We'll also need to get appropriate tattoos. Move over Thelma and Louise, you ain't seen nothing yet!

Now where is that Deli-Licious Boy and that youthful, mouthful of an appendage he has? He should be arriving soon with flowers in hand, pants full of anticipation and a smile to die for. What more can a bad girl extraordinaire ask for in one night? I must slip into a sassy little garter belt and leopard print stockings and attempt to scare the poor boy's halo off once again. He removed it last time and I played ring-toss on his weenie. Oh, it's just so much fun!

Good Advice from a Very Bad Girl

Dear Mz. Conduct,

First of all, let me say, I adore you! Now for my question. Is it a good thing not to masturbate too much? I do it about seven times a day and am twenty-three years old. Is this, as Germaine Greer said, harmful, or perhaps just coming from a feminist point of view?

Steady Stoker

> **Dear SS,**
>
> Of course you adore me, you're young, fun, and full of cum. There is no such thing, in my opinion, as masturbating too much. Now of course, if you're whacking away in the toy department of Sears, spanking the monkey under your desk at work, or would rather be stroking the man meat instead of being with a partner, then there may be a concern.
>
> I don't know about the feminist point of view being to blame, but Germaine Greer, who has said she considers herself 'to be much like Frank Zappa' may have just misplaced her silicone penis, therefore unable to masturbate to her liking. Who knows? Don't worry about it. If I had a penis I'd be downright dangerous. Whack on, mister.

Dear Mz. Conduct,

I am nineteen and obsessed with older women. The thing is that I think it started when I accidentally saw my mother with a guy. I don't think about her so much as just how older women are just so sexy. Once in awhile I see my third grade teacher in a bar I frequent. She compliments me a lot and talks to me each time I see her. I keep wondering if she's hitting on me and if it'd be wrong to try and initiate something with her?

Canadian Boy

> **Dear CB,**
>
> Nothing wrong with older women, honey. Personally, I prefer my boys to be at least a decade younger than I. Seeing your mother in compromising positions sometimes happens. God bless the glory hole, my son has seen more than his share I'm sure. As long as you're not thinking about your mother in any scenario then you're probably just fine. As for your third grade teacher, she's complimenting you and engaging in conversation, what's to initiate? Ask her out for coffee. You'll know what she's up to when she responds. Inevitably you will learn and appreciate a vast array of things from dating an older woman. Grab those nineteen-year-old 'nads and shake 'em up, baby!

Mz. Conduct's House of Sin

"A positive attitude may not solve all your problems, but it will annoy enough people to make it worth the effort."
–Herm Albright

Flowers came delivered to me the other day. A huge bouquet of lilies and roses and a card attached that read: There's no one like you. No signature or name or nom de plume even. Well, it was my ex wedding anniversary—no, my ex would never send those especially after I just wrestled a divorce out of him. It was also an anniversary of an ex boyfriend—no, he's pissed because he whipped his weenie out in the parking lot and I told people that matter. Hmmm, it wasn't the Yum Yum Boy from Australia—it's just not him. I was narrowing it down. Finally I decided it didn't really matter and it was just a nice surprise, and of course I deserve them. Thank you to whoever you are!

A beautiful blonde boy has been after me for some time now and since he's freshly back from working in Alaska and I'm hankering for a stiff one, I decided to hook it up with him. When offering up all that he'd do for me, I nonchalantly asked if I could perhaps use my strap on with him. He was beside himself and told me, to my devilish delight, "the bigger, the better!" Angels of the anus, my trustee ol' double headed dildo was going to finally get some use. I met him at the Tiki Lounge and oh la la, was he a cutie.

He bought me oodles of martinis, played footsies under the table and smooched over wet napkins and swizzle sticks. We finally we blew the joint and made a tangled dash to his car. I wanted to see what he had in his pants and wrestled his appendage out for a look-see. A decent specimen to be sure. I told him to drive, and drive like a maniac, back to his place. We didn't make it that far. We pulled over on the bridge and I got out of his car and bent over the hood, said "do me and do me now baby!" He obliged with great force and I screamed in blissful release all over this fair city.

My fabulous roommate, when he isn't thinking he's dying of some rash or head bump, has managed to cheer me up over and over again. When I'm in my funk

Good Advice from a Very Bad Girl

and listening non-stop to Billie Holiday or Jeff Buckley—drinking more than one person should and chain smoking myself into a frenzy—he brings me African violets, good coffee, leather skirts, and herb. He should have a medal for putting up with me, but instead he just loves me...and that's truly a jewel all it's own.

I had a fabulous lunch with Mister A the other day. He said he had something for me. I was wet with anticipation. Then he slowly whipped out the absolute biggest, the most beautiful, the most amazingly spectacular...snow globe I'd ever seen. He had just gotten back from New York and knew I collected snow globes. This one is in the shape of a heart, all sparkly and pink, sort of like me! He also gave me a CD with a million digital photos of Greedgirl and I doing a show together. We look pretty damn hot, if I do say so myself. Hmmm...I need to call her.

I'm off to workout, and peruse the weight room for bangable material. If I wasn't so discriminating, I'm sure I wouldn't be so frustrated today. Sometimes pumping iron isn't all a girl needs. Sometimes pumping flesh rods is what she needs, and if that doesn't pan out, then a good fantasy in the steam room will just have to do.

Dear Mz. Conduct,
What makes you so qualified to give sex advice?
Curious George

> **Dear CG,**
> **Honey, I've been around the block about a zillion times—taking turns with directions, as not to get dizzy—and after decades of helping my friends and theirs out, decided to spout my opinion to the masses. I attend many workshops, read all I can, and am continually immersed in my element; the sex industry. Simple as that. Now go grab my book, *Whores and Other Feminists*, by Jill Nagle, that was sent to me by a fan, make me a martini and then go away.**

Dear Mz. Conduct,
My girlfriend has complained, in a nice sort of way, that my penis is too thin. She said the length is great, but I lack the girth she likes. I've never heard this before and wonder what I can do to please her?
The Thin Man

> **Dear TM,**

Yeah, it can matter if a guy looks as if he could stick his wiener in a pencil sharpener. I'm not a big fan of the skinnies myself, but too much girth is not good for me either. So where does that leave you? It's all individual and since your girl has told you that this promotes a problem for her, try wearing a cock sleeve. You can get them at most any adult video/toy stores. They're inexpensive and they come in colors. It's just like a thick condom with ridges and bumps all over it and they work rather well. You can also order the Blossom Sleeve from Toys in Babeland (www.babeland.com). It's made of a soft, pliable jelly rubber and is very stretchy. It's made to feel like the inside of a vagina so it should be enjoyable to you both. Where there's a will there's a way, baby. Slide that stick-thin schlong of yours in a sleeve and have at it!

Dear Mz. Conduct,

After reading your columns, and finally knowing what kind of woman I want, how does a man like me go about getting to know a woman like you and eventually having sex with her?

Smitten

Dear S,

What is a 'man like you' all about? I have no idea, except that you show good taste in reading my columns. You like a strong and bitchy woman apparently and that can be a good thing, showing that you are secure to some extent. However, there aren't a whole lot of women like me around and getting to the bedroom (or car hood) with me takes a whole lot of chemistry, which is an entirely a fateful thing. Now leave me alone.

Good Advice from a Very Bad Girl

"When women go wrong, men go right after them."
–Mae West

The Lion King bought me a ticket to go see the fabulous *Sex and the City* writer, Cindy Chupak. It was a swanky affair held at the downtown Creative Conference Center, under huge skylights and plush, red carpet. I went solo and brought a notebook, as I always do wherever I go. After registering and getting my little nametag slapped on, I meandered around in the snob-soaked crowd. I realized my ticket didn't include cocktails or even a raffle ticket. I could do without winning a signed picture of the *Sex and the City* girls or a DVD of the third season, but no cocktail! I had thirty-six cents to my name, but figured I'd find some available man to buy me a Cosmopolitan, the featured drink of the evening, of course. No such luck. There were only a handful of men, and they looked as if their women had dragged them by the Dockers to this estrogenic event. So, I found a chair by the jazz trio, sat and observed the masses, perched from my viewpoint. Everywhere I looked, I saw perfectly coiffed heads, masks of flawless complexions, Prada shoes and Gucci handbags. I wondered, would I ever be one of these women that can afford good shoes, raffle tickets and cocktails? Oh yes, I will, but I'm also sure I'll forever have my bleached blonde pigtails and hooker-red nails, or some reasonable facsimile. And, clearly, I will always be the sassiest bitch around.

My back was killing me from waxing floors all day—my day job, I hate it—so, I was glad to have a chair, as the room was filling up fast. I had the jazz trio playing "Ding Dong, the Witch is Dead" and feasted on fancy hors d'oeuvres—or whores de ovaries, as my grandma used to say—so I was content. Then along comes a guy who looks exactly like the late John Denver, and he sits down next to me. We yakked for a bit and, when I realized he was also flying solo, asked him to buy me a drink. He explained that he was also broke and was only drinking water himself. I said he must be a freelance writer, too, and indeed, I was correct. Figures. He was a decent sort though, so we headed outside for a ciggie break together. Of course, he bummed one from me. Back inside and still a half-hour to kill before Cindy, another woman (clutching a Chihuahua)

Mz. Conduct's House of Sin

came and sat with us. The little dog was so sedate, I worried that it was dead. No, just Prozac paws and an owner who could use some too.

Finally the theatre opened its doors. Everyone else, but for us po' folk, guzzled the last of their cocktails, crammed what they could of the cheese wrapped kiwi in their mouths and headed inside. Since I had none of this to do, I waltzed in and got a seat front and center. Yay! The talk was splendid and Cindy was both hilariously lovely and very inspiring. Afterwards, as people lined up for her autograph, I jumped up (being right there and all) and not needing no stinkin' autograph, I gave her my card instead. We had a short chat and she shook my hand! I drove home, grinning like an idiot, with silly reveries of getting a call from New York to help write an episode of *Sex and the City*. You just never know!

Now, to make a booty call to one of my eager-beavered boy-toys. He better be a young, strong thing and be able to handle my raunchy, ravenous, rampage of lust tonight. Honey, his penis is doomed!

> Mz Conduct,
>
> In one of your recent columns, you told the 23 year-old that it was OK to masturbate 7 times/day. That is not necessarily true. When he reaches 40, he will not be able to get it up. The spongy tissue that soakes (sic) up blood and allows the penis to become stiff, will have atrophied. This is very bad advice you have given. Keep up the good intent though! Someday you will know enough to provide the right advice!
>
> SB
>
>> Dear SB,
>>
>> Even though my first reaction to your letter was, "Bite me boner-less boy," I realized that I do like a challenge, even a little conflict, from time to time. So, thank you for providing just that.
>>
>> I have never heard of such a thing, but decided to interview some men. My roommate, the Distinguished Deviant, told me he masturbated about that much when he was that age and he is fifty-one now and still going strong in the erection department, as well as all other areas of penile function. Asking approximately ten different men, they all came up with about the same answer. Since you didn't tell me where you got your information or toss me any sort of reference, I decided to be professional and get some for you. I contacted a clinical sexologist, Joseph Marzucco, MS, PA-C, who's been in practice for thirty-six years. He also teaches a Human Sexuality class at Portland State University. Here is what he said:

"In a human male libido (the mental desire to enter sexual activity), the ability to get an erection and the ability to ejaculate are physiologically distinct.

"First, on a psychological level, I agree with you that as long as the frequency of masturbation does not interfere with his life, relationship or cause distress in some way there is no reason not to masturbate.

"It seems your reader is suggesting that masturbation, somehow, atrophies tissue in the penis, such that he will not be able to get an erection. Emphatically not true! Stroking your penis, unless you actually injure it in doing so, does nothing bad to the inside of the penis. In fact, getting blood into the penis, regardless of ejaculating is probably good. More blood equals higher oxygen tension which produces a chemical that reducing the "Natural" aging of the tissue inside the penis.

"A mans deterioration of erectile function does begin in the forties, but by no means does his ability to have an erection go away. In fact erections suffer more from smoking, high blood pressure, medicines, diabetes, high cholesterol and heart disease, just to mention a few.

"An odd fact to most people is that a man can ejaculate without an erection. This is true because the ability to get an erection is separate from ejaculation. Another fact is that when a man ejaculates he goes into a "refractory" period were the ability to ejaculate again is impossible until a certain period of time goes by.

"The refractory period is extremely variable but in general gets longer the older we get. The reality is that we do not know a lot about the variability of ejaculatory ability in men across a life span. It would make a great research project. In my experience, talking to many men about sexual function in general, and ejaculation specifically, the ability to ejaculate more then twice per day on a regular basis is rare. Ejaculating seven times a day is extremely rare, but in no way injurious to a man's heath or sexual function...unless he thinks it is or is convinced it is by someone else."

Joseph Marzucco, MS, PA-C

Sex Therapist

So, perhaps your brain cells have 'atrophied' from lack of use and the only way for you to get an erection these days is to try your best at hacking up glamorous sex advice columnists.

Dear Mz. Conduct,

I have a quick question for you. There's a girl at work that I'm getting know pretty well. Through our "bantering" I think there's a good chance she's interested in something more physical. I must say that I'm a little nervous about her seeing my cock for the first time and being disappointed with my size. Think I should be concerned about it? Any advice?

Small Fry

Dear SF,

I think that the girl has shown that she is already interested in the person you are. Don't over-analyze the situation. If you don't stop obsessing, then if/when the time comes where she may indeed get a look-see at your little guy, you may not only shrivel up even tinier than you already are (holy prostitutes with prosthetics, I bet you can't afford that), but you'll be a lame duck in the sack too. Just relax. If you and she get to a more intimate place in your relationship, just keep in mind that there are about a zillion other aspects to sex than just your penis. Wait it out and let her see all the charming qualities that you possess. If you don't have any...then start stressing out.

Mz. Conduct's House of Sin

"Of all sexual aberrations, perhaps the most peculiar is chastity."
–Remy de Gourmont

After a nightmarish date with an over-zealous fan, which turned into an octopus-wrestling match in the parking lot of the Tiki Lounge, I decided to lay low for a bit. Okay, two days to be exact. The big bash—for the smut magazine I write for—was happening at a club downtown and I was obligated to attend. It was a huge, private party, just hoppin' with pretty strippers, pistol packin' mobsters, a couple of Dominas with slaves in tow, and a limousine spilling out scantily clad beauties. Then, of course, there was moi, in a roaring bitchy-bitch mood, and my convoluted entourage: Greedgirl, looking ravishing in a floor length black dress, slit up to the Yukon; Blue Sky Boy in smiles and motorcycle helmet; Big Bald Bouncer, in black leathers (acting as my personal bodyguard for the evening), and all of us driven to the club by The Distinguished Deviant, who wore leather pants and a naughty-assed spiked belt. I was wearing my new leather knee-high boots, black fishnets, and a wee little black dress to match.

Big Bald Bouncer had my back all evening, in case the octopus date showed his face. He even set up my protection with the guys at the door, who by the way, resembled matching Fridge-a-daires. I meandered through the crowd, the relentless thump of the Norman Sylvester Blues band pounding in my temples, and was handed martinis left and right. All Sapphire, three olives, every time. Nice. Even my son and his handsome, Spanish roommate showed up. My son was impressed with the shindig and had a whopping good time ogling the drunken strippers. I had to keep Greedgirl from molesting him though, as she had one too many double whiskeys and not enough food in her svelte gullet. Have Weenie-Will-Travel was there and took me aside to give me a V.I.P pass (whatever on earth that is good for) and to confess that I was A) the "best romp he'd ever had" and B) that he still thinks about me, "especially late at night." Tramps in Toledo, I took the martini he offered me and declared, "Well, of course, that's a given, sweetie," and strode my sleek rump into the thick of the exuberant crowd. I suppose I could have mentioned that he looked nice in his tuxedo, but I wasn't in a benevolent mood. However, I did catch sight of a gorgeous young lad who reminded me a bit of the Yum Yum Boy. And since the latter is still in a land far, far away, I just had to introduce myself to the gothic vision coming my way. He reeked of cool. He was tall, with long, shiny, black hair and vinyl pants that made his round little ass scream, 'Come and bite me, baby!' His name was Casey and I think I left some drool on his crotch. Bad-girl antics are a science, you know.

I had a lovely date with Mister Television Producer the other evening. He took me to dinner, a movie, and even bought food for my house full of critters. He didn't grope, he didn't whine, and he didn't whip out his weenie...which means he may see me again.

Fret Boy and his rockin' band, UNTYD, were on a local radio station the other morning. I meant to record it, but pushed a wrong button and ended up only recording Fret Boy saying something about sleeping with his dog. Oops!

The Lion King bought me a fab book of the *Sex and the City* escapades, took me to a happy hour that included dinner and doubles, and then to see a film called "Secretary" that I absolutely panted over. Ooooh, do I recommend that one! It's a psychological S/M love story and so very well done. It made me walk out of the theatre hankering for the sweet, stinging swats of seduction.

I had a raging workout at the YMCA and after a good steam and hot tub, I paraded my shaved, pierced, and tattooed self into the locker room, despite the evil-eyes of the Yuppie-Christian-lipstick-bare women. They are always there, looking away when they see me, muttering little prayers for me, into their gym bags of ignorant bliss. This time, there was an older Down Syndrome woman sitting right in front of my locker and I asked her if I could squeeze in behind her. She was so cute, I thought I would die. She nicely got her things together and moved aside for me and as she was turning around she looked up at me and hollered, extremely loud (as Down Syndrome people often do), "Oh, sooo pretty!" and the conglomerate of Christian housewives had simultaneous car-

Mz. Conduct's House of Sin

diac arrests. It was the funniest thing ever and made my freakin' day. God bless the uninhibited, for we surrender to hedonism, beauty and the first amendment whenever we damn well please.

I've made fast friends with a fabulous-fannied girl who wants to hook up with me. She's a dancer at some of the nicest topless clubs in the city and seeing, that she's recently left her husband, she may need some girl-on-girl comforting. Perhaps she should get her curvy self over here, feed me purple grapes, good champagne and lap-dance me into oblivion. Now, where's my damn phone when I need it?

Dear Mz Conduct,
I'm hoping you can help me with my problem. I like to be submissive to women and do what they tell me but I have found it really hard to actually link up with one. The problem is that I have a beautiful and sexy friend whom I would love to serve sometimes, but she doesn't seem really interested in it when I approach the subject. Now and then she'll kind of order me to buy her cigarettes and wine (which thrills me) but I dream of doing something more, like taking her on a shopping spree to buy clothing and get minor satisfaction from being openly used by her. I kind of like the idea of her treating me like shit for a few hours. My question is, am I asking too much or should I be asking at all?
Worm

> **Dear Worm,**
> **Well, you've "approached the subject", now ask her flat out and quit beating around her bush. If she says she's not interested in fulfilling your desires then leave it alone—if you want to remain friends. She'll let you know if she changes her mind. In the meantime check out www.alt.com or look in your local newspaper. Check out the personal ads section, and find a Dominatrix that'll rock your inflatable boat. Now, shut the fuck up and go wash my mold-covered dishes, feed the dogs and polish my thigh high boots until they blind you with glare.**

Dear Mz. Conduct,
After three weeks of marriage, my wife refuses to suck my whole penis. She just sucks the tip and I want her to do more than that. She says she doesn't like it and I don't know what to do. If you tell me I should give her oral sex, well, I do! I kiss her muffin over cellophane (because she said she gets urinary tract infections) and try to please her continuously. Can you help me, please?
Newlywed Going Nuts

> **Dear NGN,**
> **This is why premarital sex can be such a remarkable thing. It baffles me that men, or women for that matter, marry someone who doesn't satisfy them sexually. Some people say that you marry the person and not what they can do for you and blah blah freakin' blah. Titties on a tuna-melt, that's just horseshit! Let's face it, we've all been swooned into mistaken relationships, but hopefully**

we learn from them and don't repeat history. Even I once shacked up with a guy who wouldn't lick me, said he had a 'bad experience' with some girl in college or some utter garbage. I kept asking him, "Honey, have you seen my pussy?" I mean, really! In any case, I told him flat out that if he couldn't fix his sexual hang-ups then I was taking up other offers, just so he knew. He never amended his behavior, so I found someone else down the line. Granted, this was only part of the relationship problem, but it certainly contributed to the break-up. Since most people aren't as brutally honest as I am, they end up cheating because of such things. I do believe in the truth most all the time. So if I were you, I'd tell her how much it means to you—which she'd see if she deep throated you—and keep in mind that when one person gets turned on, the other feeds off of that unbridled enthusiasm. On the other hand, some women just don't like administering fellatio. Personally, that is an attitude that I can't even fathom, but still, it does remain a fact. If I were you, I'd look into some Tantric sex workshops that the two of you could take together.

By the way, get yourself tested for urinary tract infection and if you're clean, then lose the cellophane, honey. Sometimes people are asymptomatic and still contagious without even being aware of it. The point is, especially in this new marriage, you should both want to please the other, sexually and otherwise, and work through anything that is blocking that, no matter what. If all else fails, go visit a glory hole, live long, and prosper.

Mz. Conduct's House of Sin

"You can't start it like a car, can't stop it with a gun."
–Warren Zevon on the strongest of loves

Holy handbags full of Handi-Wipes! If I get one more question about incest, I will go screaming into the goddamn streets! (If someone has to ask why, then they have more concerns than Bush in the White House). Big Bald Bouncer suggests the person in question sit on a crowded freeway at midnight. Bottom line, I prefer not to dignify "I want to sleep with my sister, is that okay?" or "My mother caught me masturbating and wants to show me the right way to do it," twisted-type blather with an answer. Sick, sick puppies, is all I have to say. Fantasies are one thing, but reality is another, that's what I say!

I was steeping my bones in a gin-soaked bathtub, listening to the Stones new song "The Key to your Heart," and a thought occurred to me: If you give your lover the proverbial "key to your heart" and then later break up, is it automatically implied that you've gotten your key back? Can an ex-lover still gain access if they've secretly duplicated the key or slithered up a side window, crawling into one's life, again? Would this not be breaking and entering? Hmmm. Another thought, in the middle of a hedonistic bubble bath: Is it kosher to use the same song for a different relationship? Personally, I have theme songs for each relationship that I've been in; sometimes many songs, depending on the length of the relationship. And often it seems that the number of my relationships is almost equal to the amount of songs ever written! But I don't want to drift in to that now, honey. Anyway, I think everyone does this; a song comes on the radio and you're with your special someone, you both comment on it, oohs and ahhs, and it just easily becomes 'your song.' Well, what if you're in another relationship and your ex-lover's song plays when you're with your new lover? Should one interchange and exchange that song to go with the new lover? Or is it possible to completely forget, after time, that it was a previous lover's song? And if not, would one always feel a bit guilty for reusing it? Hmm…I'll have to think about that a little more…when I roll another.

Soon after, I went to dinner with an escort friend of mine and two gentlemen she knew. My friend was hoping to start her own business and she was looking at these fellows for backers. She brought me along for my charm and snarkiness and was confident that she and I could somehow help persuade them. We visited the Boom Boom room, noshing on oysters and gin, and had lots of each with a side of savory persuasion, then danced to Sinatra tunes and, once in awhile, my girlfriend and I slid our tongues down each other's throats. Mmmm. Naughty, I know. All in all it was a torrid little evening and she now has her business and I still have oodles of dignity.

The beautiful, blonde boy, who previously drove me in (and on the hood of) his car, called the other night and asked if he could visit. Booty call, literally! He wanted his bootie banged and was aching to try out my double-headed dildo. Who am I to turn him down? Blonde Boy walked into my house, wearing the most ultra-sexy, snappiest, fifties suit that I ever laid eyes on. It was jet black, a bit biggish on his tall, thin frame, and he sported a skinny, red neck-tie with little, black martini glasses all over it. Yummy. I grabbed him by this accessory and pulled him towards my hot mouth. I wore a long, burgundy, oriental robe with nothing but my strap-on and pheromone oil underneath. I dragged him to my candle-lit bedroom, scented with vanilla, and reclined on the heap of pillows. "Take off your clothes very slowly," I commanded him. He obeyed like a grinning, good boy. Watching him leisurely strip down to his silky, black thong was intensely erotic and I felt my thighs quickly moisten. I could see the back of his svelte body in the mirror behind him, and I watched lustily as his sinewy arms removed the thong itself, producing an outrageous hard-on the size of Florida. "Is that all for me, baby?" I drawled, and he moaned an affirmation. He bent down towards me and we kissed. We fell onto the pillows and our bodies were instantly tangled together. With our hearts pounding, we rubbed our penises together, flesh on silicone as I clandestinely poured lubricant on my hand and slid my finger up his perfect pucker. We stroked one another's stiffness. We rolled around, I grabbed his hips from behind, and slowly worked up to sliding in my silicone slice of heaven. When he eventually came, Blonde Boy growled, hollered, and ended on a high note that Tarzan

Mz. Conduct's House of Sin

would have blushed at. Christ on a crutch, how I love the absolute power! Grrrr! He Tarzan, me Jane, and jungle love is so under-rated.

Now, I'm preparing for the revolutionary return of the Yum Yum Boy, who will be flying back from Australia with lots of manly adventures to share. With new leopard sheets and two dozen tiny candles in the boudoir, we are surely going to do some celebrating. Hopefully, when I pick him up at the airport, my clit doesn't run ahead of me and get us both arrested by airport security. Nevertheless, I am planning a straddle attack in the parking garage. He's been 'down under' for so long, but I have a sneaking suspicion that I'll be the one 'down under' all that crazy Yum Yum meat, and, honey, faster than a tick on a June bug! Bring it on, kangaroo boy!

Off I go...I have strippers to interview and must self-medicate myself beforehand.

> Dear Mz. Conduct,
> My wife and I have been married for twenty-six years and, before I was married, I enjoyed anal sex, both giving and receiving it. My wife and I have never done either and, for some reason, lately, I realized that after all these years, I miss it. Can you suggest a solution?
> Missing the Tail
>> Dear MtT,
>> Sometimes a person just gets a nagging need for naughtiness, some titillating behavior memory surfaces from the 'good old days.' With you, it's perfectly understandable, since your 'good old days' are really old. I suggest that you simply tell your wife what you wrote me. Since you two have been together for over a quarter of a century, obviously something is working, so it shouldn't be a difficult task.
>>
>> I recommend watching Dr. Carol Queen's videos, *Bend Over Boyfriend* and *Bend Over Boyfriend 2,* as she offers loving, affectionate demonstrations that are specifically designed for couples. You and your wife can go (and cum) from there. It's all about communication, honey. Open mouth, speak.
>
> Dear Mz. Conduct,
> I'm a 29 year old straight man who has been told all his life that I "act like a girl." I've never played sports or even been interested in watching them. Instead, I've always had hobbies like cooking, gardening and, although I don't consider myself meticulous, I do keep a clean house. For the most part I don't let people's teasing bother me, but every once in awhile, I admit that it infuriates me. It bothers me most often when friends goad me about my "faggot behavior" right when I'm really interested in some girl. It lowers my self-esteem and I don't feel confident when I do see the girl. I

Good Advice from a Very Bad Girl

end up losing her each time and am left with the idea that she may think I'm gay, too. I don't want to change who I am for someone else, but is there something I could do to help my situation?

Het in Hell

> Dear HiH,
>
> The self-esteem issue, or lack thereof, is probably the most damaging thing I see. First of all, some men just have more feminine energy than others do. Personally, I love a man who is in touch with his feminine side and can feel comfortable enough to use it freely. You need to tell your so-called 'friends' that, although they may think they are having fun, it is at your expense. Tell them that their constant badgering pisses you off and they should cease and desist. Maybe your friends have wanted to secretly bend you over the kitchen stove, and this is their way of over-compensating. Those who protest too much, ya know? In any case, use your bitch qualities and put your foot down, mister!
>
> Just because you'd rather cook a soufflé than watch a football game doesn't mean dick. Or, with your choices, maybe it does. You need to truly figure this out. When you do (and I prefer to think positively) then you should feel secure with who you are. Remember, if a girl truly likes you, she likes the whole kit and caboodle of just who you are. A confident and secure man is a huge attraction, no matter if you're potting a petunia or overhauling an engine. Now, quit whining and go cook a fab dinner while I change the oil in my truck.

Mz. Conduct's House of Sin

"It is not enough to conquer; one must know how to seduce."
–Voltaire

Picking up the Yum Yum Boy at the airport didn't go quite as planned, but that's life, isn't it? Thank the Goddess of Guttersluts for spontaneous combustions of unpredictability. One thing that was right on target was moi getting to the airport bar an hour early, and not a minute before, as I was instructed by the boy not to cause a drunken commotion at the gates. Now, no one, and I mean no one, can 'instruct' me in the subtle, yet domineering way he can, honey! Dressed in black leather from head to toe, I swilled down a couple of double Absolut and cranberries at the airport bar and yakked with the bartender, a fun flamer named Bob. I was so excited, I whipped out pictures of the Yum Yum Boy and Bob—after announcing 'Oh, girl, he has such big feet!"—made me promise to swing on in with him as soon as he got off the plane. Half tanked, I waited for the trickle of folks deplaning, searching for some wild hat or Aussie get-up the Yum Yum Boy might have on. Nothing. Then out of the blue I saw his mesmerizing eyes, and I immediately interrupted an elderly woman who'd been expressing anxiety with all of her dysfunctional grandchildren. I dashed away in mid sentence and screamed "There's my baby!" to the Yum Yum Boy as he made his way down the maze of ropes. It was just like a movie scene, or so I like to imagine. He couldn't miss me with my newly pink pigtails and leather ensemble and swooped me up in his monkey arms to plant a big juicy one on my ready for cock-sucking lips. Beside myself, I dragged him right in to see Bob the bartender and we mistakenly stayed in the airport bar for hours. It left us to wander aimlessly through the parking garage at midnight, for what seemed hours, searching for my misplaced vehicle and paying a giant parking fee at the gate. We took a wrong turn home, a convoluted ride ensued, but no worries, mate, we made it home and he promptly tossed me on the kitchen floor, ripped out the crotch of my fishnets and banged me to kingdom come! Welcome home boytoy!

A few nights later, a New York fan of mine offered me two complimentary tickets to see his buddy and hilarious crude-man, Doug Stanhope (www.dougstanhope.com) at the Lusty Loins Lounge here in town. I took a dangerously sexy boytoy along and we passed right through the mile-long line, getting venomous looks from the folks in line, but loving every minute of it. Once in, we were approached by the door girl telling us that we were V.I.P. and needed to go through the black door behind the bar and straight up the stairs to the balcony. A balcony I never knew existed until that moment. And I had been there a zillion times. Once upstairs, we were served free, stiffer than my boytoy (well, almost), drinks all night long. Fabulous! It was a great show and even if it wasn't, how would we know, we were polluted! We shared the balcony with local KNRK radio celebrities, Marconi and Tiny and their lovely ladies. Aside from Tiny, a five hundred-pound hunka love, showing his butt on stage, it was an absolute riot. The show ended with a guy dressed as a hot dog, playing a kick drum, guitar, harmonica, and tambourine and crooning about how his wife left him for a corn dog. Too funny and free, as it should be!

Wee One, my small-penised friend, delivered a lovely care package to my porch the other day. The package contained wine, flowers, a snow globe from Amsterdam and all the things a girl really needs, aside from maybe a fat schlong and a dark chocolate truffle, that is. It was a sweet gesture and Mz. Conduct always is in appreciation of sweet gestures, let me tell you.

I went to see my friends, the UNTYD band at the Rusty Tap. Fret Boy was in fine form, as was the rest of the band and they blew the previous butt rockers right off the stage. I had too many cocktails and lost my leopard and leather gloves that night, but I did meet three girls that helped me drool over a lad in the next band. It's much more attractive to drool in a group than alone with the wrong end of your ciggie burning and your scarf in the beer. One of the girlies was quite pleasing to my slightly inebriated eye and she and I decided to slip into the men's bathroom, as the women's restroom was full of crossed-legged bimbos and whining. She went first and I said "to hell with it" and hiked my skirt to pee in the sink. Hey, it's a guys' bathroom, who washes their hands in there? We traded lipsticks and coiffed each other's hair and before long she was sucking on my neck. Pink lipstick smudged my nape and goose bumps spread over my chest and my dime-sized nipple grew to nickel size. That's where I wanted her and that's where she would be, I decided. I leaned back against a somewhat clean urinal and moved her head down to my heaving mounds where she engulfed my ringed nipples like a hungry child. The entire time we were in the men's room, not one soul came in, unfortunate for them by leaps and bounds...or heaves and mounds I should say. Anyway, with just her tongue flicking the tips of my tits, I came buckets right there on the cold porcelain. Thankfully, my sweet release was unheard through the thundering thumps and beat of the band on stage. Later, we walked out of the dark club blushing with girlie glee, giggling and smoking. At the end of the night we parted with a true sense of Cyndi Lauper-like enthusiasm. Yes baby, girls just wanna have fun!

New Year's parties, oh yay! My lovely and talented friend, Darklady (www.darklady.com) has once again thrown a wild polyamorous New Year's bash, held at a decommissioned church. Whips and chains and swings and ropes, Greedgirl did her Bukkake thang in the baptismal bath and a number of fine folks, all in various ways, worshipped in awe at her greedy gathering of gush. I, in black vinyl was escorted by a tall and well endowed lad who, in front of a hundred people, bent me over an altar and, in the infamous words of Chrissie Hynde, "when I shot my mouth off, showed me what that hole was for." Ohmagod, what a big mouth I have!

So, it's on to a newfangled new year. Perhaps it'll be a strange mix of things, but that's the beauty of it all. Things we can't control inevitably come our way, but we can never give up hope for what we need and want. We will all somehow get what we deserve and when we're bitchin' about how life is treating us, let's remember, how are we treating life! Happy New Year from the bad girl extraordinaire and all of her amazing boys and girls! Bottoms Up baby!

> Dear Mz. Conduct:
> I consider myself pretty sex-savvy. I've read personals ads since I was a little kid. So why don't I know what the terms "top" and "bottom" mean? Please enlighten me before I get into something scary like S&M!

Good Advice from a Very Bad Girl

Confused in the Middle

Dear CitM,

I'm glad you consider yourself 'sex-savvy' but if you actually were, you would know this. So quit swingin' your wiener and let me inform you. These are usually terms used in BSDM (Bondage, Discipline, Domination, Submission, Sadism, and Masochism) and is used to cover any sexual activity that involves one partner being in control and one partner being controlled. Scary? To each his own, but instead of my incessant blathering, here are the definitions and some information according to San Francisco's Sex information site—and Mister Sex Savvy Not, who could you possibly trust more in this area?:

"Bottom: Meaning varies by sexual subculture, but generally means either (1) submissive in BDSM or power exchange play, or (2) penetrated partner in anal sex.

Top: Meaning varies by sexual subculture, but generally means either (1) dominant in BDSM or power exchange play, or (2) penetrating partner in anal sex.

Switch: In BDSM or power exchange play, ability to be submissive (top) or dominant (bottom) depending on the situation and the partners they are with.

Often, BDSM activities include one of three elements:

* Role play (Example: one partner is the "master" or "mistress", and one partner is the "slave", who does whatever the master/mistress commands.)

* Control play (Example: one partner is blindfolded or tied up.)

* Pain play (Example: one partner spanks the other.)

Most BDSM "scenes" will involve a combination of some of these elements.

It's important to understand that BDSM activity always involves consent. That is, both partners in a BDSM interaction actively want to participate, and both partners have the ability to stop the activity at any time—this usually involves using a pre-arranged signal, or "safeword".

There are many theories about why people are interested in BDSM, but no one has a definite answer. People who do BDSM (both as "tops" and "bottoms", indicating power or status, not necessarily actual positions) find it enjoyable and exciting. There is no evidence that interest or participation in BDSM activities is associated with any psychological problems or that BDSM leads to abusive behavior outside the bedroom."

Always play within your ability. If you don't know how to do something safely, learn how before you try it out on your partner. Quit being a scared little loser and bend over for me, baby!

Dear Mz. Conduct,

I'm a little embarrassed, but I have to write to you concerning some perversions I have because you seem like the only person who will understand. I'm not sure if anyone else has had this experience, but ever since I was a child I've always associated the ecstasy of pissing after holding it a long time with a sort of orgasmic experience.

I'm not quite sure how to approach my girlfriend with my fantasy of having sex with her in the shower and have her ride me until she cums and then just let herself go during her orgasm to include pissing all over my dick and letting it drip out and all over my body.

Do you think women ever have these desires too? Well, thanks for any advice you can offer, sometimes it just helps to get it out of your system and tell someone.

Mz. Conduct's House of Sin

Perverted Peter

Dear PP,

Right off the bat, let me say that you are not a pervert, at least not in my book. And good for you that you're in tune with your body as much as you are! What you're experiencing is the power of your PV muscle, the same muscle that allows you to ejaculate or not. Control over it is an amazing thing. It's a very erotic feeling to have that control, bottomline. My comrade in naughtiness, Greedgirl, has been directed by her Canadian Goose as they sit through an entire movie, not to get up and pee. When they get home, he will make her shower with him, still not allowing her to pee, making her orgasm instead. After which, she can freely let her PV muscle relax and only then can she pee. That in itself is extremely erotic. That's how our bodies are made up, baby. All the childhood experiences happen for a reason, even if we're not aware of them at the time.

As far as telling your girlfriend your desires...just do it, wimp ass! If she loves who you are, she will try and encompass all your needs and maybe exchange some of her naiveté into pleasing you and maybe herself as well. You should feel free to express all of who you are with your partner. This may bring a whole new dimension to your relationship and it's a new year, honey and time to be yourself and be loved for the delicious deviance inside you! You get the Mz. Conduct stamp of approval. Now hold that bladder and go make me a martini, watch me drink it down and make me another, damnit!

Good Advice from a Very Bad Girl

"Happiness lies neither in vice nor in virtue; but in the manner we appreciate the one and the other, and the choice we make pursuant to our individual organization."
–Marquis de Sade

The Transient Trollop has again relocated her svelte buns to a cooler locale. She's already nailed a guy on the plane ride, joining the Mile High Club along with yours truly! She clandestinely slipped in a date with a chiseled-faced lawyer at the airport while her ex-boyfriend retrieved her luggage, and already has a cute little parking attendant on hold. We deviously desirable girls do need attending, and often, and preferably by someone who knows how! She's stranded in a state where there's no lottery, so I must start playing for her, she says. Our plan, if I win big, is that she'll get a laser-peel and I'll pay off the collection mongers and then we'll jet off to Paris...just to shop!

My Blue Sky Boy sped off to New Orleans for New Year's Eve and, to my surprise, came back engaged to the girl of his dreams. When I first saw her picture, she looked almost exactly like him! Well, as I always say, if I could clone myself, I would; I do so understand the mirror-like attraction. She's moving here soon and he promises that she will like me too...all of me. Something about 'when I see her tongue'. Hmmm...that should be quite the ménage a twat to look forward to, and, but of course, daahlings, I will report back with sordid details!

One foggy, crisp evening last week, I took a beautiful young boytoy out with me to hear my ex-boyfriend's reggae band. The club turned out to be on the outskirts of town, a small white trash diner. All six members of the band (including the two plus sized women singers) were squashed onto a seven-foot by eight-foot area directly in front of the restrooms. No matter, the band got rocking and before long the toothless patrons were bouncing to the beat of Jah. Red flashing lights went off in the back room and, noticeably, a drooling drunkard won big on the video poker machine. The winning alarm bells mixed right in with the bass guitar. My boytoy and I hobnobbed with the locals and,

Mz. Conduct's House of Sin

hearing that the joint had just got it's liquor license, we just had to sample a few cocktails. They were a little weak, but no worries, we had our flask! My legs had been crossed too long and I made my way to the men's bathroom. I chose to straddle the urine-splashed room because a congregation of hair-hoppers and gum chompin' bimbos were lined up at the women's bathroom. An inebriated pole-digger made rude comments as I walked in, hey, when a girl has to go. For the most part, it was an interesting night, and where else can you watch Hollywood Squares on a wall-mounted television, and listen to a live reggae band perform, all at the same time?

Not Your Average Joe called and invited me to the Ace of Hearts Swingers Club the other night. If I didn't already have a straight-boy date pouring me oodles of cabernet as we spoke, I would have joined in the naughtiness for sure. But as it was, priorities of pleasure prevailed and I made my apologies to Not Your Average Joe and resumed being pampered by the boy of the evening. He may be straight as an arrow, but so was that ample appendage peaking out of the leather/mesh shorts he wore, as he massaged my barking dogs and kept my wineglass full.

I realized something over the weekend: I can't and won't ever drink Jägermeister again. If I can pull that off then it'll surely hamper my compulsion to suddenly leave my date at a party at three a.m., in the middle of God knows where, and walk aimlessly for miles, blubbering, in twenty-degree weather. All I vaguely remember is a game of strip rummy, a dozen shots of green evil liquid going down my throat and trying to curl up on a school step somewhere in the hills. It was a crazy thing to do, and my date was furious, as he had all of the partygoers out searching for my leather-clad ass. Fret Boy was also in attendance and almost got into as much trouble as I. He did whip out his big, beautiful guitar and rock the house into a frenzy, then, somehow he slid into a heated debate with the biggest guy at the shindig, covering one of those topics that one should never discuss at a gathering of keg killers. Fret Boy at least got a blowjob and a phone number out of the night whereas I just got a frozen face and a well-deserved paddling from the Yum Yum Boy. Granted, my buns always welcome a good wallop, but not with a hangover, a queasy stomach, and shin splints! Ah, a brand new year awaits, lessons learned and oh so many to come, literally!

Dear Mz. Conduct,

So what advice would you give to a man who loves his significant other but isn't really attracted to her any more? Don't get me wrong she's beautiful, but she's boring and I can't get her to try anything new and exciting. I'm only 41 and don't want to hurt her but I need more!

Frustrated and Frisky

> **Dear FF,**
>
> It sounds like you've tried to let her know that you need more, but apparently not seriously enough. If she's really committed to you then she will find something she can do that will please you both. Sad but true, some people are just sexually conservative and need gentle prodding to open their views. I don't know what 'new and exciting' means to you, but if you're gettin' all uppity because she won't strap on a dildo and perform a strip show for your office buddies, or include her best girlfriend in your sexual escapades, then you might as well hang it up now. Subtleness is the key here. I would suggest watching some videos together. Annie Sprinkle (www.anniesprinkle.com) has some fabulous ones that may make your girl feel more confident, more adventurous. I say, take her to a strip club and treat her like a queen and/or watch some soft porn together and then role-play yourselves into a pretend one of your own. You may be sexually frustrated for wild adventures, but if you're not willing to keep working at it—this goes for her too—then quit your whimpering and confront the obvious…have an open relationship.

Dear Mz. Conduct,

I'm a sixteen-year-old girl and have been having an affair with a much older, married woman for a few months now. She now wants me to join her husband and her in a threesome and I don't know if I should do this. My lover hasn't even told her husband about me yet because she's afraid he will be very upset. What should I do?

Girl in a Mist

> **Dear GiaM,**
>
> Well, little Miss Jailbait, for one thing, I think it's irresponsible of this woman to be having an affair with a minor in the first place. I also think you're way too young to even be asked to join a married couple in a threesome (pssst! it's illegal!) This woman, your lover, has been cheating on her partner as well as committing illegal acts with a minor, gee she must be a real peach. Enjoy your youth while you have it and steer clear of this whole shady deal. Always remember lil' tootsie, never do anything with anyone that you don't feel entirely comfortable with. Now go yak on the phone with girls your age.

Mz. Conduct's House of Sin

"Life is clay, honey, and I have a Deluxe Play-Doh set!"
–Mz. Conduct

Wet me down and call me slick chick, it's a hot, hot summer here in the Northwest, and I've been up to a heap o' trouble. But what's a girl with pigtails and too much body jewelry to do? The other day, the Georgia Peaches and I had a tad too many cocktails—oh that strawberry lemonade and vodka makes for a mean summertime memory—and what started innocently enough in a booth, early afternoon at the Labia Lounge, crossed into an evening of debauchery at the Sinferno Bar and Grill. We headed out to the Labia with a hankering for a cool drinkipoo, and after several games of pool and a very happy hour, we made our way across town in a cab, paid for by a fan of mine. At Sinferno, we had oodles of beverages sent over to us by a distinguished, dark skinned stranger in a pale gold suit. He promised me the moon and stars and everything in between, but I opted for girl lips instead. The Georgia Peaches and I smooched up a storm, which seemed to gather even more attention from all the boys. We soaked up the attention, and all the booze we could muster—while still maintaining our ladylike dignity—and ended up in a girl-pile at home on the sofa!

The Yum Yum Boy and I have been romping at the river every week. We found a secluded spot nestled between the trees, right on the sandy riverbank and declared it ours from now on. The last time, we were partaking in our usual water wrestling and got ourselves all worked up and romped in the water until we laughed so hard we almost peed our pants. Oh, wait a minute, we did pee our pants...in the river! After swimming out to the middle of the river, we found a giant rock in the exact shape of a big chair, where we sat for a good portion of the afternoon, browning our bulges. No sooner than I had started to relax, listening to the squawk of bald eagles in the sky, than the YYB grabbed me and dunked me in the clear, cold water. I was still laughing when he flipped me over, tossed me across one of the huge rocks, and sunk his submarine deep into my tunnel o' love. My screams echoed all the way down the river, around the curves, and got buried somewhere amongst the pines. After swimming back to the shore and smoking ourselves into oblivion, I decided I hadn't had enough of that meat whistle yet. After swallowing every bit of yum yum substance, the YYB tells me in a whisper, "Don't move, just look really slowly to my left." I did just that, and to my delight, saw a picturesque fawn and doe standing only ten feet away. They had watched our whole show! The animals had such a beautiful curiosity on their faces! They looked as if they were going to come nudge us, but decided instead to graze in the blackberry bushes that surrounded us. The YYB lay there nibbling my nipple berries in the setting sun as the deer nibbled their berries. We felt like stray stoners on National Geographic. Amazing!

A week earlier, I attended one lame-ass party that consisted of a bag of chips and a keg of Coors. Most people at the shindig displayed the intelligence of a Lincoln log, which made conversation a true challenge. One pretty, bucolic boy told the same story of washing his car with his nephew, and repeated it consistently throughout the evening. I would ask him to go fetch me another cocktail, just to hear him shut his trap…and look good walking away. I did meet a spanking-cute boy with a blue Mohawk who almost proposed to me right there alongside the bonfire. Was it my charm or was it the Coors, one may never know. Fret Boy was there and whipped out that big guitar of his and played us all into the sunset…and that was the highlight of that night.

Another weekend, another party, but this was fantastically fun. It was a camping party on top of a mountain, overlooking a vineyard. As far as the eye could see were grapevines and forest and the most beautiful sunset ever. Homer K. Simpson's reggae band played until the wee hours, and the piggy on a spit seemed to rotate to the beat of the Congas. The Yum Yum Boy and I danced and smooched under a zillion stars that lit up the night sky. There was a limbo bar, which forced us to bend in ways we hadn't done since, well, the night before. It was big fun. Shrek, our large and lovable friend, miscalculated the distance of the pole and ended up hilariously crawling on all fours right under the bamboo bar. We pitched our tent near the grapevines and by the time most folks had passed out, shirtless and inebriated, halfway inside their tents, the

Mz. Conduct's House of Sin

YYB and I were snuggly zipped into our own tent and tearing it up, as only we can do, honey! The next morning, to explain the unidentified howls coming from our tent, I told stories of mating coyotes. No one bought it. We did all agree that the hair of the dog was much needed and immediately polished off the beer that was left in one of the kegs. Sunrise on a mountain vineyard, birds singing like mad, and a tummy full of carbonated cheer...what a beautiful morning.

Sordid sex in a hair salon waxing room? You betcha! All those mirrors and massage tables, the naughtiness of getting caught, how could I resist? Well, when the YYB plied, I didn't resist (but I never do), we never got caught, and let's just say that now the waxing room takes on a whole new meaning of strippin'!

> Dear Mz. Conduct,
> I want you, yet I hate you. What is my problem and what the hell is yours? You think you're hot shit, but then again, you probably are. I know for a fact that we would absolutely tear each other up sexually, but then again, when the smoke from the bed sheets start to clear, would 911 get there before we strangle each other? Or, if I'm still in a loving sort of mood, would I be able to escape the black widow's trap?
> The Fly
>> **Dear F,**
>> **Of course you want me and it's no real surprise that you find me unnervingly seductive. In your feeble little fantasies, you explore the fact that we would tear up the sheets. Most likely it would never reach that point in person. If you are young and hairless and like to be bitch slapped and butt-fucked (and I doubt if you own all of those prerequisites), then perhaps there's hope for you yet. In the meantime, keep flying close to the web, sugar!**
>
> Dear Mz. Conduct,
> I met a wonderful guy via the Internet. We met the other night and it was really great, although we were both very nervous. That same night we had sex and I noticed that his penis wasn't totally hard. So, of course I assumed it was because he wasn't into me, now that he met me in person. I figured maybe his interest was gone and that I wouldn't hear from him again, but he still emails me just as much as before and he says he is looking forward to seeing me again. So, my question is; what's up with the lack of hardness of the man? I have never experienced this before.
> Oh, and by the way, you are very sexy!
> Pajama Girl
>> **Dear PG,**

Good Advice from a Very Bad Girl

Yes, I know I'm sexy, and thank you. Remember that true sexiness comes from within: attitude, confidence, experience, and humor. You could use some of this now.

There isn't anything to worry about at this time, as men have lots of reasons for not being completely hard when approaching intercourse, i.e., If you guys had been drinking, if he was on medication, if his grandma just died, if the Giants just lost, if his buddy is waiting to hear about your date, and the list is endless. Don't fret, baby doll, he's wanting to get together again and obviously still interested. If you like the poor guy, give him a break and be patient. Maybe you weren't wet to your knees as you should be either, eh? Seriously, it's nothing to worry about this time. Get to know the man behind the limp weenie and you'll both feel more comfortable. Then and only then, you can make a decision as to remain with him or not.

Mz. Conduct's House of Sin

"Okay, I gotta be honest with you. I only listen to you about half of the time and the other half I just nod and smile and wait for your pants to come off."
–from King of the Hill

It amazes me, the amount of men that continuously feel the need to send me pictures of their hairy schlongs. Do they actually think I'll say to myself, "Wow, that's the man for me!" Instead, I just tell them to find a razor and send themselves their own pictures. After all, they seem to be quite pleased with themselves, and what better way to boost their egos, by gazing at their appendages like it's a pot of freakin' gold. I am not the one to send them to, believe me!

I got stuck for jury duty and I was not so happy. I tried to get out of it, but to no avail. For two solid days, there I was, in a huge sealed room with two-hundred people, on a hot summer day. "Kill me now" I thought to myself. The round, old woman who narrated our 'day in hell' explained that we were free to use our cell phones and laptop computers and when we break for lunch, in five hours, the snack bar is in the lobby of the courthouse. Well, being that I own no cell phone, laptop, or money for lunch (let alone the parking meter in which I was sure I had a ticket by this point), and didn't even bring my reading glasses, yeah, I was livid. People seemed content to knit, yak away on their cell phones and after pacing around for what seemed eternity, I finally decided to plant my svelte buns and settle in with the television watchers. I stomached my way through a gossip show and then onto Oprah.

The best part of each day was when we got to go outside and smoke. Fresh air and nicotine, what a great combination! On one of these breaks, I was bitching and smoking with some of the other unhappy folks when I heard my name called from behind. I turned around and there was an ex-boyfriend from twenty years ago, no bull! Wow, how crazy to recognize me after so long and I asked him how he did just that. He exclaimed that I looked even better than ever, and of course I knew that, but it was nice to hear. He looked as handsome as ever and I was glad to see he still had a head full of blonde, curly locks. He's called and admitted to me that he has fantasized about me over the years. Of course he has, and even though he's soon to be married, he is after all just a red-blooded man. Who knows, I may have to refresh his memory before the big day of rice and doves and marital bliss, just because I can. I think it might be an immoral imperative.

My cerebral boytoy, PolyCarp, is pushing his book, and I promised to plug it... and him as well. As he reminds me, he's clever, witty and not completely against drinking human blood in social situations. His book is called *The Treasure in El Alameda's Belly*. He says it's much like a comic book for perverts. I know some of you fit that bill, so check it out!

The Yum Yum Boy and I had an evening under the summer stars when we saw the über fab Ben Harper perform his multi-tasking arrangements. What a talented man he is, especially when he crooned Marvin Gaye's "Sexual Healing." The YYB and I held each other tight and smooched up a storm under the sparkling night sky. And as Ben Harper sang another Marvin Gaye tune, "Let's Get it On", the YYB hiked up my skirt behind a closed down snack bar, and we got it on...and on...and on!

The YYB is waiting to paint my nails and I mustn't keep him.

> Mz. Conduct,
> How do I let my boyfriend know that I want to have a threesome? I also need to know how to tell him what he can and can't do. And how would we go about picking the right girl?
> Please help me,
> Girl in Need
>> **Dear GiN,**
>> Love your acronym, ahhh, you need gin and lots of gin...Sapphire at that! Seriously, communication is the first aphrodisiac that comes to my mind. When you're lying in bed, try sharing some fantasies and then telling him yours. Believe me, unless he's a mutant mundane sexual midget, he will be yahooing under his breath when you reveal your desires. Then, you discuss what the rules would be...even in theory, discuss them and cement them and if and when you decide to proceed, be sure to abide by the rules you've set. You can place an add in the personals or go to a swinger's party or club (and there are

oodles, honey!) and see what works out. You can't be impatient, as you want this first experience to be a good one together.

Good luck to you and your future ménage a twat!

Dear Mz. Conduct,

I have read your articles with amusement and wonder. In many ways, the freedom and innocence of your sexual explorations is refreshing, and mind-expanding. Thank you for sharing them. I admire your cheery abandon, and cheeky wickedness. Like you, I am an animal lover. I appreciate the gift you have for noticing and celebrating the fact that we humans are animals, too, with all of the predicaments and joys that flesh and hormones bring.

I've been celibate for most of my life and have just recently begun to explore my sexuality with other people. I feel like a baby navigating through adult waters. I didn't join a convent. I'm not a prude. I don't have hang-ups about sexual pleasure or positions. I'm in my early thirties, entering my sexual adolescence a few decades late with a more developed sense of self, a wiser skin, and a fragile, curious heart. And, Goddess of Guttersluts, I am clueless! Sometimes, it is hard to not feel like a circus freak.

I read articles like yours and feel like an unskilled laborer in a highly, sophisticated marketplace. I want to explore with other people, but I'm not sure I know exactly what kinds of relationships/encounters I want to have. I have been independent for so long, I'm not sure I want a conventional, one-to-one relationship.

I'm intrigued with the open way in which you are sexual, but am afraid of the pitfalls (STD's, emotional fallout) of not having a committed partner. I have already had a few mishap blunders and one burning question I have is whether or not it is a good idea to share with potential partners my lack of experience with sex and relationships. I'm afraid of judgment, and outright rejection. But, I wonder if withholding the information creates misconceptions.

Another difficulty is that while I can be flirtatious, I have a hard time initiating sensual encounters, and sometimes I am afraid to engage with others when they do, even if I want to. It's easy for me to keep things in the platonic realm because it is familiar, but I want to learn how to move beyond it. You are obviously a passionate trailblazer of your own desire. Do you have any tips, advice or words of sexual wisdom for someone who is just coming out of her closet and wants to explore in a fun, light-hearted way?

Signed,

A Long-Winded Late Bloomer

Dear LWLB,

Thank you for all the support, first of all, and secondly, for seeing into what I try to portray to people. Suzie Bright (susiebright.com) said, "Sexual self expression and sexual honesty may be rare, and they may often be repressed, but there's no real health, real ethics, or real pleasure in life without it." I believe that to every inch of it's core!

I think you should gradually open yourself up, literally, to people. When you do meet someone you choose to be with sexually, even an exploration venture, I wouldn't mention anything about your lack of sexual history. Wait a bit and be sure this is someone you can trust. Most men, initially hearing about your virgin-esque self will be all worked up over that alone. It seems to be in a male's genetic make-up to find a challenge in just about everything, especially sexually.

Personally, I have a list that I carry with me at all times. I have ten things that I want in a person and ten things I absolutely don't want. Sometimes we get caught up in a lusty love thang and forget or dismiss these things. The 'list' is a good reminder. Needless to say, we may not find all the things we want in a person, but we can strive for as many as possible.

Bottom line, keep hold of your standards and the search for a trusting and committed partner. When you get to know someone of this caliber, only then can you let him know about your past. Hopefully you'll feel secure enough to truly just be who you are. It's all a risk, but if we don't venture out there in those rough waters, full of sharks and blowfish, we may never know what pleasures await.

We all have different points in our lives when we hit a sexual peak, just because it's not average doesn't mean it's wrong. I am an exception, as I have been sexually charged since kindergarten. You seem to be an intelligent and vibrant woman, and whomever you capture will most likely be a lucky individual. Don't fret so much, just have fun, explore your desires and the rest will come.

Mz. Conduct's House of Sin

"It was so cold I almost got married."
–Shelley Winters

To start the New Year, the Yum Yum Boy and I have moved in to a cozy little bungalow all our own. It was my greatest challenge yet at cramming a house full of eclecticism and erotica inside this cracker box of a love nest. We were exhausted the day of the move, even with all the help that we had. By the evening, we decided to take a break and check out the neighborhood. Lo and behold, there were two of the seediest strip clubs in town right across the street. Well, it was perhaps an immoral imperative to give them a visit. The Swingin' Sassycat was a dive and a half, but held a certain charm that only some of us could understand. The bouncer, a huge round-faced man with a shaved head, knew who I was and came over and introduced himself. I explained that we were now his new neighbors and he bought the boy and I a pitcher of something supposedly alcoholic and carbonated (PBR I presume). We watched the miniscule stage area as a flat-chested crack whore swiveled her non-existent hips to and fro to the beat of a Bob Seeger tune. The next dancer was just as mundane, with her stringy hair and cellulite thighs, so we downed our pitcher of suds and moved on to the next club.

The Frolicking Fanny was a tad better, more spacious, with a pool table and a couple of fun pinball machines. The dancers had slightly more stage, this time, to display their tried talents, and soon, an obese black girl with pink, light-up heels got up to jiggle her jelly rolls. Okay, we agreed, time for a game of pool. As the YYB was slamming balls in the pockets, a cute and curvy little dancer came sashaying my way. The charm wore off however; as I noticed she was a pants-less inebriate in pigtails. Drunk as six pigs and lipstick smeared from here to the moon and back. However, she recognized me and told me how adorable I was (not flattering, as she could barely see three inches in front of her), and insisted I write about her in my next column. Well, here you go sugar buns! Drunken dancers are just not attractive...unless they're in your bedroom. After that conclusion, the YYB and I headed home. Home again, home again, jiggity jig, where we proceeded to christen every room of our new abode. We started, soaped to the gills, in the shower and ended up with me arched and spread across the kitchen table. My face smashed on the table, staring into the avocado plant, I thought what a joy it is not to have roommates for once! Intimacy can be a true jewel!

A few weeks back, it was a full moon and a lunar eclipse, just like the one that occurred on the Yum Yum Boy's and my first date, a year and a half ago. Without realizing the irony, the YYB noticed that the tenth anniversary of Quentin Tarantino's first screenplay, *True Romance*, was playing at a funky little local theatre. This meant we absolutely had to go, as it's always been 'our' movie. There are so many parallels it's almost creepy! So, off we went, I in my leopard jacket and handbag and the YYB in his Elvis shades and cowboy hat. This attire wasn't only 'us', but outfits befitting of the movie itself. We had an awesome time and later found out the lunar convergence happened while we were whooping it up inside the theatre. True magic, true romance!

One recent afternoon, at the Yum Yum Boy's mother's hair salon, proved as uncomfortable for us as a squeamish person at a suspension piercing show. YYB, his dad, and I were all at the salon cleaning up a storm, as we do each week, when his dad decided to go to a store across town for light bulbs. He had to replace the old bulbs—a specialized sort—and only available in a few select places. Thus, across town he drove. Figuring he'd be awhile and bored with sweeping, the Yum Yum Boy and I got tangled in a smooching session right after ol' dad left. It wasn't long until I had the YYB sitting at a hair dryer chair, my pants around my ankles, and the reverse cowgirl was riding the range. Yee-haw! All of a sudden I heard a grumbling sound, only to look up and see the YYB's dad watching the whole show! He sort of hollered, I sort of screamed and twirled around to accidentally give him a panoramic view of my bald-below self. Panicking, I quickly yanked up my pants as he jogged away, red-faced, to the other end of the salon. Well, the YYB just sat there with his beautiful boner and broke into hysterical laughter. I've never been caught shagging

Mz. Conduct's House of Sin

by someone's parent before, so this is a first for moi! Oh, I live for those little surprises life can toss you!

So, my new neighbor boy across the way, casually informed me that the woman who lived in this dwelling before me was an insane prostitute (our conversation had begun by him asking me if anyone had been knocking on my door late at night). Bianca the Bilingual Bisexual apparently entertained men and women throughout the night. Sometimes she would string the hose out across the road and wash various neighbors' cars at three in the morning, and occasionally throw a little sugar in a gas tank or two. Wow, so I have to revamp the energy of this place and fast! In a more positive mode than Bianca, I'm going to bless and plant our living Christmas tree outside the front door and keep the YYB's hose and my sugar inside the house! But, Goddess of Guttersluts, bless all us bad girls!

Dear Mz. Conduct,
I am a 23 year-old woman who is extremely submissive sexually and wonder if it's normal to be that way. I don't seem to ever get enough degradation, and worry is there something wrong with me?
Sad Sandy

> **Dear SS,**
> As long as you are aware of your submissiveness, I think you're okay. Some folks are just basic subs and must have a dominant person to be involved with. I am a switch myself, but understand the desperation of your need, as it is a definitive need. There are communities that may benefit you though. Check out this site for more information that may help you understand/find your way /answer your questions http://www.dungeonnet.com/weblinks/SupportGroups/, and now go make me a bone-dry martini and paint my nails, you subhuman wench.

Dear Mz. Conduct,
I've gone out with a guy, twice now, that I really like. He is handsome, seemingly honest, intelligent and funny. Toward the end of our last evening together, we started discussing some serious issues that each of us thought we have. I guess we've decided that we're interested enough to share some things and I like that. I have some issues with rape in my past and we talked about that for a while and then he told me he has Priapism. I have to admit that I don't exactly know what that is and maybe made him feel uncomfortable with my non-reaction. I guess I thought he'd explain and he must've thought I was okay with whatever Priapism is, and we skipped on to another topic. He hasn't called me and I feel like I should have another chance, but I desperately want to know if Priapism is a contagious disease or if it's a hair loss product. Can you help?
Girl in a Fix

Good Advice from a Very Bad Girl

Dear GiaF,

I had never heard of this ailment before either, but I found a few things out for you that may help.

"Priapism is a condition in which a male develops a permanent erection. If the erection lasts for an unusual period of time and is unrelated to sexual contact, one should go directly to the emergency department of the nearest hospital.

Although this can be a potentially embarrassing situation, waiting to correct Priapism may result in permanent damage. There is penile injection therapy for impotence, physical trauma to the penis or surrounding region diseases, which thicken the blood like leukemia or sickle-cell anemia, a cancerous growth around the penis preventing outflow of blood. In some cases there is no known cause

The physician may choose a different treatment depending on the severity of the Priapism. Medication, or minor surgery to remove the old blood from the penis, are the most common treatment options."

Yikes, a constant hard-on sounds oh so lovely, except it's not in this case. This looks serious. Perhaps you should wait until he gets a handle on his malady before you secure another date. Unless you simply want to be supportive and enjoy his non-sexual company, then that's my suggestion.

Mz. Conduct's House of Sin

"Good judgment comes from experience, and often experience comes from bad judgment."
–Rita Mae Brown

The months go by so quickly, and straddling that bench at the dental school has seemed to take up a huge chunk of my time lately. My assigned dental student, Master B, a sweet-faced thing with an ass just begging to be bitten, likes to exchange naughty flirtations with me during each visit. He'll whisper to me to open up wide so he can get in and drill me, or when he lifts the suction tube to my mouth, insists I 'wrap my lips around it', it's adorably hot. In one instance, where I had just climbed into the dental chair, Master B grabbed for the water hose and accidentally squirted it all over my chest. I teased him about premature squirting and that perhaps that was a window into his performance technique, or lack thereof. And I can't count the number of times I needed to remind him that I should have the goggles on so that he won't get into trouble. He shouldn't be looking at my blue eyelashes...focus on the open mouth, boy! Honestly, it sure took my mind of the discomfort of it all, but since I'd never even had a cavity in my life (now suddenly I had four), I need all the distraction I can handle.

Being that it is a dental school, even the smallest of procedures takes nine times as long as at a regular dentist office. After each procedure the student leaves you helpless while they go try and find some misplaced tool or a supervisor to moderate their work so far. Once under the hideous fluorescent lighting, and three feet away from the next poor sap choking on a new pair of false teeth, I admittedly freaked out. I didn't just have metal gadgets crammed into several of my upper back teeth, but tubes, cloths and dental dams filled my breathing space. Holy nuns on Novocain, I quickly learned that I do have a gag reflex after all! After a half hour of tedious preparation, with the unpleasant taste of manufactured coconut numbing my gums and sharp metal pushing against the roof of my mouth, Master B, once again, left me to go hunt down a drill bit. I waited, chanting the mantra "mind over matter". When he finally came back to me, the tears started streaming down my face. I knew I couldn't deal with this. Not being able to talk, I motioned to him that something was wrong. He asked if I was going to hurl and I nodded yes. He whisked me right away down a corridor, a hall and around to a stairway, and into a men's bathroom which he quickly cleared for me. Master B pulled back the dental dam enough to allow me to vomit, which I did. That was lovely...but everything was still wedged in my mouth, so I frantically motioned and moaned to remove it all, and now! We scurried back up to the next floor and into my little exam chair where he took everything out and comforted me sweetly.

I had a half dozen or so visits after that, and although none were quite so freaky, Master B did his best to make things better. Several fillings and one root canal later, I banked on having ended my visits to the dental school for some time, or so I thought. Master B called me the next night to tell I needed to come back again, apparently there was some form I had neglected to fill out. What he failed to mention on the phone was that it was his form I would be filling out.

Two days later when I arrived, still hopped up on Vicodin, Master B was waiting for me in the parking garage. As I got out of my car, he grinned mischievously, and walked over to me. Just as I smiled and turned around to lock my car door, I felt him press himself up against me and whisper in my ear, "This is the way I want you, baby." I instantly felt his ample bulge prompting my cheeks apart, his hands on my wrists, and my juices flowing down the inside of my thighs. He turned me around and took my hand, leading me inside the large brick building, filled with students in purple scrubs and oral fixations.

Master B had me flustered with anticipation, and since it was late in the day, things were winding down and closing up...except for the two of us that is. We walked down a dark hallway, apparently emptied for the day, and into a private exam room that by the sign on the door was reserved for oral surgery. The only light in the room was from a dim overhead hall light somewhere faraway. Master B steered me to a large exam chair where he sat down, pulling me towards him for a deep, and long awaited kiss. I straddled his scrubs and lifted my black

Mz. Conduct's House of Sin

lace skirt to my waist, showing him my metal and smooth flesh. He told me it was the prettiest cavity he'd ever fill, and we made use of that chair in every way possible.

An hour and ten minutes later, we slinked out and down the hall, back to the vacant school lobby. He walked me back to my car and plastered me against it once again for one more tooth polishing. My drive home was oblivious to say the least. That night I slept like a coma patient instead of a dental school patient, yes I did! I have another appointment next Wednesday…also known as hump day.

> Dear Mz. Conduct,
> I've been seeing a guy casually for a couple of weeks. We both just want sex and friendship and we both see other people as well, that's been clear. We have fun and the sex is okay too. I like this guy, he's smart, cute, funny and sweet, but one thing he did just made me feel disrespected. After a night of partying, we came back to my house ready to jump each other's bones. He started licking me and that was really great, but when he put his penis to my lips I tasted something nasty. I asked if he had bathed since his date the night before and he said nonchalantly, no, he hadn't! I made a big deal out of it and he got upset and walked home seventy blocks in the rain. The next day he emailed me with a vague apology and then blamed me for wanting more out of the friendship and said it wasn't working out. Was it wrong of me to make a big deal about him not washing and loose his friendship?
> Bitchy Bubbles
>
>> **Dear BB,**
>>
>> **Christ on a crusty one, you have no reason to think you did anything wrong! It's a matter of respect, and obviously he didn't have enough respect for himself let alone you. It sounds to me like that was a bit of drastic behavior, walking home miles in a monsoon. With any luck, all that rain washed his dirty dick off, but in any case, if he would have handled the uncomfortable situation differently, I'll bet my candy apple wrist restraints that things would have turned out better. Perhaps if he would have intensely felt the downright shame, maybe asked you to shower with him, scrub him and make him worthy, you would have gotten over his double-dippin' ass and moved past it. However not taking five minutes to shower the last girl off before going out with another is absolutely disgusting. And if you tasted her pungent pooty, it means he certainly isn't using condoms either! Good riddance, I say.**
>>
>> **It sounds to me as if he was embarrassed, and knew the extent of his unworthiness, so he ended it to save face. This, girlfriend would be a deal breaker for me as well, so you just keep your self respect and bitch about anything that tries it's best to soil your soul…or your mouth.**
>
> Dear Mz Conduct,
> I want to know if you think that's it terrible to have fantasies about family members?
> Pervert in Providence

Good Advice from a Very Bad Girl

Dear PP,

As I always say, fantasies and reality are two very different things. Keep them that way and to yourself and no one will care. I sure don't.

Mz. Conduct's House of Sin

"Everything has cracks, that's how the light comes in."
–Leonard Cohen

New Year's resolutions, not for me! Valentine's Day, bah humbug! Why is it that we pick just one commercial day a year to promise ourselves we'll change bad habits, profess our love, make our lives better, or wipe the slate clean? The slates are not clean, honey, they are full of messes and junk from the past that we should be working each and every day on, learning and listening to the inner voice. Without all the crap we've waded through in the past we wouldn't know what we want or where we want to be in the future. Even if we don't know exactly what or where that is, by reviewing our past we can at least rule out what we don't want or where we don't want to be...that's what we can control, and that's something, damnit!

I woke up this morning after a convoluted night sleep, tossing and turning with freakin' hot flashes and memories of female ejaculations the night before (one out of two ain't bad.) I had a dream that I was on some sort of expedition in Moscow. Everything was stark white, covered in ice, and snowflake crystals the size of dinner plates were falling all around. There were about six of us, a mix of women and men, all comfortable in a huge snow cave complete with several big round beds with crimson blankets and a million pillows tossed on top of them. (Interpretation: even when things aren't warm and fuzzy, one can still find comfort) The premise to that dream was something about getting to an ice cave and researching crystals in exact shapes of penises. Hot verses cold, interesting. I woke before we found the cave or the crystals, which I suppose can mean I was still on the search, yet comfortable and open to whatever my heart allowed.

Then, with the divine, universal energy, and the order I put into it, I met my Romeo in Black Jeans and have discovered after all these years just what real friendship and connection is. I won't be writing about this private part of my life, as it remains the most sacred element I've ever encountered, and deserves to be held in that light.

So, meanwhile back at the ranch of raunch, the girls came over for cocktails the other evening and, as some of us enjoy, we watched gay porn and painted each other's toenails. I demonstrated the best oil and way to shave one's pubic hair completely off and when the girls felt how smooth a cooter can actually be, the girlie painted mouths got involved. We ended up in a pile of moist girl flesh on my big, leopard bed sheets. It was sensual warmth that curled our toes and touched things deeper than flesh. Heaving breasts upon pierced nipples, teeth on necks, mounds pressing against mounds, round asses in the air, double headed dildos pleasuring simultaneously, and lip locking labias. We took turns demonstrating different boys that we knew, their kisses and cunnilingus performances, and we laughed, screamed, orgasmed like chainsaws...then made more cocktails. Now, that's a cum-passionate girl day!

A few nights later, on a warm, rainy spring evening, I attended a friend's birthday bash, held in a giant Victorian house sewn with tiny twinkling red lights throughout. Lighting is everything, baby! The faint crimson glow illuminated everyone's faces just enough to cast a devilish ambience to the night.

After mingling and meeting people (many I didn't know), I decided I was heating up like a Bunsen burner and looked for a room to toss my black velvet coat in. As I wandered through the massive halls, the decadent howl of Diamanda Galas pulsing through the house, I walked into a large darkened bedroom with five huge white candles burning on the fireplace hearth. My nose detected the sultry scent of sandalwood and cedar. The rain beat down against the leaded windows and I suddenly got a shiver down my spine. I slipped off a sleeve of my coat when suddenly two arms held my hands behind my back, and the deep voice of a man I couldn't place, whispered, "Let me show you to the coat closet, beautiful girl." Then he quickly garnished that statement with, "Don't turn around, it'll make this better."

Something sounded remotely familiar in the depth of his voice, but I couldn't quite place it. He took my coat and still bound my hands behind me, standing so close I couldn't turn around to see him. I played along, as the moisture between my thighs started soaking my black lace bloomers. As he held my wrists, he slowly moved them up his flat, bare stomach. I could smell his soap, something clean and comforting. I ran my fingers over his chest, or as much as I could reach, and lingered when I touched the happy trail. Not much hair, but enough to guide me, wanting to grip farther down. The stranger threw my arms in front of me, wrapped his arms around mine, holding me tighter. Then pushing my body, I felt his substantial stiffness as he walked me into a huge closet and began kissing the back of my neck, his lips dragging across the ink on my shoulders until I was shuddering almost uncontrollably. His moans and mine mixed in the motions until I came undone. My knees buckled as he caught me and gently turned me around, his mouth on mine, demanding more. The flicker from the distant candles danced vaguely on a dark haired, handsome face, but I still couldn't recognize the man. He was right, it was better this way.

The stranger lifted my skirt and dropped to his knees, breathing, sucking, and licking in my juices as I cried out in a hedonistic holler. He sprang to standing, his hand shot to my mouth, muffled the sounds of my pleasure. With his hand still over my mouth, he banged me like a cheap screen door...until I took over, grabbing his hips, I pounded myself onto him, over and over, then my hands reached his biceps, held them down, above his head, until we both released, one after another in a mad craze. Zapped of energy, we crumbled, right down in a pile of coats and handbags. Breathing hard for what seemed like hours, we finally gathered ourselves and walked out to the candlelit room where I could see his face. Well, what do you know; it surely was the birthday boy! He told me he had always had a fantasy of doing that to me and what a perfect opportunity. Amazing. After all it was his day, but became mine too.

Speaking of birthdays, I have a big one coming up, which my friends have planned some sort of surprise shin-dig for. I'm excited and will embrace all that I'm given, most likely in more ways than one!

Good Advice from a Very Bad Girl

Dear Mz. Conduct,

I have a very small penis and although my wife has never complained, it still and always has bothered me. Is there anything you could tell me about this subject that would help ease my mind? Are those products really helpful?

Mini Me

> **Dear MM,**
>
> A lot of men are obsessed with their penises, no matter what size—just the biological nature I suppose—but I think you guys are much more worried about that than we women, for the most part anyway.
>
> First off, no, the products don't work. Don't waste your money. When you stroke yourself try using a warming oil and see how big it gets, you may be shocked. I have an organic clove and blood orange oil that makes all the difference in the world. You could try using a cock ring as well, as they can keep the stiff in stiffness and make it appear larger, as well as enhance your orgasm. All that blood is trapped and expands the skin to the fullest. They make all sorts of cock rings, but a leather adjustable ring I found works the best. You can take it off easier if it's uncomfortable and the leather is less pinching.
>
> Keep in mind, I have had fabulous lovers with wee appendages and horrid lovers with huge ones, so it's really all about tantra and what you do with what you have. Your wife doesn't complain, bless her heart, so shut your hole or I'll be compelled to bitch slap you and snip off whatever it is you do have.

Dear Mz. Conduct,

My boyfriend doesn't seem to like fellatio. I like to give it to him, but he always changes it up so that we end up in another position. I wonder if I'm not good enough at it or is it something else. What do you think?

Sucking Sara

> **Dear SS,**
>
> Christ with a crowbar, has it ever occurred to you to ask him about this? People don't communicate enough in this lifetime and that's where trouble begins. Maybe you aren't good enough, maybe he just isn't into it, or maybe the sky will fall on you. My point is that you should ask him about his needs, likes, erogenous zones, and tell him of yours.
>
> Some men don't really like getting head just as some women don't like getting licked. Some men say their penis is too sensitive for fellatio, or some say they'd rather eat pussy, or some love it, it's just a crapshoot. You won't truly know until you ask them, not me! If you care and respect your partner then you talk about these things, and take into consideration what they like or don't like. Either live with it happily or move on, silly girl.

Mz. Conduct's House of Sin

"Art has treated erotic themes at almost all periods, because eroticism lies at the root of all human life."
–Edward Fuchs

Happy birthday to me, happy birthday to me, happy birthday dear me, and tra la la la. My birthday month is here again, and with the catch and release of the Yum Yum Boy behind me, I can now be seen tooling around town with a doctor, a tugboat captain, a television producer, and a financial consultant. Not all at one time, mind you. It's all about the juggle. There's also the various others that slip into the mix, and damnit, if I'm not having fun being treated like the queen that I am! After all, I deserve all the lobster, champagne and outings that I can possibly handle. It does get a bit exhausting, but I figure that this is the beginning of the second half of my life…and I'm going at it with a vengeance.

With that in mind, while at the gym the other day, vigorously sweating all the previous night's vodka out of my skin, I decided to charge up my workout. It proved to be too intense after I almost launched myself right off the cross-trainer machine. I started to laugh at myself, thinking how it would look to actually catapult oneself across the weight room, and land spread eagle, on the back of a macho dead lifter. Something out of the Cirque du Soleil, sans the grace and dignity, of course. When I was finished exercising my thighs and imagination, I showered and hit the steam room. Once in awhile, if no one is in there, I have to turn on the timer and crank the fat, red hose to get it going, full steam ahead. This time it was already churning out the steam, crowding the little room with a blinding fog. I sensed another body in the midst of it all, and heard a woman tell me she would scoot down so I could stretch out. I thanked her, finally catching sight of the voluptuous strawberry blonde. I lay down and stretched out long, covering my face with crossed arms, as the ceiling tends to drip with interspersing plunks of hot water. A couple of drops hit my knee and my head, and then an unsought drop fell, with a hard kerplunk, directly on my clitoris! I sat straight up and exclaimed, "Ooh!" when my strawberry blonde steam mate asked, "What happened?" A little embarrassed, but more stimulated, I told her what had happened, and pointed out that since I shave it was probably inevitable. We laughed and discussed the at-hand shaving topic, body jewelry, and relationships in general. The steam was starting to overwhelm us, so we decided to continue or conversation in the hot tub. I told her, I liked to take a cold shower in between, as the skin adores that. Strawberry agreed she should start doing the same and asked if we could share a shower. Parts of me were throbbing uncontrollably and suddenly the word 'no' was not in my vocabulary.

We slid into the last shower stall, one that the light had burned out over, and turned on the cool water. Strawberry put her hands on my waist and I combed her long wavy hair with my fingernails as she tilted her neck back, begging for my lips on her nape. We had an intensely passionate make-out session, which led to an exploration of each other's every crease. After what only seemed like an hour, we rinsed the slickness of our release from between our legs, and sprinted to the hot tub. Too many people in the tub, but I felt the total relaxation of the tub for maybe the first time ever. Strawberry got out before I did. I gave her a wave and a smile and knew I wouldn't see her again. Never say never though, as this life tends to hold spontaneously combustive surprises all the time…and I do so love this life!

The Transient Trollop, still nesting temporarily (and complaining daily) in the deep South, has been sent a gift of appreciation from a grateful client in Paris. Rosary beads, most likely, wouldn't be the TT's gift of choice, but that's what she got. She tossed them around her neck, cracked open a PBR, and called me to tell me that she had a Parisian Jesus tossing about in her cleavage, and they're both doing well, thank you. Bless her alcohol-drenched heart!

My Brother Juniper, the rock star, and his family have moved back here to the constant rainfall of the Northwest. They've been in sunny California for the last decade and I've missed them! He and his Juniper Queen arranged some music gigs at a club downtown the other night and the gang was all there. Punk Girl, who, still upset (the only one perhaps) over losing her voice due to a recent flu, and her Hungary Man were swinging from the rafters when I arrived.

Mz. Conduct's House of Sin

The Yum Yum Boy was there, professing his undying love for me and showing some major life changes in the works. We shall see. I met oodles of my brother's friends, most of who, thought I was his baby sister. I always enjoy explaining (and watching facial reactions) that I'm actually half a decade older than my brother. Okay, ego sufficiently boosted and ready to rock!

Homer K. Simpson, my ex from eons ago, headed up the first band on stage. Three chefs calling themselves The Cooks, broiled up the stage with remnants of Nirvana and songs about golf carts with bongs built in them. Then, Monkey Fur, Brother Juniper's buddies started grinding notes with gusto. They wear different masks and costumes and have a number of scantily clad chickadees parading about. Big guys with gorilla, pig, psycho kewpie doll and wrestler masks on. Wife beaters and tighty whities, black fishnet body stockings, codpieces and Daisy Dukes. Quite the ensemble and an earful of parody to ingest.

Oh, and word out to the men that continue to send me photographs of their appendages; please stop putting the 'ick' in dick! Cease and desist! What do you think I'm going to say to you? "Oh what a gorgeous penis you have and let's hook it up, baby!" Give me a freakin' break, and go far, far away!

Now, time to shake up a martini, put on some James Brown, and slip into my birthday suit and celebrate the way only I know how!

> Dear Mz. Conduct,
> I did two stupid things and now I'm paying for them. I went to a party without my boyfriend, only because he didn't want to go, and while I was there, I got trashed and made out with a guy I work with. Okay, that was the first dumb thing, but when I got home, I told my boyfriend. He is really pissed off at me and I feel very shameful. Is there anything I can do to make it up to him? He hasn't spoken to me in two days!
> Guilt Without Grace
>
>> **Dear GWG,**
>>
>> **First of all you're about three bus rides away from being stupid, honey. You're just human and you've been honest! Nothing wrong with either, however, after reminding your partner of that, you should allow him to blow off steam, as he does have that right. Is it easier to get forgiveness than permission? Sometimes, but the truth is always the best route and you took it, so yay! Things can**

always be worse, and I'll bet my nipple rings that you'll both move on, as understanding and intelligent people do, in no time.

Dear Mz. Conduct,

I was engaged to the greatest woman ever, when I got cold feet and backed out. I know I broke her heart and I don't know why I chickened out! I'm 44 years old and have no excuse! She has moved on now and has a new boyfriend, but I find myself consumed with her still. I really think, now, that it was meant for us to be together, so what can I do?

Perplexed Without a Plan

Dear PWP,

There was most likely a reason that you didn't have your heart completely into the relationship in the first place, whether you are aware of it or not. Always go with your gut instinct, it is there for a reason, believe me! Your 'plan' should be to move on with your own life and leave it be. If it were in fact truly meant for you two to be together, then you would be, bottom line. If the Goddess of Guttersluts brings you back at some point, then that too, shall be. In the meantime, it's out of your hands; consume yourself with other things, such as listening to The Pixies while rock climbing. That always does it for me, honey!

Mz. Conduct's House of Sin

"I never write in the daytime. It's like running through the shopping mall with your clothes off. Everybody can see you. At night…that's when you pull the tricks…magic."
–Charles Bukowski, Interview *magazine September 1987*

Sitting up at three in the morning, I listen to Coltrane, Monk, Miles. All the great ones. I'm on my second bottle of Spanish red and my ciggie burns a thin line of curly smoke above my pigtails. I've turned on the fan, realizing that it's still warm and very humid. The whistle of a train haunts in the distance and my mind gets onboard. I think of the Bukowski film that I saw last weekend. Ever since the Yum Yum Boy read one of my Bukowski books, the heroic rogue has fascinated him, as many people are on their first read. So, when the film on Charles Bukowski's life came to town (seven years in the making), we rushed right out to see it. I think of his life's agenda: to drink, write and fuck. That's mostly my agenda too. Bukowski was misogynistic, no doubt, but he also had a deeply sentimental and passionate side. I suppose I feel some sort of camaraderie with him, as a great part of his fame grew from writing a column called "Notes of a Dirty Old Man" for an underground newspaper. In another time, I may have been that dirty old woman who would have happily dunked her liver in the same bottle he was after.

Ahh, that glorious scarlet liquid and my imagination take hold, and I realize the sun will be up soon. Different times, different dreams. The Transient Trollop always reminds me that in a past life I was surely the madam of a chi-chi brothel, and 'tis nights like this that I can feel a definite decadence surround me.

It's been an interesting onset of summer, and one evening, hotter than Georgia asphalt, the Lion King took me to the Tiki Lounge. We hadn't seen each other in ages and it was long overdue. It just happened to be happy hour when we arrived, and we made good use of it. The club was loud and hoppin' that night, and one of the best things about the place is that they always have a wide array of unique folks that drop by. Thus, we noticed two BBBW (big, beautiful, black, women), raising eyebrows and other things, three sheets to the wind. We thought them amusing…from afar that is. When several Absoluts took hold of my bladder, I ventured through the crowded room of palm trees and coconut lights, and into the tiny bamboo-lined bathroom; my immediate destination. There were the big girls, sprucing up their lipstick and do's. They were just yakking, not waiting, they told me and waved me towards the hula skirt toilet door. I flew right into the stall and took care of business. Just as I spread my thighs to wipe, I looked up to see one of the BBBW staring through the hula grass at me. Bold as a pro-life cheer at a pro-choice rally, she said loudly, "Oh weee girl, you sure is pretty, are you a dancer?" I told her no, and shaving everything doesn't necessarily mean 'dancer', if that's what gave her the idea. Then I told them, "But I write for a dancer magazine!" When my identity became clear, both of them chimed, "oh girl, we love the shit outta you! You're so funny and naaasty!" Thanking them for reading me, I washed my hands and tried to squeeze by them, when one of the large hands grabbed my arm and did it's best at convincing me to stay. I was in the middle of not so politely declining when the other BBBW grabbed my waist and tried to hold me. I was thinking to myself that being molested by two larger than life, drunken women (with the Ebonic plague) was surely not the way I wanted to spend my evening. Right then I angrily grabbed a wrist and twisted it until it removed itself from me and spouted, " Don't mess with this biotch!" and I escaped out the bathroom door and back to the Lion King.

Luckily the Lion King and I had selected a secluded table that sat behind two oversized oyster shells and a fish tank, and were hidden from view. I later saw the girls get booted out the front door for causing a racket. Something involving a tampon, a poker machine and a skinny, white man with a cane. No telling. The Lion King and I ordered another cocktail and toasted to life or something on that order, and called it a night.

Then came the Fourth of July. The Yum Yum Boy and I were celebrating our two-year anniversary, and after a private gift and bodily fluid exchange, we drove out to our friend's house for a dinner of crab legs and lemon pasta. Our friends are another couple with an age difference you can barely count on your hands and toes. They have a remarkable relationship that's been working for well over a decade, so it was the perfect inspiration for our celebration. They presented us both with congratulations and champagne, and then humorously bestowed on me a medal. It hung on a gold ribbon and was my reward for being, in their words, the only woman on the planet that could ever tame the YYB. Tame? I never thought of it like that, but that reminds me, where's my horsetail whip at anyway?

We all made stiff cocktails and sat on their wrap-around porch, which overlooked the Columbia River, and awaited the fireworks show. It was a fabulous display. In the midst of a gigantic purple and silver splash, the YYB and I smooched up a storm, and he said softly, "I don't know about you, honey, but when we kiss, I still hear fireworks." Ditto. After two years, and a zillion hurdles, we've reached an amazing point. I kick his ass when he needs it, and he writes me poems, and most days we fornicate (ways that are illegal in most states) so much that I'm almost swollen shut! Thank the Goddess of Guttersluts that I finally found a man who has my libido. So, I'll keep those pelvic muscles tuned to the hilt, baby, and welcome whatever the next year will bring.

It's summertime, here's to: laying in the tall grass, listening to the Golden Palominos at midnight, cranberry lemonade (with a splash of vodka, please), picking blueberries (and seeing if they fit up a nostril), wearing skimpy outfits and Brando boots, sneaking in to baseball games, water-gun fights, laughing until your kidneys hurt, and big ol' fireworks...even after July!

Dear Mz. Conduct,
Could you tell me if my girlfriend is a freak? During sex, she likes her hair pulled. Now, I don't mean just yanked a little, she likes me to pull chunks of hair right out of her head! I love her and don't want to hurt her, but she assures me I won't. It makes me pretty uncomfortable, what I should do?
Harvey the Hair Puller

> Dear HtHP,
> Yes, your girlfriend is a freak, so what? Goddess bless the freaks! I like my pigtails pulled during sex too, because it's that thin line between pain and pleas-

ure, honey! Your girlfriend may be a little extreme in my book though, as having bald spots on your head isn't real attractive, but hey, that's her thang. Maybe she has lots of hats, I don't know. In any case, she may have some sort of deep-seated past that she hasn't worked through yet, or she's just into a little S&M. I'd suggest exploring the latter with her, and who knows, you may discover another side to you too! I can suggest a couple of books the two of you might read. One really good book is *S&M 101*, by Jay Wiseman and another outstanding informative read is, The *Ties that Bind*, by Guy Baldwin.

Now when you're through with that assignment, go shake me up a bone-dry martini and don't make me want to pull my own hair out!

Dear Mz. Conduct,

I am a 20 year old man with a secret desire. I'm too shy to discuss this with anyone, so I thought you could help. I work in an office and sometimes the women that work there make me so crazy, but not like you might think. They wear suits and blouses of nice fabric and I find that I can't stop wondering how that would feel to wear. I get fixated on the fabric and how it would feel against my skin. Would it give me that sense of power that the women seem to get? I want to ask the girls I date to let me wear their clothes, especially when they have something shiny or soft looking on, but I haven't done that yet. I'm afraid they'll think I'm gay or some kind of a nutcase. I really want to wear a pair of nylons under my pants to feel the sensation. I don't know how to go about even buying any. Can you please give me any advice on this subject?

Shy in Seattle

Dear SiS,

Gee, I don't know, was this acronym appropriate? Probably not so much. You sound like a sweet, blooming, little crossdresser, and when you say 'please', well I can't resist. One of my best friends is a straight (most men are), manly and wonderful guy. He just sometimes likes to wear women's bathing suits and fishnet stocking under his jeans and tee shirts. While a lot of women aren't actually turned on by this, or even understand the whole concept, this world has someone for everybody, babydoll. Not to worry! Like him, I'll bet my silk-ribbon thigh highs that you can find a woman who respects this need in you.

However, you are a young thang, and I wouldn't suggest telling every girl you go out with. Wait until you find someone with kinks of their own and one whom you trust. That will all evolve over time with the right person, as in any relationship. In the meantime you can order some things online, and just experiment from there. You may just look stunning, daahling, in a pair of silk stockings and red leather pumps!

Mz. Conduct's House of Sin

"Dancing is the perpendicular expression of a horizontal desire."
–A. Nonymous

Aside from sitting in dog crap and accidentally vacuuming up my last tampon, what a wickedly wonderful hurricane this last month has been for this happy hoyden! As promised, my report on the second annual Masturbate-a-Thon is here! With around two hundred and fifty folks in attendance, it was one raging party. Just like the last year's Masturbate-a-Thon, it was hosted by the fabulous Darklady herself (www.darklady.com), but instead of being held at a dungeon, this year an enormous old church provided a home for the festivities. Say your Hail Mary's and get down on your knees, baby!

I attended the shindig in drag, as I wanted to get a different perspective on things. I got rid of my omnipresent eyelashes and lipstick, slicked back my hair, and wore a vintage men's green suit. Big Bald Bouncer went with me, dressed in leather from head to toe, and looking quite dashing. Upon our arrival, we saw lots of naked men sauntering around, some with their appendages just flapping in the breezeless night. Many of these men were gay, but most were heterosexual boys showing off their stuff. It was also a night to celebrate selected people's birthday fantasies, such as kisses by both sexes, spankings by leather-gloved men, drag queens blowing other men, and lots of flogging devices on red-assed girls.

Blue Sky Boy and his Southern Bella Donna were there. She put on a strip show and displayed her unique erotic artwork and he went to peruse and support. They are always fantabulous together, regardless.

There was a Spit-or-Swallow contest where people were blindfolded and fed anchovy paste, hot sauce, and marshmallow crème, and challenged to see if they guessed correctly. A big blue tarp sectioned off the 'anything goes' area where bare butts bounced and slapped, and bodies received more floggings. A tasty little redhead whipped up two men into a foamy frenzy. A very long line of girls formed for the Thrillhammer Orgazmatron trying their best to break porn star, Corina Curves', record of something like fifty-seven minutes. Big Bald Bouncer got blown by a Dominatrix while watching some hot tamale hump the stuffing out of several guys, and he was one elated leather daddy! Pyrex dildos and porn tapes were given as prizes for various games and absinthe was being poured down everyone's gullets.

Dr. Carol Queen (www.carolqueen.com) was the guest of honor. She was constantly surrounded by fans all evening, and I didn't get a chance to talk with her, but I'll not be in drag this weekend when I do get my opportunity at Darklady's Parlor of Passionate Prose night. I kept myself incognito through the rest of the evening and slithered out right after midnight.

The Yum Yum Boy, Homer K. Simpson and I were hanging out at the Boom Boom Club on karaoke night, when to my delight, they got up and sang Tom Jones' "It's Not Unusual" to moi! Bring it on, boys! Needless to say, many cocktails were under their belts by then, and no offense to their voices, but under their belts is where my attention remained.

We have two new roommates that rule the rockin' world. The Georgia Peaches are two sweet and naughty girls (a requirement of course) that have backpacked their way across the states and landed their pretty butts in our house for a spell. We've been tooling them around town in our not-so-new '61 Ford pick 'em up truck. I promised to take them to all the best lesbo clubs in the city and I intend to fulfill all my promises...and soon!

My friends, the UNTYD band, almost won a gig at a huge music festival, opening for Korn, but lost out to some shoddy adolescents that voted more than us, damnit all to hell and back. UNTYD is still numero uno in my book though!

The Yum Yum Boy and I backpacked in the mountains for a few days in search of some rumored hot springs. After miles of uphill climbing and hours of hardcore hiking, we finally discovered the amazing place deep in the woods. We stripped off our gear and our clothes and filled a hollowed out log with

Mz. Conduct's House of Sin

boiling mineral water. While it filled, we hiked down the mountain to a cold-water creek, scooping up buckets of ice water and dumping them in the log-tub to make a comfortable temperature. At last, it was purrfect and we slid our naked bodies into the steamy log. Heaven. A group of Asian Lutherans were in some of the other tubs, grinning from ear to ear, but I couldn't help drooling over the Yum Yum Boy's ample erection. I egged him on until he could stand it no more and he boned me right there under the blue sky and pine trees...and Asian churchgoers! I think I heard them praying as we left. All I know is that it was a religious experience for me! We hiked back up to our campground and cracked open the beverages and made a bonfire next to the river.

Then right after I decided that I felt confined with pants on, two flashlights came into view. It turned out to be a couple of handsome hiker boys that had made their way from the Mexican border and were looking for some company. We welcomed them into our campsite and after indulging in various vices for a while, we all got in the tent. I ended up screaming like a whore on nickel night, through the forest and louder than the ravens, all night long, honey!

The next day, we shoved off, and hiked (or in my case, swollenly hobbled) back to the truck. We drove up the mountain until we happened onto some friends that were at a makeshift shooting range. I got my first chance to shoot a .44 and a 9mm semi-automatic rifle. Let me tell you, after a lifetime of having a fear of guns, it was a very powerful experience and I loved it like crazy. One of the targets was a picture of Osama Bin Laden, taped to a cardboard box, and I shot the left cheek right off of him! Not bad for a skeptical neophyte.

We had a big, sacred celebration on the fourth of July, a big-ass BBQ at my house. Dozens of people toasted the Yum Yum Boy and I, long into the night. He was the barbecue master, and I, of course, was the hostess with the mostess. Everyone fell at least once. Only two chairs were broken. I designed a spread of food that will be talked about for a long, long time. Lights were strung all over the yard, and the Closet Queen played his dulcimer. Oh, I absolutely looove parties!

Good Advice from a Very Bad Girl

Dear Mz. Conduct,

I lost my sexy, gorgeous soul mate to nightlife: martinis and the bright lights. How do I bring a lost lamb back to the fold?

Three years ago this month I meet this wonderful, wild and passionate woman, a princess she is and, well you can guess the challenges. Myself, a know-it-all, demanding but very passionate man is having a difficult time. We have had two years of ups and downs and back and forth about career, lifestyle, goals and objectives. Sex was always great and passionate but I always felt that my gal could be bisexual. Recently this seems to become more real for her but I know that she wants her man (me?) because she is at heart a princess who wants her prince.

How do I convince this princess, whom I adore, to return to the nest for love and babies? How long can she do the nightlife and martini scene without going too far? Do I pretend that I don't care for her and see if she comes back? Well that's not easy because she seems to be living out her 20's again with a different man or woman on her arm every night. I am not going to wait much longer for this girl to wake up and grow up.

Advice please?

Prince Charming

> **Dear PC,**
>
> I think you should get off your high horse and pull your royal head out of the steed's ass. It seems your princess is doing what she wants to do and you want to control her lifestyle. And martinis, nightlife and dating aren't just for twenty year olds, honey, it's for anyone secure enough to know that they want it, and she seems to. She doesn't want babies and she doesn't want you. You cannot 'convince' this princess to be anything she doesn't want to. Perhaps you are just two different souls, and you should leave it alone. If she decides it is indeed you that she wants (and I wouldn't hold my breath), then she'll return on her own. Or maybe she'll figure out that you're really more like a frog than any kind of prince she ever dreamed about.

Dear Mz. Conduct,

I was thumbing my way through an SFX magazine and read your column. It was interesting reading. After a 12 year relationship/marriage that recently ended in divorce and me with the shirt off my back (no children), I find myself, ready and eager to please and explore another relationship(s). The thing is I cannot seem to meet a woman that I really want to have fun with sexually. Also, I haven't yet found a good place to hang out and meet potential "dates". I sometimes find myself just wanting a beautiful woman's company, smell and taste without the baggage, say for an evening or two. Can you help?

Getting Back on Track

> **Dear GboT,**
>
> Christ on a crack whore, cry me a river and then drown yourself in it! Of course you want to bang as many beautiful women as humanly possible, you just plopped out of a very long relationship. You're chomping at the bit and getting all frisky. A real relationship takes time and you'll meet someone compatible when the universe and the Goddess of Guttersluts is good and ready for you to. But I don't think that's what you want right now, so keep thumbing your way through SFX magazine until you find the escort section. Ring up an expensive call girl and be happy with your pitiful self.

Mz. Conduct's House of Sin

"What really makes us is beyond grasping, way beyond knowing. We give in to love because it gives us a sense of what is unknowable. Nothing else matters. Not in the end."
–Josephine Hart from the book/movie Damage

A train trip to Seattle, one hundred proof vodka in my purse, crotchless underwear, the Yum Yum Boy...this could only mean one thing...trouble. After a bit of fancy-assed canoodling in the tiny train bathroom, repressing laughter and kissing in between, we were buzzing heavily by the time we clamored off the choo choo and stumbled in to the big city lights. A quick cab to the hotel, a little spruce-up, and we were off exploring as many clubs as possible. We had a hankering for the Lava Lounge, which is why we ended up there for hours on end, smoking cigars and drinking whiskey. Realizing we needed food in our gullets, we set out blindly on our mission. Our quest was hampered each time, as we seemed to get sidetracked by yet another cocktail. We were bar hoppin' fools well into the night. After all, it was a different city, full of life, lust and libations and we were, after all, on holiday.

Our final stop was a glamorously swanky place, a black and gold draped lounge with Tony Bennett coming through the hidden speakers. This was more like it. I wanted food not set loose from a can and perhaps some lovely, romantic eye gazing with my baby. Well, the Yum Yum Boy was entirely trashed by this time. While I perused the late night menu, he excused himself to go to the restroom. I was sipping a ten-dollar glass of wine when the YYB strolls up, entirely oblivious to the several other men sitting at the bar, puffs out his chest, continues to stand, straightening up his leather coat. With a comically serious expression on his face, he excitedly bellowed, "Hey, I was just looking at myself in the mirror and I was thinking that, wow, I look really damn good!" and if that wasn't enough, he proceeded with, "And I know you were just going to tell me that, baby...but I beat you to it!" Always a riot, that's my sweetie! I then figured that the only romantic eye gazing that would occur that night would be with the YYB and himself. As snickering from the guys behind him broke out, I raised an eyebrow and said, "Actually, I was going to ask if you wanted to order the cheese platter." "Yes" he said simply, and finally sat his inebriated ass down as I ordered a platter of Asian pears, Spanish blue cheese and baguette slices. I ate. He picked and complained that blue cheese was too stinky. Full and satisfied, I carted us back to the hotel. The next morning, the Yum Yum Boy had no recollection of anything that happened (after midnight), and while in the shower, he hollered that his cranium hurt and his dick was sore. Well, I figured I'd put that good lookin' weenie to use, by gawd. Whether or not the Yum Yum Boy could recall any of it, well, that's just his misfortune!

With the holidays upon us, I was thinking of the spirit and our spirits. I thought about materialistic habits, feeling obligated to buy gifts one really can't afford, shopping like maniacs for more useless crap, and forgetting that love is not buying stuff. Lately, it seems I've come across many lonely people. Some whine about not having anyone to love or love them. One man wrote me, asking where all the available women were and why couldn't he ever meet someone special and blah blah blah. Well, I told him that he should remove his fat ass from the computer chair and get out into the world and socialize. I do realize that there are shy and introverted individuals who use the computer to interact with, these days especially. I'm not saying it's necessarily a bad thing, just that we depend on technology for so much these days, maybe we should have more human interaction too.

Then, still on this thought and the season, I was walking my fabulously full-figured dog (in her thrift store pearls), noticing the amazing tutti-frutti sunset, and thinking that these were the things that filled me with love. Dogs in pearls, sunsets, being offered a bunch of crimson dahlias from an old woman gardening in her yard, a hug from my neighbor, a smile from the postman, etc. I believe that we truly have to love ourselves before we can love anybody else completely. It's our responsibility as human beings. With a world full of war, hatred and anger, we need more love, and we need to start with ourselves! I think we forget sometimes that there can be love in everything, and it comes in many different forms. If we own a spirit of unconditional love within then we automatically invite it into our world. It can come back to us in so many ways! Let's

Mz. Conduct's House of Sin

keep that thought and work on loving ourselves a little more this year, because when we do we will never really be lonely. Putting the ho ho ho in holidays, may all yours be happy!

> Dear Mz. Conduct,
> What is the nutritional value of sperm? Is it true it makes a good moisturizer?
> Curious Cookie
>
>> Dear CC,
>>
>> Here is what I know and learned, just for you and any other sperm curious minds out there. First of all, sperm, despite what you may think, is neither loaded with calories nor is it particularly nutritious. The amount of sperm in an average ejaculate is somewhere between 100 and 500 million, but the little swimmers actually account for a very small percentage of the ejaculate. What about the rest of it? Well, that's made up of sugars, proteins, some naturally occurring acids and minerals. Calories figure extremely low. No worries, you won't be going off your diet if you decide to swallow. As far as being a good moisturizer, it's subjective. I love it rubbed into my skin and face, or wherever it lands, but I suppose some people don't. If you remember the movie *Something About Mary* then it could possibly make a good hair gel!
>
> Dear Mz. Conduct,
> I am very verbal when it comes to sex and always have been with my partners. The trouble is that the girl I'm seeing now won't even moan while I'm boning her. I sort of get lost in my own ecstasy and have to admit not paying attention to what she's feeling at all times. It would really make things hotter if she would let me know how she feels. I have asked her, or tried to tease her about it so she wouldn't feel bad. Is there a better way or are some people just quiet and boring?
> Tarzan
>
>> Dear T,
>>
>> Yes, monkey man, some of us are more vocal than others, but if you're really troubled by your mute Jane, talking to her about it can be good. Explain that it'd be hot if she could open her mouth as well as her snatch (and no, not in those words, you dolt! Use your own seductive speech, if you can muster it.) Don't persist though, as this may put too much pressure on the situation. This is something that should be felt and not demanded, or it wouldn't be real.
>>
>> Maybe she has inhibitions and insecurities stemming from some unpleasant past experience; something involving a wolverine, a flyswatter and Uncle Rupert, maybe a finger wetting outburst that left a classroom of adolescents in mad hysteria, or perhaps an intense vocal release on Mount Hood that triggered a fatal avalanche. I don't know, but whatever her reasons, they need to be respected and you should be patient. In time it may get better, the more she trusts you/feels comfortable with you, the more she may want to join you in those jungle cries. Then again, maybe not. Leave it alone. Maybe she's not having a good time at all and you should be paying attention to her needs and desires instead "getting lost in your own ecstasy." Quit beating your chest and focus on hers!

Good Advice from a Very Bad Girl

"Never let a domestic quarrel ruin a day's writing. If you can't start the next day fresh, get rid of your wife."
–Mario Puzo

Virgins on a Vespa, the holidays are over and we can all concentrate on a brand new year! Christmas brought me joy, I must say. The Yum Yum Boy not only gave me a gorgeous garnet ring, but an orgasm marathon day as well. Not often does a girl get a garnet and a pearl necklace all in one snowy afternoon! Ahhh, the boy does know how to turn on his carnal charm. His gift from me was a pair of long-awaited Chinese dragons tattooed on both his forearms—and the fact that I allow him in my bed each night. The fabulously sexy and talented Paul Zenk, at Infinity Tattoo (www.infinitytattoo.com) did the work. He's done several tattoos for both of us and we are continuously loyal and amazed. Bend over Pauly, we love you!

On New Year's Day, not only were my pink flamingos covered in lovely fresh snow, but also a local radio show called to tell me I had won their Sexy Artist contest. I had never entered this contest, but sure wasn't going to open my mouth about such trivia now! I suppose someone else entered me and my website, and for that, whomever you are, I appreciate your faith in me and am grateful. It seems my prize is a much needed massage and a dinner at a swanky joint downtown. Ooh la la and shish boom bah, what a nice little surprise to bring in 2004.

Okay, so as Valentine's Day approaches, I hope all of you are going to proceed accordingly. Some women adore flowers, such as I, but being a florist for eight years, I know that it is the absolute worst day to buy them. Prices are tripled and the quality usually isn't quite up to par. If you're a wealthy sort, then have at it, but for the working class, try for something different. This is, of course if you want to keep the best piece of ass you've ever had!

Mz. Conduct's House of Sin

Here is Mz. Conduct's Top Ten Sexiest Ideas for Valentine's Day (based on my absolute most favorite things the Yum Yum Boy has done for me, which is why he's still around...get it? Good!);

1) $$$ Take the little woman to an art gallery and clandestinely buy the piece of art she likes the best—this should guarantee a damn good meat massage.

2) $ Surprise your sweetie with a new piercing and a six-pack of Guinness—good for a grope and a burp.

3) $ Fill the entire house—and run a bath—with candles and rose petals awaiting her. Champagne helps greatly—prepare for tears of joy and anything you want.

4) $$ Most cities have a horse drawn carriage that you can always finagle into a spur of the moment ride...preferably with the destination of a swanky restaurant in mind—The reverse cowgirl should be more than happy to ride her stud after that.

5) $ Chocolates are nice, but not the discount drugstore drabsters. For the love of labia, invest in a nice box of Godiva or something equivalent. It matters, believe me. If we're going to delve into the week of feeling bloated and beyond, we at least want it to be worth it! – Be content with a hug and maybe a big smooch.

6) $$ A surprise getaway to a favorite beach or mountain cabin with no communication whatsoever. Hot tubs are a plus and the animal in her will more than likely let loose!

7) $$ Tickets to see an upcoming show, i.e. Sandra Bernhard or Elvis Costello, and never you mind if it's not someone you want to see! Attach the tickets to a bottle of wine and lay it on the bed with an always-phallic anthurium (that's a

tropical flower, genius!)—Appreciation, gratitude and a handjob in the parking lot before the show are a shoe-in.

8) $ A favorite CD and a handmade card can go along way, really. It's sweet for the po' and you'll get laid on general principle.

9) $$$ Lobster dinner, a new pair of leopard heels, and one long-stemmed rose...sigh. Her mouth will be searching for that bouncing beautiful boner, baby!

10) $ Last but not at all least, a heartfelt poem, being extra nice to that obnoxious friend of hers, doing the dishes and making her a coffee table with your own manly hands. – A good recipe for everyday and a sure-fire way to always get sex and lots of it!

Granted, variations and different tastes must be taken into account and if you're paying proper attention, you will make it your business to know her interests. Get creative and when you get naughty, do it right, honey! Now, I must go, as the Yum Yum Boy has been leaning over my shoulder rubbing my neck, and in my peripheral vision I see that his pants resemble a pup tent. So, off I go to hone my sword swallowing skills, not that I need it, but a girl must practice practice practice!

> Dear Mz. Conduct,
> I have been trying my best to avoid a woman who is stalking me and it just isn't working. I dated her three times and realized she was very needy and shallow, so I broke it off. I never return her calls (which come weekly by the way), and in no way have I shown any more interest. A neighbor told me he has seen her car outside of my house on numerous occasions and I keep finding (not so) anonymous balloon bouquets and such nonsense on my porch. What is with her and what can I do?
> Freaked-out Fred
>> **Dear FOF,**
>> The skin-crawling subject of stalkers, ugh! I welcome any of my readers to comment or share suggestions on this, as I too, feel the need for input from others who may have shared a similar experience. I had an insane Dominatrix threaten my life a few years back, claiming I stole her husband, and after I called the police, that was a done deal, but now I seem to have an unstable

woman living half way around the world who can't seem to get it through her head that the man she wants, wants me. She is obviously mentally unstable and unable to decipher reality from fantasy and hopefully by bringing this to a public surface, she will retreat. I have only compassion for these people, but contempt brews eventually, doesn't it? Indigence is so unattractive, and ironically in some cases, such as mine, the more the stalker pursues, the closer it brings my lover and I.

I can't even fathom how the mind of a stalker works. When one makes it clear that they don't want anything to do with you, how can one humiliate one's self by making themselves a nuisance to their so-called heart's desire? Why would anyone in his or her right mind do that? Well, that's what we need to remember; these people aren't in their right mind. Here are some descriptions that could be fitting:

Schizophrenia

Schizophrenia is the most severe of the major adult psychiatric disorders and interferes with the ability to think clearly, separate fantasy from reality, manage emotions, make decisions, and relate to others.

Personality Disorder

A personality disorder must fulfill several criteria. A deeply ingrained, inflexible pattern of relating, perceiving, and thinking serious enough to cause distress or impaired functioning is a personality disorder. Personality disorders are usually recognizable by adolescence or earlier, continue throughout adulthood, and become less obvious throughout middle age.

The National Mental Health Association website is http://www.nmha.org/ in case you feel the need to understand your stalker's disorder, as I did. I realize this is not a solution, but it helps sometimes to know just what you're dealing with. In your case, I don't know how long this has been going on, but obviously 'avoiding' her isn't working and confronting her may be what you need to do. You may need to be brutal and direct and if that doesn't work, the police in most states will convey your message to her, acting as your agent. Then if she continues, they can arrest her. Restraining orders are there for a reason, honey!

Dear Mz. Conduct,

First of all, may I say that I met you once at a magazine party, and you are one of the sexiest women I have ever met. The way you carry yourself and your smile were the biggest turn-ons for me. Anyway, back to why I wrote you.

How can I get my wife to masturbate? She thinks it's naughty and dirty, etc. I've told her that I would love to watch and even participate in playing, but she refuses and gets very upset with me. Dirty talk is out too because she gets equally upset. I'm seriously thinking of playing around with someone else. I've been married eight years to my wife whom I love dearly, but I am so frustrated! Do you have any suggestions?

Pent-up in Portland

Dear PuiP,

Thank you for your flattery. It will get you nowhere. Meanwhile, back on the ranch, you are in a frustrated fix now aren't you? This is a frequent subject with men, especially. It seems that when you marry someone, all of your standards, sexual ones as well, must be met, but for some reason some people think their significant other will change or that they can deal with certain inhibitions in time. Not a reasonable state of mind, as it almost always comes to this.

I'll bet my strap-on that she's had some sort of sexual trauma making her feel uncomfortable with her own body. Perhaps she's been raised Catholic and hasn't recovered from that yet, as some of us have. In any case, I suggest that you sweetly sit your wife down and seriously tell her that her sexual inhibitions are ruining your marriage. Maybe some counseling would be in order, if she were willing to try that. There is also a wonderful book called *The Clitoral Truth* by Rebecca Chalker that she may benefit from. Susie Bright has a swell site www.susiebright.com and if that's too much for her, then a tame and informative site can also be found at http://lovingyou.com/.

So, before you tangle with infidelity and canoodle another clam, deal with these issues directly with your wife. If she loves you and wants your marriage to work, she'll get some much needed help, for her sexual health as well as yours.

Mz. Conduct's House of Sin

"If you love something, let it go. If it comes back, great. If not, it's probably having dinner with someone more attractive than you."
–Bill Grieser

Yes, the glorious month of hearts and hard-ons is upon us, and damnit, if that little flying baby isn't hovering around with his archery equipment in hand. He can just point that arrow at someone else's body part, love hurts! If I swatted him like a fly, would that be considered child abuse?

I've been thinking a lot about love lately. The Buddhists explain that there is sex, then love, and above that, compassion. Sometimes that can be a difficult thing to see or even feel especially if some asshole just cut you off in mid traffic and you're not really feeling the Zen thang. But thinking calmly, it makes sense.

Sex, great sex, can blind you. It takes a long time to really get to know someone and have the balance of give and take work out. Communication is always my number one key, but it should continue to be an ongoing work in progress. Each person involved in a relationship usually has individual issues. We all have work to do within ourselves, and the responsibility of working on the relationship as well. Where am I going with all this? I'm not really sure, except that I've been experiencing drama in many couples' lives lately and I think that it's important to keep these thoughts at the forefront for any sort of healthy partnership.

Our past history is important to inspect and hopefully without regrets. Rather, be aware of all we've done makes us the person we are today. Okay, so we got involved with a liar, cheat and/or married person, or someone that takes us on a first date using coupons. Maybe we remained in the same abusive relationship year after year with the excuse that we could at least go shopping at a whim, or we shamelessly stayed in the closet far too long (closets are for gowns, honey), or oops, we married the wrong person partially because our astrology charts suggested it. It's all lessons learned and we'll just be careful these things aren't repeated, right? Well, we try anyway. We can look for those red flags next time and if we're lucky, by the time we reach ninety-seven (which is lucky anyway), we'll have it down pat! It's life and it's love and it's not love and it's enough to make you want to jump on a slow boat to China with a case of vodka, a tube of lipstick and the Oxford dictionary. But it's been an introspective year so far, for so many of us, and I'm just sharing and reminding.

Then there is this morning, when I woke up to an ice storm and my full figured dog unknowingly flailed herself down the ice covered front steps. All four legs went in separate directions. Poor old bitch. The wind was whipping so hard, I imagined wee small bandits rattling my windows—which I couldn't see out of because of the freakin' ICE slathering the outside! My head throbbed and my groggy brain cells screamed, Escape! In a New York minute my reveries sent me straight to a tropical beach. My toes curling in the grit of white sand, the slight rustle of palm trees, sweet nectar of guavas running down my face, and boys (who put the sin in sinewy) wrapped loosely in loin-cloths, painting my toe nails. Oh la de da, back to reality and the realization that ice isn't nice unless it's in my cocktail, honey! So, here's to the month o' love and staying warm, if only in our heads and hearts, and striving for compassion above all! Remember, Shakespeare said, "To thine own self be true." Amen, baby!

Dear Mz. Conduct,

The onset of Valentine's Day makes my girlfriend get all goofy and this drives me nuts! She's normally not materialistic, but she always reminds me that it's on the way. I refuse to acknowledge it. Each year it's the same argument and I don't feel as if she respects my views. I believe it's just another day for consumerism to rear an ugly head. Marketing ploys try their best at making a guy feel as if they need to buy diamonds and roses (that are tripled in price just for that day), and spread all sorts of mush on one single day instead of finding random days all year through. How can I get my girlfriend to shut up about this ridiculous day?

Boycotting Bob

> **Dear BB,**
>
> **You know what? You're name should be Boob. Boob the Boycotting Babe Bonker...that's it! What is your freakin' problem? Okay, so we are all well aware of your opinion on consumerism, holidays, and your girlfriend. You can own whatever view on things you want, it's absolutely your right, yes indeed, but when you choose to be in a relationship, there are rules of respect. I'll bet your girlfriend does respect your views, however, it's in everyone's best interest to put your opinion to the side in order to please your partner. Just the way it**

works. That's respect, honey, and it should be mutual! I didn't read that your girl was pestering you for diamonds, furs or dozens of roses. Cupid on a crackwhore, perhaps she just wants to be acknowledged with a card, a tulip and a pair of crotchless undies. If you were smarter, you'd realize that when you give in just a bit to make your sweetie happy, it comes back to you in buckets…buckets of your favorite un-boycotted liquid at that! Now, I'm boycotting you.

Dear Mz. Conduct,

My husband and I have discussed trying some new sexual positions, but that's as far it's gone. It seems as if we are both too inhibited to initiate any, or maybe it's that we don't know where to start. Can you help, please?

Moot Maria

Dear MM,

Talking about this is the first step, good girl! There are plenty of good books out there that can help make you feel more comfortable. Keep in mind that you should be having fun. You don't want to put too much pressure on each other, get frustrated and have a sudden need to race to the mall or something. Start with sharing a warm bath. Light some candles and/or incense and focus on the other senses. The Kama Sutra Company has made a heavenly clove scented oil for years, but now has a new line called Love Essentials with an amazing honey dust that you can dust on and lick off. I use the random flying goose down feathers that constantly seep out of my comforter, so you can be creative even if you aren't able to get those fancy kits. They are worth it though. The Love Essential line also has sexy, spicy cinnamon oil and when massaged it into the skin—and especially the genitals—it's torrid, baby, and feels wonderfully crazy. They also have a fabulous water based lube that slippery slides nicely through all those curves and crevices, and with a light jasmine scent, really tickles those senses…and yum, they're all lickable! You can find these at most adult shops or online at Toys in Babeland, http://www.babeland.com/.

Speaking of the *Kama Sutra*, I suggest reading Anne Hooper's *Kama Sutra*. She brings the ancient masterpiece up to date and easy to explore. She's also a licensed sex therapist and interprets it all in her own way. You can get her book on Amazon.com if going into an adult store isn't your cup of tea.

Tantric sex has great aspects and my suggestions on where to go after the senses have been stimulated romantically are:

(1) Sex positions, both from the *Kama Sutra* and other ancient writings, help introduce some variety into your romps, and can teach you new ways of bringing consciousness to the experience of it all. The powerful thing about trying new positions is what happens when we break out of those old molds and become enlightened with something new. It can bring us lots of power, not only for our bodies but our psyche as well.

(2) When you do get ready to try some new positions, keep in mind that the essence is more about what's going on emotionally and in your "interior" than about the mechanics of a new position. Make a mental note how each position feels, then you can explore from there. Use different rhythms and pump and squeeze your pelvic muscles with each position. Lift your leg or turn around, whatever, just don't be afraid to let those creative juices flow along with the vaginal juice, honey! It's fun, okay?

(3) In some positions eye contact, breath connection, heart chakra connection, and deepened intimacy are all facilitated through facing your partner. Don't think 'Man, he could sure use a shave' or I never realized how much his nose

resembles his mother's nose,' just focus on the attraction and let yourself feel. Some positions are better for increased G-spot stimulation and female orgasm, others lean towards the man and how he can master his ejaculation and pleasure. Exploring as many different positions as you can in a lifetime is surely rewarding, believe me! You tend to learn a huge amount about yourself and your lover.

As I always say, communication is the best aphrodisiac and the basic rule to everything. Talk with each other about what you liked, thought, felt and what you may not have. Once you get on a roll, honey, the inhibited nature will fade away and I'll bet my double-headed dildo on that!

Mz. Conduct's House of Sin

"The proper behavior all through the holiday season is to be drunk. This drunkenness culminates on New Year's Eve, when you get so drunk you kiss the person you're married to."
–P.J. O'Rourke

Sometimes Santa brings just what you ask for, even if you are a very naughty girl! So, maybe what I asked for wasn't my favorite reoccurring dream of giving Ashton Kutcher some silicone love up the ass, but close enough.

Punk Girl and her Hungary Man met the Yum Yum Boy and I at a downtown holiday function, and what a spectacular shindig it was! It was a rock 'n roll fashion show complete with oodles of hair hoppers, nearly naked models (love the hat, scarf and shoes, daahling), and a definite pinch of serious eye candy. Punk Girl was sporting a teeny tiny leopard skirt and fabulous biker boots. The girl is all boobs and eyes, I swear. It looked as though she were hugging two small bald men in that tank top, lined with rhinestones and silver. I was draped in black velvet and fishnets, and the boys were clad in black jeans and leather. Yumm! Models in the bathroom fussed and mussed over some invisible flaw and refused to go out without a hissy fit first. The shallowness dissipated as I swilled my fourth vodka/rocks, then somewhere towards the end of the show, Santa came strolling through the sea of glamorous bodies, handing out candy canes. When I turned to grab one for myself, Santa pulled out a massive, barber-pole candy cane just for me! I proceeded to wrap my lips around it and suck. This caused a bit of a commotion and before I could get another lick in Santa picked me up and threw me over his manly Santa shoulder. He made his way through the crowd, announcing that this was a very bad girl that he was whisking away. I was giggling all the while, wondering just what Santa had in store.

Santa carted me up a small flight of stairs and we ended up in a back stage semi-private dressing room, full of brightly colored wigs, feather boas and empty bottles of champagne. He promptly bent me over his knee and landed a couple of good, hard swats on my rule breaking round rump. I screeched joyfully and he swung me around and onto his bulging lap. When he pulled off his long, white beard and kissed me, I knew my suspicions were true, it was indeed my imaginative Yum Yum Boy. That night I sat on Santa's lap and got more than I could ever ask for…well, all except for that Ashton Kutcher thang, but I'll get over that in time.

Later that week, I woke to the sound of the garbage truck beep beeping it's big-ass self right past my bedroom window. Infuriating! Realizing that I was now officially awake, I wrapped myself in my new leopard robe and padded towards the kitchen. I made my coffee and checked my email. The first thing that came into view was an advertisement telling me I should 'give someone a facial for the holidays!' Hmmmm. Well, I was feeling quite benevolent since Santa had delivered his special package to me, so I found the big candy cane and slipped back under the covers. The YYB was still trying to sleep, but I slid that cane between my thighs and worked it for a good twenty minutes. The movement of the bed woke him up and I whispered in his metal-clad ear that I was ordered by MSN to give a facial for the holidays. Without a word, only a series of moans, he slid his face down to suck the end of the unattended cane. Pushing it with his mouth and hand, he found the spot 'o love zone. When I yelled "Now!" he yanked it out, and voila! He had his facial. Female ejaculation is such a wonderful thing! As Mae West so salaciously said, "When I'm good I'm very good, but when I'm bad I'm better."

Ever since the YYB and I went to the premiere of *Beyond the Sea*, the new film about Bobby Darin's life, I've been listening to his music non-stop. I've been replaying the song, "More" so much that I'm making my neighbors feel homicidal. Even my faithful, loving dog looks at me as if she would like to harm me. Bobby just put that cocktail swing into everything, baby! Sometimes I think I was born in the wrong era. And isn't *more* such a lovely word? So, on that swingin' note…cheers to another year ahead! Clink Clink go the martini glasses and here's to: even more hair colors to experiment with, more marriage proposals, more direction in life, more spontaneous adventures, more choco-

Mz. Conduct's House of Sin

late macaroons, more singing and laughter and sex. Here's to more compassion and love and constructive criticism. Here's to more, more, more of all the good stuff!

Dear Sexy Mz. Conduct,

My husband and I have been a little tense lately. I can't get into having sex without kissing and he has this big gnarly cold sore on his face. Usually they are in the corner of his mouth so we can smooch carefully enough that I don't touch it, but this time it's smack dab in the middle of his lip! As far as I know, as long as there is a visible mark, it is contagious, is that true? If so, how can I get into it without the smoochies? We exchange hand jobs to appease the monster but it just isn't enough.

Sincerely,

Gotta Lick It Before We Kick It

Dear Licker,

You're kind of a whiner too, aren't ya, sweetie? Your husband's herpes is very contagious when he has a sore on his lip, but it can also be passed along when he doesn't have a visible sore too. You're probably screaming right now, but you did ask. A person with herpes can notice an itching or tingling before they actually see anything on their skin and it's sort of a warning that the virus may be present on the skin. If your hubby is aware of these sensations then you can still take precautionary measures and he won't spread it to you.

Perhaps a compromise on your end is necessary, avoiding the smooching and just having sex, by some role-playing. Maybe pretend you're a high-class call girl or a Dominatrix. Use your imagination, honey! Remember though, that herpes can be spread through oral, anal, and vaginal sex. Another option you can experiment with is to get out the saran wrap and cover his sore with it. You then could kiss and do whatever else your heart desires. That in itself can be quite fun! Wrap on, smooch girl!

Dear Mz. Conduct,

I'm a married man, age 30, and have been married for 8 years, but with my wife for 12 years, since high school. She is the only woman I've ever been with and I guess I'm curious about some things sexually. There is a lot I've never done or experienced and there are things my wife either can't or won't do. Basically I'm looking for a female friend and possible discreet relationship. I'm relatively new to the online thing and never attempted anything like this before. I wanted to be honest and upfront, so I'm sorry if this is awkward. Do you think you could point me in the right direction?

Stuck and Frustrated

Dear SaF,

I'll point you in a direction all right. Oh gee, is my finger pointing towards the bowels of hell? You write that you 'wanted to be honest and upfront' with me, Christ on a crouton, your wife is the one you should hone these skills with!

When you marry so early without experience it almost always comes back to bite you in your ass. You made a vow to your wife and you should tell her what you've been thinking...bottomline. She deserves your respect, damnit! As your life partner, she should want to take the steps necessary to fulfill your desires, as you should hers. I can't say this enough, *communication is the biggest aphrodisiac*. If you open up with your wife and let her know that you need more, she may just surprise you. Any little deviant fling you may have with someone else will only lead to trouble in some form. And here's a task, put yourself in her place! How would you feel if she were searching for another person besides you for intimacy? If after you hash it all out with her, make some decisions. Maybe you and she shouldn't be together anymore, but your vows to each other deserve truth and respect. That's my advice…sneakiness is so unattractive to women of worth. Now go away.

Mz. Conduct's House of Sin

"You live but once, you might as well be amusing."
–Coco Channel

It's 3:30 in the morning and I woke up to a light blue clarity. One of the best friends I'd ever have, my Wise Ol' Yippie Mentor, left this world three nights before, at just this time. When I looked at the clock, it made sense that I was awake at this hour. Stew Albert is the reason I write today, and I knew somehow I had to write.

When I first met Stew, fifteen years ago, I had no idea of who he was. I just cleaned his house for his soul mate, Judy, his daughter Jessica, and him. Judy went to work each day, and Jessica went to school. It would just be Stewy and me. We would talk as I cleaned. He would follow me around from room to room, his favorite being the kitchen where Stew would sit with his coffee and bread, and I would scrub and yak about endless ideas. He was an old hippy who initially thought he had met me at some point before in the fog of the San Francisco sixties. We established that it probably hadn't been possible, as he had twenty years on me. When he was storming the Capital with the Black Panthers, I was locked inside a group home for very bad girls.

As the months turned into years, I continued to discover who Stew Albert really was: an incredible chunk of history, a fearless rebel, a subdued celebrity, a master of the word (both written and spoken), the wisest man I'd ever met, and the dearest person to ever touch my heart.

One day, sitting at the table with Stew (as that's how it had become, he would ask me to just sit and talk), and the hours would drain by without me cleaning anything but my own soul. I remember the day I was ranting about this and that and blathered to Stew about how I'd always written, but was afraid to actually present anything anywhere. When I told him I'd always had a dream of putting out a fanzine (a self-published, minimal paged musing for the literary subculture), Stew simply said, "Kimsters, we all carry around dreams and ideas, but until we put them out into the world for people to see, they don't mean anything." He told me stories of the zines that were spread around Paris in earlier days, and of the zines that were put out all over in the sixties, how they were an outlet for poetry, politics and ranting. My fear vanished and turned itself into the excitement of making my dream real. I published my zine for three years after that, with constant praise, constructive criticism, suggestions, or unthought-of perspectives, depending on the issue, from Stew.

He always listened, he always made me think in areas I never knew existed, we made each other laugh and sometimes almost cry. Stew is the reason I write, and without him I wouldn't be all of who I am today. I will miss looking into those wise, blue, and loving eyes, but I will carry him in my heart for always. Stewy, the last thing I said to you when we talked about my next column, was "I won't let you down." This one's for you, Stew, with untellable love.

Holiday ho-downs and shin-digs were celebrated in any way, shape and form that I could possibly muster, as it's been an emotionally tested year, and I am so very ready for the new year.

My dear friends, Cocoa Bean and her Heady Hubby, came out west for a two-week visit and we made the most of it all, especially on New Year's Eve! A large group of my bosom buddies and I decided to spend New Year's at the Tiki Trouble Lounge. This included the aforementioned members: Punk Girl and her Hungary Man, Homer K. Simpson, Lola de Luscious, and a sort of other folks. One of Punk Girl's friends was hoping to be my date for the evening, but whoa mama, no date for me. I wanted to keep my options open for a floodgate to freedom on this brink of a new year, damnit! Punk Girl's friend asked to smooch me at midnight, and I told him "sure, only he'd have to wait his turn, as Lola de Luscious was my first choice, and I hers." Then, out of the blue, our hotter than Georgia Asphalt, punk boy waiter asked if he could kiss me at midnight, and I just had to say yes, hence the line. Midnight struck with abundance and as Lola de Luscious and I locked our ruby lips, I felt her hand on my loins, and I was instantly moister than a snack cake, honey.

Mz. Conduct's House of Sin

Next was Punk Girl's friend, coming in for the kill. That kiss lasted way too long, but was nice nonetheless. Two minutes later, our hot little waiter swooped down and lingered a long, sweet kiss upon me. Left me wanting more.

Lola de Luscious asked me to go to the restroom with her and I was happy to. A line a mile long was too much for her and her full bladder, so I suggested we go to the men's room, which is usually empty. It was, and we dove into the only stall, smooching and grasping at body parts until my nipple rings were being tugged by her tongue. I reminded her that she had to pee, so she sat down to do so. All I had view of was her kinky maroon hair with my fingers holding her head, crotch at her eye level; she untied my belt and, licked my baldness with a vengeance. I was tossing my head back in ecstasy when a knock on the door yells, above the lounge music, "You girls need any help?," in which we both simultaneously coughed out, an emphatic "NO!" We pulled ourselves together and walked out blushing only to see a line of twelve guys waiting in line. I'm not sure how long we'd been in there, but it was amazing, and back to our table we went. The rest of the evening was a bit of a blur, as it consisted of karaoke, champagne and people wrapping Hawaiian leis around my pigtails.

Two nights later, throbbing with lascivious thoughts, I decided to grab the bull by the horns, or the bull by his horny thorn. In any case, I called up the Tiki Trouble Lounge and asked for the waiter. He got on the phone and I hadn't time to explain whom I was. He remembered me clearly. I asked if he wanted to go out sometime, he blurted an excited, "yes!" It so happened that the next night was his only night off, so I invited him out with Cocoa Bean and Heady Hubby and I. We were to meet at the Fast Bar, a very cool bar seeped in blue neon and tall, red leather booths. We all met and that's where I found out he was twenty-three years old! Christ on a cheese ball, I thought. I asked if he knew how old I was and he replied in the suavest of suave, "It doesn't matter!" I was in lust! We had oodles of cocktails and then went to my place, where my lust got the best of me and I straddled the Hot Boy and gyrated on his lap. Cocoa Bean had her video rolling the whole time, and being the exhibitionist that

I am, it got me hotter still. Soon, everyone left at my insistence and Hot Boy unleashed his ample, pierced member into my clubhouse.

Mz. Conduct's House of Sin

"Penetrating so many secrets, we cease to believe in the unknowable. But there it sits, nevertheless, calmly licking its chops."
–H.L. Mencken

The Fourth of July produced more than fireworks for this girl! Just when I was considering going on a penis embargo, I acquired a brand new boy toy, or this time, as it seems, a man toy! My Rockabilly Man has become my own personal Elvis, baby! Tall, and dark, with sideburns to die for, he and I have found a whole new meaning to misconduct. I'm his queen about town, but when we get home, I'm his fair maiden, his personal slut, his naughty schoolgirl, and anything else we're feeling at the moment. The future holds unusual sexcapades to unravel…and tell!

Getting to know someone new is always exciting yet curiously unsettling when relinquishing trust. Some people feel they can trust no one until they give them a reason to, but my motto is the opposite. I trust until someone gives me a reason not to. Just how I am, and I like it that way. Rockabilly Man has told me many of his secrets, he has been lied to in a past relationship, but haven't we all at some point, so he's still in a scary place with all of this. He will soon learn—if he doesn't know already—that I am not like any other woman he has met or will ever meet. We agreed to keep slapping each other's ass, making out in the moonlight and communicating at all costs. And that's a perfect start.

Thinking about this new relationship (and the old one too), has led me to delve into the subject of deception in this society. I hear so many stories from people confused by this topic as well, lately it's been a virtual downpour of break-ups, fighting and miscommunication…all based on deception. So, investigative nature in tact, I interviewed many different couples about infidelity, and it remains an interesting and eternally unanswered topic.

I know couples who are involved in polyamorous relationships, open marriages and closed marriages, swinging, monogamy, and every variation in between. It seems that in all of these relationship types, that age old cheating element is still so prevalent. This fascinates me. I guess because I've experienced and been involved in each of the aforementioned relationships, and answer so many questions pertaining to the subject of cheating, it piques my interest to no end.

I started talking with women, most of whom admit that they do see the signals, red flags, or suspect behavior at an early stage, but confess that they either don't want the conflict of accusation or they don't want to believe the truth in front of them. Some are indifferent, said they just don't care. None of these things are healthy in my opinion. And it seems that the women who cheat in these relationships have entirely different reasons than the men, for the most part.

The women that I spoke with about why they cheat or would consider it, say either it is—or would be—because of the lack of attention in their own relationship, stagnant sex or next to none, and/or the lack of love and sexual desire for their mate, a lack of libido, with no interest in the intimacy department. Many said they no longer were in love with their mates at the point of having an affair. Whether they feel 'stuck' in the relationship financially or because of children involved, they choose not to leave their mate. This is when the biological factors come in to play I think.

When I spoke with the same number of men, the reasons were somewhat different. Most said that a sexual fling, with someone other than their mate, didn't mean they didn't love their significant others, it is more like a, 'I'm a man, I can't help it' state of mind. Although I do believe there is a biological validity to that, I also believe we make choices. In there lies the deception of being truthful to oneself and to another.

Several young men told me that as long as they "didn't get caught, no one gets hurt" and that amazed me, because in most cases people get caught. Part of the thrill may be in not getting caught, but it's not so thrilling when you do. I was told that if a guy is honest and tells a woman he's involved with that he wants to date other people, most women don't want anything to do with them. Okay, I get that to some extent, but when you meet the right woman she will respect the honesty above all else. At least that's my thinking.

Sadly, some men explained that they usually tell whomever they're involved with anything they want to hear just to keep the drama down. And then some men told me that they just stay unattached emotionally so that they don't get cheated on themselves.

Why is it that we have such a hard time telling truths? Fear. Fear of getting hurt, hurting someone else, being alone…basically. Fear is the opposite of love and a negative energy that we allow in our lives. We live in a country that's run on deception, and all around us in our daily lives, and it's time we took back our power as individuals, and deal with all truths, inside ourselves first, as we are all connected. And so are our actions. Loving someone wholly involves respect. Enough respect for truth. It builds integrity, character, and love enough for oneself. We all have that responsibility as human beings.

I am having a rant of sorts, but want people to think about these things, and since I have the floor, I can tell my truths…always. Now, where is my own personal Elvis with that big ol' microphone he carries in those black Levis?

> Dear Mz. Conduct,
> My girlfriend confided in me that she has a crush on a friend of mine. We have been together for over a year and this really hurt me. I asked her if she wanted to break-up and see other people, my friend (who is unaware of her crush), to be exact, and she told me no, she was just explaining about a silly crush. What should I do? Should I break up with her before I find out that she's cheated on me with my buddy or just wait until she does and then dump her?
> Dazed and Confused
>> Dear DaC,
>> Christ on a crumpet, just simmer your freaking jets, mister! Your girlfriend obviously had enough respect for you to be truthful and you're getting your boxers in a bunch! If she were seriously considering canoodling with your friend (who, by the way, may not be interested in coveting his buddy's girl), it sounds as if she would have told you that too. Quit being insecure. If you have a rela-

tionship based on trust then you have nothing to worry about as long as you keep it that way. Instead of whining and plotting to 'dump her first' why not thank her for being so honest and don't make more of this than it needs to be!

Dear Mz. Conduct,

I dated this guy three times and we had such a blast on every occasion. We had sex twice and it was great for both of us. I haven't heard from him in over a month and wonder if I should call him and see what's going on. I really want to keep this going, but don't want to seem pushy. Should I call him?

Grabby Girl

> **Dear GG,**
>
> Avoid the desperation, honey! Obviously, he's not that interested in 'keeping it going', so move on. All sorts of things could have happened: he flew to Norway to study the mating call of the Egret, he met the love of his life and they're planning a wedding, he's banged so many girls that he can't keep them straight, or he just doesn't care about you. No big deal, sweetie, let it go and find someone who mutually cares.

Mz. Conduct's House of Sin

"Love is a fire, but whether it is going to warm your hearth or burn down your house, you can never tell."
–Joan Crawford

The smoldering summer has arrived, but I started celebrating early this year, and then catapulted into bit of a break...literally.

I started the tail end of spring out with a trip to San Diego to visit my son before he makes like a baby and heads out...back east to law school that is. I bought fabulous new purple luggage, re-filled my Dragon's Blood oil, and was all revved to go when the ex (Yum Yum Boy) called, wanting to see me and have cocktails. With a few hours still before my plane left, I agreed to meet him. He's had a new girlfriend for months now (at my insistence), but has been confessing his thoughts, love, and penile needs to/in me on a regular basis. It's wrong, we repeatedly say, and I swear not to let it happen again, but I do. We do. We are pornstars in bed, what can I say? I would elaborate much more, but it weaves itself in later.

I made it to the airport with twenty minutes to spare. Tearing apart from the Yum Yum Boy can be difficult especially when he throws me up against my truck and sends his tongue down my waiting throat, then complained about having a boner at the bus stop. With that visual (and a wee feel of the throbbing member, just for kicks) I headed to the airport bar and slammed down a double vodka rocks. I was about to have some fun, honey. Sashayed my knee socked and short skirted self onto the plane and found I had a whole row to myself...right smack behind first class. Yeah, that'd be me! When I looked across the aisle, to my pleasant (and half intoxicated) glee, there was a hot little hunk of manmeat who asked about the newest tattoo covering my back. He turned out to be a tattoo artist who knew lots of people I knew and used to work for Infinity Tattoo, where I get most of my ink work done. We had the obligatory "it's a small freakin' world" chat for the next two hours, and yakked about our upcoming adventures in San Diego over oodles of those ever so adorable little airplane booze bottles. Hic. Ironically, we had the same flight back, so vowed to find each other again.

When the plane spilled me out at midnight in the middle of beautiful downtown San Diego I was ready for some city fun. My son picked me up, driving us straight to Ocean Beach, where the scene was rocking with crazy surfers in wife beaters, muscles and testosterone. We bar hopped our way around the beach community and made it back to my son's place just as the sun came up. After sleeping sufficiently the next day, and visiting the Hustler store, a moral imperative, I got a call from one of my dearest friends, the Distinguished Deviant, asking us to come join him in Mexico. We hopped a bus to Rosarito Beach and celebrated in a gorgeous hotel courtyard, toasting to old times and meeting his fabulous friends, such as the sweet and talented artist, Paco Garcia. The D.D. purchased one of his paintings from him for me and I adore it. When I whined about my hunger, the next invitation was to pile into the D.D.'s friend's clunky, old truck and drive to a nearby town to chow lobster. No way in hell's red kitchen could I ever refuse lobster. We risked life and limb rumbling at a speed limit unacceptable in the states, complete with a screwdriver for a stick shift, a cracked windshield, and an uncomfortable engine noise. Horses were everywhere! We saw soldiers with machine guns, poverty, garbage, beauty, ocean waves crashing against giant rock formations, stray dogs wandering the streets, until we whipped down a winding street filled with happy people and parked. The five of us climbed to the roof of a canary yellow restaurant across from the pounding shoreline, gathered around a long wooden table, and inhaled the salty ocean air. It was amazing to be spontaneously in another country and I was taking it all in. I was glad my son is fluent in Spanish, so as to avoid me ordering gawd only knows what, we were promptly served freshly made tortillas, beans, rice, big fat lobsters, and free tequila and beer. Viva la Vida!

Hours later, when we were stuffed to the gills, and six sheets to the glorious Mexican wind, we drove to a nearby town to watch the Oscar de la Hoya fight on the big screen. There I had the best tequila and mucho kisses from a handsome Mexican man, which was okay by me! Oscar won the fight, and the shabby, dark bar erupted into the best kind of chaos. We left there in a sea of hoopla and spent the night at the Distinguished Deviant's lovely friend's beachfront condo. Two o'clock in the morning on a Mexican beach was where I finally felt all my cares wash out to sea.

The next morning, my son and I walked about a mile through the streets of Rosarito to the bus station. Not a soul was about except for the occasional thin dog, and the bar owners hosing down their patios from the party spillage the night before. It didn't smell so great, but that's part of the deal.

Getting back across the border was tedious and long, but once back in the states, our rights returned, we slept like babies until it was time to get up and celebrate Cinco de Mayo in Old Town. We feasted on Ahi tuna and steamed clams and more tequila. We spent a day at the world famous San Diego Zoo, ate as much seafood as humanly possible, and had just under an hour to scoot me to the airport for home. Well, lord love a lapdance, there was my tattoo artist buddy I had met on the way. I had forgotten about him and now we shared a row of seats and our stories. He bought me tequila while I rubbed his feet and he told me about his girlfriend. Damn, guess the mile-high club wasn't going to happen, but I made a new friend, even better than that, a faithful boyfriend…albeit someone else's. It was the principle I admired.

Speaking of which, and back to that subject, the Yum Yum Boy ex and I have been hanging out entirely to much I've decided: the Fourth of July (producing our own fireworks once again), an entire weekend together drinking, talking and humping every which way but loose—no, well there was that too—in any case, then another Reverend Horton Heat show with all the trimmings of trouble afterwards. We always have an incredible time together, but what the hell am I doing? I'm being selfish, as I wouldn't take him back for a million bucks, but I get the good parts and then send him home for his poor girlfriend—has no idea—to deal with. I feel the shame, the guilt, as I've been in her place, not to mention my whole take on deception to begin with. Okay, this has got to stop! Christ in a convenience store, even I need a bitch slapping and butt-fucking sometimes! So, YYB, deceitful sodomite, I will be the stronger one, as I usually am, and stop this carnival ride...I want to get off (so to speak)!

Lately, I've had time to be very introspective. Here's why: One night, soon after returning from my trip, I experienced another kind of trip, one that involved too much tequila, leopard heels, and a gravel road full of potholes. Need I say more? I did have a large and in charge gentleman take especially good care of me that night, and for that I am grateful. Although sore and banged up (literally), I ventured out the very next night with a wild boy sporting a two-foot blue Mohawk. Great in the sack, but if I had to suffer through another twenty minute conversation dedicated to his Camel ashtray collection, or how he head-butted a guy ten times, I knew I would become homicidal. Sometimes it just isn't worth it, ya know? Someone once said, "While a girl waits for the right man to come along, in the meantime, she can sure have fun with all the wrong men." Got that covered!

Here I was, strangely still sore, my side bruised beyond belief from the fall a few nights before, but oh no, that didn't stop me from going out on a date with a boy I really liked the very next night. That turned into a three-day date involving wonder drugs, sex toys and oodles of canoodling. Wild, crazy and intensely gratifying...that is until I realized I should put a hold on my party-girl parade and go see a doctor. I did, and unpleasantly surprised, I had snapped two of my ribs right in half from the fall! So, it's been weeks upon weeks of good pain pills, no motivation, bad television, charity baskets from friends, and a ton of forced opportunity for exploring the contents of my silly head. I may take a break from dating for a while, a break from participating in deceptive behavior (forever I hope), and concentrate on my future, my book, and my own general health, both physical and mental. I'll be fifty years old on my next birthday, and although I still get asked for I.D. when buying cigarettes—however flattering that may be—I am what I am. It just may be time for a penis em-

Mz. Conduct's House of Sin

bargo, or at least changes bigger than I've ever expected! No dumb-asses, not a boob jobs...just some growth within.

Dear Mz. Conduct,

I had a date with a guy, whom at first I wasn't attracted to, but after an evening of good conversation and shared interests I decided I really liked him. We had sex that same night and it was really great. A few days later he called and asked me out again. I told him I would like that. Okay, here's the catch. I told him I had to take busses all over town on the day he proposed for our date, and explained that I might be too tired at the end of that day. Instead of offering to pick me up in his car, he said, "Well, you can just hop on one last bus and come to my place, hell you'll be on your back anyway." Even if he was joking it would have upset me a little, but he wasn't! I told him we'd have to get together some other time and we left it at that. Should I give him another chance since the first date went so well?

Bussin' Bonnie

Dear BB,

For the love of labia, woman, the first date went so *well* because you gave up the cooter to this undeserving loser! He got you the first time, apparently assumed he was just so goddamn manly that you would leap at his any lurid suggestion. He ultimately has no respect for you whatsoever, sorry. Sometimes if good conversation and common interests are present it's better to linger on that for a while and get to know someone even better before giving up the gift. I get it, sometimes we just get horned up and want the heat-sinking missile, but this guy doesn't deserve the saliva it takes to spit on him with. Don't let anyone talk to you like that, not without a swift kick in the peanuts. The next guy you go on a date with, take a little more time to figure out his character first and just to be on the safe side, duct tape his mouth shut. A friend once blurted, "God likes it when you don't speak". Amen to that, honey!

Dear Mz. Conduct,

I am not gay, but I sometimes fantasize about sucking my own dick. I've seen pictures of guys that do that and it just makes me horny to think about it, even cumming in my mouth. Is this unusual and any tips on how can I actually do it?

Peter Pondering

Dear PP,

Auto fellatio is the name for that, and it's not all that uncommon to fantasize about it. I mean who knows your body better than you? Of course it'd be hot! I had an ex boyfriend who would lay on the bed, put his legs up over his head against the wall, then gradually lower them to his ears. He was able to suck the tip and stroke it that way. It was pretty smoking to watch, I tell ya! If you're into yoga and/or fairly flexible, that can be helpful, and even if you don't have a long penis you can still accomplish it if you're in decent shape. Now go suck yourself.

Dear Mz. Conduct,

I'm a twenty eight year old straight guy who has been seeing this one girl for almost a month now. The first night we got together we made out and fooled around. She almost let me get further, but then changed her mind when I brought out the condom. Ever since then she won't even let me kiss her. We go out, have fun and she even spends the night, but she still won't let me do anything with her. This is driving me crazy! I am trying to respect her, but I also told her I want more. She says she's not ready and wants to just cuddle in bed. I have to get up in the night and head for the bathroom to take care of myself and she gets mad, not understanding the male body I guess. I'm leaving town in another month and don't have time to invest in any sort of 'meaningful' relationship and I was honest about this with her. What should I do about this unfulfilling situation?

Blue Balls in Boston

> **Dear BBiB,**
>
> You poor thang! I can understand wanting to wait, but if she knows you will be leaving and still isn't ready for more, then it's just not fair to either of you. I would at the very least quit letting her spend the night. Go out and have fun with her as you've been doing, but keep the sheets for the girls who'll use 'em! She sounds as if she really doesn't understand or respect what she's doing to you as a man, geeze! She may have a butt load of baggage, and I'll bet my Baby Jesus Buttplug that you don't need any more baggage than you've already got packed. Might as well get some action before you go, so buff up those blue balls and be a man about it! Say Bon Voyage to this one.
>
> *This column is dedicated to Greedgirl, who left this world and some of us with very special memories. May you finally be at peace, sweetie.*

Mz. Conduct's House of Sin

"Razors pain you; Rivers are damp. Acids stain you; And drugs cause cramp. Guns aren't lawful; Nooses give. Gas smells awful; You might as well live."
–Dorothy Parker

La de freakin' da, the sun has been out, and me, being the hedonistic sunshine girl that I am, the feel of warmth from that big ball of sky fire on my skin makes me so gloriously happy! It spells mischief. On one such day, Cinco de Mayo, Fret Boy, the Yum Yum Boy and I all went to the infamous Labia Lounge to masticate black bean quesadillas and swill as many cocktails as need be for the holiday at hand. At the Labia Lounge, you never know just what tunes will be spinning, anything from old television hits, to European dance beats, but happily, and befitting to the night, it was Los Lonely Boys we heard as we entered the dark and kitschy club. Colorful piñatas hung from the ceiling, and the spot that usually held a pool table was turned into a confetti-covered dance floor. Everyone joined in and before long it was a regular Mexican hootenanny! Needing to catch my breath, I sauntered up to the bar to get a shot of Patron, where I met a very depressed looking man. It pained me to see such sadness on a festive evening, so I asked the sad sack why he seemed so down. He mumbled something about "some days suck more than others", so I dug a little deeper, asking him why he thought that way. We had a strained conversation over the next few minutes, as he seemed not to be in much of a social mood, but with him sitting at the club, on this particular night, it led me to believe that somehow he did want more. I have great instincts. Determined to get a smile of some sort out of him, I told him that this day must be a less sucky day, because after all, he got to talk to me! With that, I actually saw the corners of his mouth turn up just a bit. I supposed that was as good as it was going to get with him, and feeling gratified by his slight mood swing upward, I took another shot, gave him a peck on the cheek, and headed towards the dance floor. The Yum Yum Boy and Fret Boy were waiting for me with open arms, as if I had been gone for days. I kissed them both, they kissed each other, and we blurrily rocked on into the night. Later, our waiter placed a drink in front of me, telling me it was compliments of a downbeat fan. The napkin under the drink had something scribbled on it. It simply read, 'thank you'. I looked around, but he seemed to have vanished into the sultry night. This time, the corners of my mouth turned up and I thought, life is what you make it. Via con Gutterslut, mia amados!

The next week, the Yum Yum Boy and I took off to parts unknown, as we always do when we go camping. A toss of the coin, a blindfolded point at a map, and away we go! Our first trip of the season proved that it wasn't quite summer yet. It was raining and chilly, but my pornstar cowboy and I were determined to get the hell out of Dodge. Towards the ocean we headed, found a little tucked-away island and pitched our tent. I guess we were the only ones brave enough to tough it through the drizzle and Pacific Ocean wind, as there wasn't a soul in sight, and the sequestration was a good trade-off on any day. We discovered a nature conservancy on the island, so we hiked for miles along the moss-covered trails, leading us right down to the water. Breathtaking in the mid-morning quiet, all we could hear were strange birdcalls and the crash of the ocean waves against the rocks. With no worries about my carnal-burning screams there, we almost ran out of places to have illicit sexual romps. There's nothing like being tossed over an enormous tree stump on the edge of the forest, opening your eyes (upside down and after seventy-two orgasms), and seeing your lover's spectacular, protruding profile against the green-gray sea. Anchors aweigh, baby!

All that relaxation and decadence was much needed and when I returned home to my computer full of questions, for some reason, one question seemed to be overwhelmingly asked: "how did I get started writing advice in the first place?" Well, babydolls, I have no degree, no academic experience, and no title, except for what I give myself, so I thought I'd touch on this subject.

My life seems to have been threaded with survival mode, and though I've wallowed and struggled through things that most people haven't, I've always tried to see the bright side of things. It just makes sense to me. Life can be a bitch, but I can be a bigger one, and besides, what's the alternative?

Mz. Conduct's House of Sin

As long as I can remember, I've been one of those little-miss-know-it-all girls, whom I partially blame my friends for, by their constant wonderings of "what do you think?" Somehow, I just elicit people asking me advice. Now, I rarely asked advice from anyone. I guess I just figured that if I looked inside myself long enough, I would have all the answers right there...and usually I did. Growing up in an orphan asylum, full of eighty black girls and three white girls, and more or less forced at an early age to stand up for myself, be brutally honest, good or bad, that became a large part of who I was. I was a scampish young thing who grew up in San Francisco in the early seventies, with peace and love and experimental everything taking place. I tried everything at least once, so I could form my own opinion on all subjects. As it came to be, most of the people I knew, would ask me advice on relationships, knowing they would get my truths. Then the beauty of the Internet came into play. I decided to share my opinion with people all over the world. After all, everyone is entitled to my opinion! My endeavor took off, and I developed an ever-growing fan club and viola! Mz. Conduct was born! Helping people see the truths is my calling, this I believe. Thus, this next question was a perfect way to help express why I do what I do. Granted, the truth doesn't always make one happy or feel good, it is what it is...the truth. My truth, nothing more, and nothing less.

Dear Mz.Conduct,

I need help! I recently went to a local strip club, and before the night was out I had the invitation from a dancer to go toy shopping, skinny-dipping in her pool, and wine together. I'm supposed to call her at the club and she will have a surprise for me after her working hours.

I usually take a taxi, but this beautiful seducer said she would take me in her car. Problem #1: I'm just out of the hospital and have bills to pay (I spent several hundred in a night of titillation at that club.)

Problem #2: I've been married for decades...no excitement there. The dancer also gave me her name, club phone number and the name of another dancer who I really enjoyed. I'm in my early 50's and these ladies are in the early 30's. They say it's no problem to them. These ladies also gave me a little extra at the club, especially in private table dances. I'm crazy about these ladies and want to throw caution and money to the wind, and possibly my marriage.

I apologize for this short notice, but I'm desperate. This situation is moving too fast for my brain to grasp over my sexual urges. So I put out a desperate plea to the one and only Super Mz. Conduct, in hopes that she can help in the nick of time.

Thanks.

Man in a Dream Drama

Good Advice from a Very Bad Girl

> Dear MiaDD,
>
> No matter how beautiful these girls may be or how much they seem to enjoy your company (you're most likely a gentleman, which can be refreshing in a strip bar), remember that these girls are 'giving' you this opportunity only because they can see visions of their rent being paid and possibly a new pair of shoes. You are an easy target. I have a feeling that you're a decent guy who is simply bored in his marriage and along comes this fantasy and well, of course, you are tempted.
>
> I won't tell you what to do, except to think about what you will venture from this escapade, and what you might lose. A thirty-year marriage is something to treasure, especially if you still love your woman—and I think you do. The money and energy you're spending on the young beauties is a fleeting thrill and could be put towards strengthening what you already have. Nothing fleeting about that.
>
> It's important and healthy to have fantasies, but remember that fantasy and reality are two very different things! There aren't many brain cells, no matter what it seems, in a penis. Quit thinking about the beauties and their Spam purses, and focus more on your own purse. Now, stick a fork in me, I'm done!

Dear Mz. Conduct,

You are fantastic! Thanks for responding so quickly. Your reply came in enough time to contemplate the consequences of my adulterous actions. Very hard choices: beautiful women and lustful pleasures or ruining/destroying a 30-year marriage. I almost called the girls' number, got stomach knots (guilt or money), still not sure!

In short, I hope to renew sparks in my marriage. It may turn into a full-blown bonfire and I'm excited for that. Thanks for thinking that I'm a good man. I used to be in the eyes of others, and was concerned about other people's needs. Lately, only my own pleasures are tarnishing that image.

I don't want to bore you with my past history. Just want to say thank you and that I appreciate what you said. The advice was right on…hammer on the nail. I consider you a special person. I would like to send you something…an appreciation gift. What do you like? When is your birthday?

Thanks again,

MiaDD

> Dear MiaDD,
>
> This is the main reason I write my column. I could ask for a bottle of champagne or a new pair of black boots, but then I'd be in the same category as the girls you steered clear of. Your thank you letter is gift enough for me. Sometimes we just need a little kick in the ass to realize what we truly have, and decide if it's worth a little sordid pleasure to lose it. I always figure we can have both if we communicate in the right ways.
>
> One of my favorite quotes is "Sometimes on your way to a dream, you find a better one." That's my truth, there you go!

Mz. Conduct's House of Sin

"A liberated woman is one who has sex before marriage and a job after."
–Gloria Steinem

I hope you all had a fantabulous Valentine's Day and are ready for the season of new beginnings! The crocuses are sprouting from the warming ground, the birdies are chirpin' and good things are poppin' up all around. Speaking of which, I had a seriously sated Valentine's Day with the Yum Yum Boy. I was showered with tongue baths, my favorite Merlot, the most decadent dark chocolate ever, a beautiful, mushy card o' love, and the biggest leopard pillow in all the land! Now, mind you, my rooms are filled with leopard print, from the toilet seat cover to the sheets and bedspread. I have leopard print gloves, boots, and even a toothbrush! The YYB told me that he snapped up my new, giant pillow because he immediately pictured my bountiful buns bent over the spotted splendor. He was right, 'tis indeed a truly fabulous square of fluff for fornication, honey!

Thank you to all the fans that sent me cards and emails, and for the lovely and saucy poem from my die-hard fan, and talented writer, Mister Coyote.

A few weeks ago, the Yum Yum Boy and I trotted off into the rainy night to see a friend's show at Cargo, an art gallery in the downtown Pearl District. It's always such fun just being me, hob-knobbing with the snooty gallery crowds and swilling red wine like there's no tomorrow. While I was there, warmed by the crackers and spirits (and the YYB's hand), I did a little networking, chatting with the gallery owner herself, and somehow finagled an art show for another friend. I've been pushing hard for him to show his shamanistic Central American paintings and it looks like it'll happen now! Oh, la de da, some people do so love my mouth, in more ways than one!

Later that night, after the show, the Yum Yum Boy and I headed across the street to Touché, a restaurant and bar that we'd heard rumors about their wickedly wonderful martinis. Well, right off the bat, we could tell that it wasn't our crowd, with the chronic cell phone users in their slacks and pantyhose, all coiffed and neck-tied, on a Friday night, no less. Nevertheless, we sidled up to the bar and ordered a pair of martinis, when suddenly out of nowhere, a small animated Greek man, wearing his glasses on his head, whisked our drinks away from the bartender and set them down in front of us, introducing himself as the owner of Touché. He told us he had never seen us in his place before and he liked our 'look', so the drinks were on him. Basically, we stuck out like a sore thumb in our 'let's dig in the trunk and mix up the ensemble like a harlot meets a cowboy' attire, and we caught his eye like a fishhook on a tennis shoe. Cocktails for free is a good reward for individuality! We introduced ourselves, chatted and sipped our martinis. The little Greek man loved my name, as that was his wife's name and he proudly stated that he'd been married for twenty-four years. I said something to the effect, that it was probably even a longer marriage for his wife, and he chuckled. I asked his advice on a lasting marriage because I love to hear these stories. He delivered one of the best things I've ever heard: "Once you've decided that the person you are with is the one you want for life, everything else will fall into place." He said that so many problems arise because people are waiting for something else to come along or are unsure of what they do want, and from that, always stems trouble. Very wise words, in my book! Shortly after that, he moved on to another restaurant owner task, but told us the next time we come in, drinks and desserts would be on him. We left the bar with a buzz in our breath and a bee in our bonnets, getting only as far as the car where my king bee stung his honey, right there on the leopard-covered car seats!

During the recent blizzard, housebound with cabin fever, Punk Girl and her Hungary Man saved our night. They hoofed it through the ice and snow just to visit us—all the while, the Chihuahua in tow, skidding and barking down the entire road. Seventy-five feet away, Punk Girl was holding a large jug of something homemade and screaming about how much she missed us. We hugged and slid in the ice and watched the Chihuahua sail under the parked truck. Once inside and warmed up, we cracked open the home brew and decided to play strip Scrabble. Punk Girl was inebriated before any of us, but still man-

Mz. Conduct's House of Sin

aged to beat the pants off us all (literally) by fifty points! Weenies and whistles, was that ever fun!

The Royal Diva is packing up and relocating to the warmer climate of California, intent mainly on broadening her horizons in the world of jazz. I know that she will absolutely bring sunshine to a whole new group of fans. She's been celebrating it up, having her so-long shindigs by the score and while on the phone with me, narrating one of her eventful evenings—in glorious mad cackle—smack dab in the middle of a miasma of martini madness, she dropped her cell phone into the mix. End of call, bye bye. Didn't hear back from her until the following day. No worries, Omar, her own personal cabbie, made sure the precious princess booty got home all safe and sound. Oh, do those Californians know what's coming?

So, it seems we're all merging into the new. Let's do our best to become better people and careful lovers. We should face whatever challenges come our way, take them on with soap and confidence, lust in our loins and a love-fest in our hearts!

> Dear Mz. Conduct,
> I am interested in swinging…and I don't mean dancing. I've been trying to find ways into the life style, but I'm single and that's the way that I want to go in to it and stay!
> I live in Seattle, can you suggest some single swing clubs to attend?
> Single Seattle Swinger
>> Dear SSS,
>> Well, okay already, mister weenie swinger, I wouldn't worry that you won't remain single. Tempting as it may be for some gorgeous bombshell to snap up a witty one like you, staying single shouldn't be a problem.
>> I consulted my friend, the truly tasty Darklady (www.darklady.com), and she told me of an on-premises club in the Seattle area called New Horizons. It's in North Lynnwood, about 20 miles north of Seattle and their website is http://www.horizonsclub.com/. Also there is a site, mostly geared toward couples, but you may find more information there as well. It's called Bay Couples and their website is http://www.baycouples.com. Good luck, something tells me you'll need it, and swing on sailor!
>
> Dear Mz. Conduct,
> My boyfriend and I have been sexually active for 8 months now. He complained to me at 2 months that he wanted to try something new because it was getting boring. He's the only person I've had sex with, but my boyfriend has had a couple partners.

Good Advice from a Very Bad Girl

He tells me to come up with new methods, when I'm the one who is inexperienced! I found new methods of styles we hadn't tried but that was months ago. My problem now is, that I just am not interested in having sex anymore. We need to find something new to spice up our sex life. We need some new methods, whip cream and chocolate, or anything will help us. Can you please give me some advice? Thank you.

The Vapid Virginesque

>**Dear VV,**
>
>Where do I start? Oh that's right, I'm the one answering questions, damnit! If your boyfriend has been demanding and pressuring you into being the sole supplier of the next mind-blowing sexual position, no wonder you don't even want to bother with sex at all. I'll bet my leopard vibrator that he's not a mental giant in the first place, and probably fails miserably at any imaginative tasks, so he's simply lumped it all on you. That way he can also put blame, which is entirely unfounded, on you, the dolt!
>
>Good sex, really yummy sex, starts with intimacy. Maybe instead of focusing on each other's orgasms, you could just lie around. Insert Enigma CD (not penis), light candles, and talk. You can start with something like: What three sexy things would you choose to take on a deserted island? Stuff like that. Yak about your wildest fantasies, even if they seem embarrassing. Opening up and honesty are the biggest aphrodisiacs ever known. The more comfortable you both get with one another, the more ideas that will come to you naturally.
>
>I would leave out the food-play for now, as you're not truly into each other's mind-set yet. There is always Violet Blue's *Ultimate Guide to Adult Videos*, which you can get on Amazon.com and great for figuring out what turns you, and your significant other, on. I recommend it highly, if you're willing to watch some porn. "Oh look sweetie! That looks like it might be fun!" Honestly, I would suggest specifically focusing on getting to know your boyfriend more intimately. Hey, you may just decide to kick his lame ass to the gutter-lined curb and find yourself a nice, shiny new one!

Mz. Conduct's House of Sin

"Life is rated X. It is not rated R."
—Ice-T

One afternoon, as I trotted my healthy package into the Rose City post office, I saw a tall, cutie-pie-and-a-half who was yakking on his cell phone. He had bundles of large envelopes under his arm and was pacing around the lobby, obviously in deep discussion with whomever was on the other end of the phone. I kept stealing little glances, as he was extremely edible looking and, on the fourteenth glance, I happily noticed that it was my all-time favorite local comedian! Wow, Dwight Slade right there in the post office. I wondered if he was gathering new material, as it was certainly a motley crew of folks who stood in the non-moving line that day. I tossed my letters down the chute, then wrote on the back of my business card, "You're the funniest man in town. Perhaps you'll find my column amusing!" He was still on his cell phone, so I clandestinely slipped my card to him and smiled as he looked up, grinning back. A few days later he emailed me, and said he found my column "not just amusing but intoxicating". Whoa daddy, I thought, I'd like to lick his stamp and go postal with this guy. He invited me to be a guest at his next comedy show, which I attended. I was thrilled to get a special comfy chair, unlike the rest of the crowd's, and then to my surprise, voila! a sapphire martini showed up, with three olives of course, courtesy of Mr. Slade. Now that's just what a girl like me needs to start the lubrication process on any given evening! Mister Comedian Extraordinaire went into his hilarious routine about getting a super-charged, triple caf, ultra-whammo espresso and then stalled in freeway traffic for hours, at the butt-crack of dawn. I almost peed my non-existent panties when he went into a rant about being stuck behind the yuppie family driving their SUV on the way to the outlet mall. The family was driving a ripping forty-five miles per hour in their swanky vehicle, complete with perfectly coiffed children with names like Forrest and Sunburst. Dwight Slade (www.dwightslade.com) is a funny, animated and talented man (and don't forget to drool for!) I see big things to come for him (and maybe his big thing will come for me, honey!)

Good Advice from a Very Bad Girl

A few nights later, the Lion King, his beautiful tulip of a girlfriend, the Yum Yum Boy and I, all attended a fabulous fetish party. I was in black vinyl from head to toe, black feather boa and gloves to match. I was named the 'eye candy' of the evening…but of course daahling! I also had a dashing gentleman approach me, kiss my hand and tell me I was gorgeous, which was absolutely delightful, but another drunken slob felt compelled to drape his sleazy, beer soaked bones all over me, slobbering such indecencies as "Oh, you're Mz. Conduct and I'd like to misconduct myself all over you!" To my rescue, the Yum Yum Boy had the insipid inebriate tossed right out of the party. Quite satisfying, I must say. The party held spanking fests on one stage. A girl with an ass the size of Kansas was getting walloped by a slim, hairy man in a lime green speedo. A pretty woman was doing body painting downstairs next to the table full of snacks, and wild screams were coming from the Pleasure Room, a red-curtained makeshift area in one corner of the church. I dragged all of my cohorts into the PR and we ended up performing quite a saucy little show for the onlookers. My vinyl came off, the boys' leather pants came down, skirts were hiked up, smooth mounds were exposed and boa feathers were flying everywhere. We heard lots of moaning around us and had fun with it, swilling red wine and snacking on each other. Boy breath on boy appendage and the crack of a gloved hand on my ample behind. A dollop of girl mouth on girl flesh and the sweet-as-honey ooze of approval. The next morning, with slutty snickering, I surprisingly pulled a simple boa feather out of the Yum Yum Boy's nether regions! Now being of Dutch decent, that's what I call a delicious buffet in the Netherlands, honey! Another smaller stage area had giant velvet pillows thrown over it and what looked to be an extremely flexible man, lying on his back—or shoulders at this point—with his feet over his head and his own long erection in his own wide mouth. Hmmm…now, this was cause for further investigation. I watched eagerly from a corner, and not too surprisingly, found myself to be moister than a snack cake. Okay, this brings me to one of the questions I received recently:

Dear Mz. Conduct,
Is it strange for a straight guy to want to be able to suck his own dick?

Mz. Conduct's House of Sin

Wanting My Own Wand

Dear WMOW,
Holy straws in a screwdriver, no! I don't think this has anything to do with one's gender preference, as we're all very interested (if not obsessed) with our own genitalia. I'm of the belief that if we were all as ultra-flexible as the bloke I saw at the party was, we'd never leave the house! It may seem a bit freakish, and unfortunately even if I were Gumby on crack, I couldn't establish such a feat, but for me to watch such a thing is definitely a major turn-on. If you master the technique, send me a picture, baby!

A round-assed boytoy and I celebrated Elvis Presley's birthday at the appropriately kitschy Lo Brow Lounge. We sat at a tiny table right beneath a giant blue neon martini glass. The eerie glow of the neon hit our faces like a stage light. I plugged the jukebox and chose some Elvis tunes, while we tossed back different drinks, as we didn't know what Elvis really drank. We figured he pretty much consumed everything, which is what we ended up doing that night as well. In mid-swill I felt a tap on my waist and turned to see a friend's husband holding a half-empty beer glass. He was accompanied by of his co-workers and apparently had been in more bars than one this evening. This guy is a doll, and I imagine a wicked little fuck, I'll give him that. Needless to say, I've let my sordid little mind wander there on more than a few occasions. So, he stood smirking at me, his hand never left my waist, and he barely acknowledged my boytoy, whom I immediately introduced. Now, I know that he loves his wife, my friend, and I also know that I could have taken him into the bathroom and rode him 'til the cows came home, but I pulled his hand off my waist and asked him to tell his wife, my friend, to call me soon. That seemed to sober him up and he went back to his buddies at the table across the room. So, here's another question that pertains:

Dear Mz. Conduct,
Well, I am no sex freak, but I figured you, of all people, would have some insight into my issue. I had been hanging out with this woman, we spent a few weeks together but she had a boyfriend. Now, one day we got drunk at her house when she grabbed me and stuck her tongue in my mouth. I became extremely aroused and it showed, however, I pulled away. Her boyfriend was on the way over. Was I stupid for retreating or was that retarded of me for not going for it? There was another day when we were in her car and I could have become affectionate, but once again, I did not make a move. For future reference, I want to know if I should avoid this type of

game or should I relax and go for it. What do you think? What is her game? Should I avoid these types of women in the future?

Yours Truly,

Too Sensitive

> **Dear TS,**
>
> Honey, the grass is always greener because that's where the septic tank is! We all have desires and we all want what we don't have…at least some of the time. Monogamy is only a choice, not a design of human nature, and a lot of us struggle through the in-between. You should think about the worth of the romp at hand, little man. It may be rockin', it may blow your feeble mind, but is it really worth the complications that most likely will occur when someone is being a big, fat, flirty sneak? As you can tell, I have issues with sneakiness! If a person wants to see other people, then just say it, don't try to sample the salami around town and then swear that you're true. In my estimation, sneaky people are subhuman scum and, with any luck, will become a bad smell in the basement one day soon. We can so easily put our brain (remove plastic first) in a microwave in exchange for a couple of hours of exchanging bodily fluids. Sure, it's difficult and sometimes people make mistakes. Then they choose to work through them or not. We have so many choices. Think of the consequences of your actions and then make your own decision.
>
> I think you were right to avoid any further involvement with the slutty strumpet and should steer clear of this woman altogether. She knows you're interested, she knows you want her, but let her know that until she is boyfriend-free, you're off-limits. In the meantime, ask yourself this: would you truly want a girl like her anyway? Whatever you decide, you may indeed find some integrity when you remove your brain from the microwave.

Mz. Conduct's House of Sin

"I may be the outlaw, darlin', but you're the one stealing my heart."
–Brad Pitt as J.D. in Thelma and Louise

As the nicer weather approaches and more people are out and about, I'm finally seeing the likes of this ever-so-lovely neighborhood I live in. Between the fifty-six constantly barking dogs in the alley, the call girls coming and going next door, the omnipresent police activity at the strip club across the street, and the drug dealers buzzing around on little motorized scooters, I find that I can either bitch about it or find sordid little stories to write about. I choose the latter.

The other day, I was out planting some ixia bulbs, when my Yum Yum Boy pulled up and said "Baby, I just got out of jail and haven't had a woman in a long, long time...and I ain't never had a woman like you!" I looked at him, thinking he had lost his last marble, and I see the sly smile slide across his handsome face. I snapped back with something on the order of how I'd always wanted to wrap my legs around a 'hardened criminal', and he promptly bent down and scooped me right up in his Popeye arms, making me drop all my gardening tools. YYB carried me into the house and for a few sweaty hours, my make-believe jailbird made me forget about dogs and cops and even flower bulbs!

The Transient Trollop couldn't make it down for the Tom Jones extravaganza, so my Yum Yum Boy took me...and it was fabulous! The crowd—contained in the fanciest-pants show place in town—consisted of octogenarian couples clenching hands, twenty something girls with matching tee shirts spelling out the showman's name, gay men all aflutter, and every sort of person in between. Then there was YYB and me, decked out in matching red and black retro wear and looking quite smashing, if I do say so myself. Tom, though, he was da man! At sixty-three years old, he was moving those hips and feet and singing his big ol' lungs out and still, women's panties were flying on stage left and right. If I had been wearing any, they would have joined the stage full of lingerie in a New York minute. Hilariously, Tom was in the midst of crooning, "She's a

Lady", when some woman tossed a gigantic white girdle at his feet. He stopped singing, the band still playing, picked up the girdle and asked, "She's a…lady?" Everyone rolled with laughter and he smoothly resumed the song.

My favorite highlight of the evening is when he was talking his way into "Baby Put Your Red Dress On"—the band in the background, with that sultry saxophone soulfully slippin' in notes—and Tom seductively said, "This one's for the ladies. Men, we need to remember that we need to give the ladies what they want" (and the crowd goes wild) "and when they want it" (the roof is raising now), and then he gets wickedly nasty and runs his hand over his ample crotch, and in the lowest voice ever, simply says, "and how they want it!" and the women were in conniption fits from balcony to stage front. This included me, of course. I felt a bit of empathy for the straight men in the audience, looking as if they knew they were going to be delivering some penis pleasing that night and not any of them could quite measure up to ol' Tom. Yum Yum Boy and I had a marvelous evening. Quite a man with quite a package…and Tom wasn't bad either!

Speaking of men with ample appendages, I have a video recommend! I'm a huge fan of film and watch an eclectic bunch of movies each month, but *Wonderland* is truly worth watching. Val Kilmer stars in the amazingly poignant life of Jon Holmes, the famous porn star who died of AIDS, and the film wasn't about his thirteen inch lingam or his claim to have had sex with over ten thousand women. Instead, it covers his turbulent life otherwise and his struggle to survive in a world we can only imagine. *Boogie Nights* was a parallel of his John Holmes' life as well, but *Wonderland* is better.

I've been working out at the oldest YMCA in the city, where the drinking faucets are like the ones I remember in Kindergarten and the only folks there are one hundred and ninety years old. It's the cutest thing to have sweet little prune women tell me how cute my pigtails are or ask if my tattoos are real or the temporary kind. They're so non-judgmental and it's really a hoot. Some

Mz. Conduct's House of Sin

old broads share inside information on the best times to swim in the pool, not to flush the toilets when anyone is in the shower—at least not without yelling "flush" first, and who the best towel boy is (none of which are a day under sixty.) The other day, there was a morbidly obese woman who embarrassedly asked me if I could dig her bra strap out of one of her back folds. Lord on a lamppost, I cringed a bit and managed to dig and push and pull until I could square the old girl away. I figure that was my good deed for the week, and it motivated me even more to get my buns on that Stairmaster! I was determined, that day, to climb as far as the stars. I swear though, if there were only a place to put a cocktail and ciggie on that evil contraption, I'd sure be a lot happier. Perhaps I should put together an old women escort agency of some sort. Call it something like 'Old Broads R Us' or 'Wrinkled Wenches for Fun'; hey, it's an entrepreneurial thought!

Dear Mz. Conduct,
Men in general seem to want more sex than women. It's a supply and demand thing, 99% of men and 3% of women. This causes a huge shortage of product and driving the price right through the roof. The balance of power and ability to control any situation sucks. I once traveled 3000 miles just on the chance of getting laid. Tell me why pussy is so valued and cock is not?
Broke Commodity Seeker

> **Dear BCS,**
>
> I don't know where you get your statistics, perhaps you are Mormon or hang out in gay bars, whatever the case, you are so wrong! Maybe the women you know are taking medications, which inhibits their sex drive, or gee, I don't know, maybe, just maybe, you aren't taking into consideration that women like to be thought of as people and not a "commodity"! If you're walking around with this attitude then it's no wonder life is rendering a great big zero for you in the romance department.
>
> Aside from your obvious shortcomings and shallowness, pussy has had power from the beginning of time and it always will…and believe me, cock has its value as well. It's our biological make-up, and the difference in hormones between men and women; women having 40 some odd hormones running around within (causing emotional priorities and such), and men having about six (basically simpler minded and more visually stimulated.) Fair or not, it's just the way it is. What has true value is a person! Until you learn the meaning of this, you'll be doomed to travel thousands of ridiculous miles in hopes of laying pole, and then constantly complaining about it.
>
> Some men are controlled their whole life by the pursuit of the pooty, and that's a sad factor to me. They complain that they've shelled out their life savings for some women only to be turned down in bed, or they marry some woman who promises them the world, in hopes that they will have more and better sex. Those men are idiots. Get everything you want ironed out first before you

choose a partner for life, bottom line. That's brings me to 'choice', which is what intelligent people do. Just as monogamy is not in human nature to follow, some of us make a choice to follow that, and the same goes for chasing pussy all your life. Breaking it down into a "supply and demand" description is cause for bitch slapping and butt fucking, honey! At some point in life, all men are faced with a choice of either pursuing some hot thang over and over again, or to venture out in a more spiritual and/or career oriented direction and perhaps meet someone likeminded along the way. The ones who truly are men of worth will choose to put greater things before a constant focus on getting laid. It's all about choices, and personally I have no need for an insecure horn dog, not many women do!

Dear Mz. Conduct,

I am 18 years old and a virgin in the strictest sense, but I've done about everything except penetration. I'm waiting until I get married. Anyway, to get to the issue, my penis is curved. It's pretty obviously too, especially when I'm hard. It curves about 45 degrees to the right. I've only done 'stuff' with one girl and she never said anything about it, but I'm sure she noticed it and just didn't want to embarrass me. Based on your experience, how rare is this condition, and is it a turn-off? I know that every girl is different, but how big a problem do you think this might be? Any advice would be appreciated.

Pointing Right or Wrong

> **Dear ProW,**
>
> First of all, kudos to you for wanting to wait until you are serious with someone. Whether you stay true to that or not, you shouldn't worry about the shape and curve of your penis. "Based on my experience", I've seen hundreds, honey, and it's quite common to have some sort of curve: right, left or sometimes upward. Penises are all unique and for the most part, beautiful for that sake alone. I wouldn't worry about what a girl thinks of your penis. If it's a concern of hers, she most likely either doesn't realize that penile curving is very common or she just doesn't like you, and that should be what it's really all about. Don't allow it to be a problem because it isn't, believe me. You and your pretty, curved meat whistle, just rock on!

Mz. Conduct's House of Sin

"It's best not to be too moral—you cheat yourself out of too much life."
–Maude, from the movie Harold and Maude

Alert! There's been a vicious rumor going around that I am a man! At first I was appalled, as I've been told by a handful of sackless suitors that I am more woman than any one man (or ten men, a woman and a couple of hermaphrodites) can handle. But on second thought, I decided that I kind of like the wonder behind it all. Mystery can be a very good thing, and since my life is an open book, perhaps this will tangle up the true tale of Mz. Conduct and add a tad bit of enigma to my life. I don't have penis envy, I cause it, honey!

About a month ago, my computer committed suicide, logged off and went to the big Internet in the sky. I was forcibly reminded that one cannot always be in control of things. I ended up doing things I needed to do. I read more books, updated my journal and wrote some handwritten letters, which are largely becoming extinct in this society. (I owe a special thank you to the Lion King who bought me a brand new computer out of the sheer love in his heart. Smooch smooch baby!)

Then one morning, feeling my oats, I grabbed the Yum Yum Boy and headed for the saltiness of the seashore. I told him that he would be my slave until further notice. He smiled and nodded in his yum-yum way, got behind the wheel of the truck and started the engine. I said, "Stab it and steer it, baby!" and we roared off into the foggy hills. Destination: Trouble. Gazing at his handsome profile while he drives always turns me on, so we managed to travel only about a half an hour before I felt compelled to release his ample appendage from those snug fitting Levi's he wore and do some damage. As he drove us down the road, I drove his flesh down my throat. Though laughing like a hyena, he yelled over the music that his slave-time was taking a break, then whipped the little truck off the highway and down a bumpy logging road. He drove faster than common sense allowed until we encountered a sudden and formidable roadblock. YYB ordered me out of the truck and "Bend your ass over." Together, we were hotter than Georgia asphalt during a heat wave, and soon screams of animal delight echoed through the thick of the woods. This all gave new meaning to knotty (naughty) pine! Later, with limp limbs, we climbed back in the truck and drove off. An hour later we finally made it to the coast. We hiked down a path to a secluded cove, then fornicated over the giant rocks, smoothed to a polish by the tide, both wetter than a bucket of suds in a rainstorm, in more ways than one. Afterwards, we started collecting interestingly-shaped rocks and China hat shells until I had a conniption fit, as I screeched with sheer delight finding a piece of driftwood in the exact and perfect shape of a ten-inch penis! I proudly carried it down the shore, waving and stroking it, snickering at how it must look to any faraway eyes. It now resides in a shrine in my living room, surrounded by candles and sandpaper.

Hours later, still on the sand, the sun went down and so did my boy. Looking at the heavens, I felt I was there already. We drove to the nearest coastal town and, following oodles of cocktails, we decided to get a cheap motel, the cheaper the better (as cheap motels are the soul of America, in my book), found one right away at the Scarlet Starfish. In a wee-hour sex bout, I inadvertently yanked the plywood headboard right off the bed and in my unbridled orgasmic enthusiasm (the norm for me where he is concerned) I managed to clobber poor Yum Yum Boy right smack in the back of the head! It's safe to report that he not only lived, but also forgave me. I then made peace with both his heads. Just a day at the beach, honey!

One fine evening, I strolled downtown to my absolute favorite bookstore, Powell's Books—the largest bookstore in the Northwest, maybe the galaxy, which occupies one entire city block—to hear Susie Bright (www.susiebright.com) read from her latest *Best American Erotica* series that she annually compiles and edits. I truly recommend it to all of you, as she is a true Goddess. She read a story aloud called "Courtney Cox's Asshole", written by Jill Soloway, and it's the funniest thing I've heard in a long time. After the reading, I plowed my way through the crowd to get my book signed and boldly introduced myself. She got googly-happy and told me how great it was to finally meet me, which tickled me down to my painted "Ride Me Red" toenails! She reads my column on royal occasion and I consider her the Queen, honey!

Last week's trip to traffic court proved amusing. One guy, clad in a bright orange parka and a cornrow hair-don't, described his entire driving history before the judge and tried to connect the fact that the demise of his father had to do with his driving blunder. He was armed with a death certificate and multiple insurance records (for all other cars except the one he was driving, of course). Another fine specimen, wearing overalls and a pair of thongs on his feet, did his best to describe in copious detail why his car didn't have a rear license plate or working taillights. His reason being, he was in the hospital from another car accident and couldn't get it taken care of. He was supposedly on his way to get everything fixed when pulled over, but when the judge asked for proof that the repairs were made, he came up with a whole other story. Slam went the gavel and off he went to the stockade, or at least to pay his non-reduced bill. Another bloke informed the judge that "if I only knew that was a police car next to me, I'd never have made that turn!" Holy hobo on a hooker, people can have the IQ of a butt plug sometimes.

The Distinguished Deviant has moved on to Las Vegas to pursue his writing-slash-acting career and I miss him terribly. No longer do I shuffle into the kitchen each morning and smell my coffee brewing or a fresh pack of ciggies and my favorite chocolate lying on the table. I will forever long to see his handsome and lanky profile hovering over a stove full of meat and grease. No more are the visions of a two-inch long ash at the end of his cigarette as he bends to wash the dishes. Sigh. It's funny how some of the seemingly most disgusting things can become so endearing. We'll keep in touch, I know, and he'll forever be in my heart.

The Blue Sky Boy and his Southern Bella Donna came over for a night of divine intervention. It was a turbulent night and they calmed and soothed the Yum Yum Boy and me. We tried on fetish gear and Southern Bella Donna danced for us to the beat of the latest Johnny Cash CD. Quirky and sweet, and bathed in vodka, she tasted just like a Georgia peach. All I know is I want more more more and, of course, I'll get it.

This month the second annual Masturbate-a-Thon will be held at a local dungeon and depend on me to report all the sordid details! If I end up riding the Thrillhammer Orgazmatron, I will indeed be wearing the crown! You can take that to the bank, bucko.

Dear Mz. Conduct,

Over the last few months, I've gotten to know a local Dominatrix. We've played a little and She's done a pretty effective job of taking control of me. Currently we are seeing each other every few weeks, but we've talked about turning our relationship into a 24/7 one. The thing She's made clear is that, in a long term 24/7 relationship with me, She would want to have me castrated and me be her eunuch. I have mixed emotions about this, but have not ruled it out. What do you think? Have I totally lost it?

Could Be Balless

> Dear CBB, Lost it? Not yet, mental midget man. Although it isn't just the balls on a man that make them one, I suggest that you seriously reconsider this option. I mean, aside from actually having the surgery, the pain of recovery and the hormonal disruption, what happens when She is tired of you and/or decides that She wants to move to Venezuela to grow coffee and leave you with the house payments, hmmm? Think about it long and hard (ahhh, now there's a vision), and whatever you're in search of, this is not the answer. Wieners on white bread, I'll hack 'em off myself if you don't grab yourself by those 'nads and realize how nuts this is. Okay, pun intended. You might consider a less radical alternative on the order of a chastity belt. They make some dandy models that render you effectively effectiveless. No harm, no foul, I always say. Now go away.

Dear Mz. Conduct,

I rather doubt you can help me, but as I do have a dilemma of sexual nature I'll submit it for your critique. Essentially it's that my girlfriend has just about the lowest sex drive of any woman I've ever known. We've been together for almost 2 years and she's been gradually losing interest in sex. This might be an even greater tragedy, but we are in an open relationship so I can at least have sex with friends or other agreeable persons. Unfortunately, the other people I sometimes copulate with have increasingly tended to live out of state or are getting into monogamous relationships of their own. That's just my own problem, but it has highlighted the infrequency to which my girlfriend has been a willing party. The problem is she only wants to have sex with me after we've gone to bed, and even then it would be fine, but she now has to spend sometimes almost an hour before we can even perform any act at all. Since I have to wake up early, sometimes I just pass out right before she's ready, which pisses her off in turn. It's just really frustrating she can't seem to get into a mood to have sex with me except when it's most inconvenient. The only other times she wants to have sex is if I have to leave her house to go do homework or something. Then she seems to suddenly develop a desire to fuck me, exactly when I can't again. She admits this is a problem, but can't arrive at a solution. Anyway, that's a rather poor excuse for a sequel quandary, seeing as how I am free to indulge in other arenas. Do let me know if you're aware of any scheme that might assist me.

Befuddled.

Dear B,

Two years is a very long time to be sexually frustrated with the one you choose to be with. I'm not sure if you deserve a medal or a smack in the head. I would first learn if she's on any sort of medication, as that would be a definite source. There are all sorts of meds that interfere with one's libido and if that's the case, you could work with her on seeing if her doctor could substitute another that would work as well but with lesser side effects. Secondly, if that isn't the scenario then I would probably just ease out of the relationship altogether because continuing it as it is will just drive you into a frantic frenzy and do either of you no good in the long run. It's so important to make sure that the person you're committed to has an equal sex drive. Move on and find a girl that will be ready for your rod whenever you are. You have plenty of material to pick from, or so it sounds. Also, diet, drugs and alcohol play a part as well and maybe that's an area to think about in your relationship. So, Einstein, experiment and see what unfolds!

Good Advice from a Very Bad Girl

"Generally, by the time you are Real, most of your hair has been loved off, and your eyes drop out and you get loose in the joints and very shabby. But these things don't matter at all, because once you are Real you can't be ugly, except to people who don't understand."
–Margery Williams, The Velveteen Rabbit

I've been away for a smidgeon, but PLEASE, even I need a vacation sometimes! And take one, I did! I had a fabulous sojourn down to sunny California to visit my lawyer-to-be son, and the always headed for mischief, Royal Diva. First order of plan: my handsome son whirled me around the city like mad. We took in the orchid gardens, swilled martinis on sidewalk cafes, sunk our toes in the sandy beaches, visited a wild animal park where I was compelled to smooch several African deer. We crammed a lot into one wacky week: Thai food, a wine tasting, ostrich jerky, sushi, coastal drives, seal watching, surfer watching (yummy!), and hot tubbing under the stars. The next week, it was off with old fans/new friends. We shopped for arcane accessories in the splendidly sordid Hillcrest neighborhood, and absorbed the nightlife with luster, honey! Later, with a looming view over the sailboat-filled marina, I polished off a gigantic bucket of chubby clams with a lovely bottle of 2002 Macon white burgundy, at one of the swankiest seafood restaurants in town. Ooh la la! All courtesy of my new friends! It was heavenly, my darlin' ones!

Next, a jaunt up the coast for a visit with the Royal Diva. This did indeed bring a tad of tawdry trouble! She greeted me in tiara and towel. Flashing her fantastic smile, we hugged, kissed and laughed as we compared our past year shenanigans. It had been a warm drive, so I freshened up in her beautiful Spanish tiled bathroom, with the view of the ocean snatching my attention. Still awing over the ocean view, I walked out to the kitchen and was handed a to-die-for platter of homemade crab cakes, tabouli salad, salted pork kabobs, fresh asparagus, and of course, champagne! What a treat. After our feast, we cocktailed and yakked up the night. We wound down with more champagne, accompanied by fat, crimson strawberries, dipped in dark chocolate. Licking our fingers, we decided to stroll down Ocean Boulevard to have random discussions with strangers whom we thought needed to be graced with our presence.

Mz. Conduct's House of Sin

Our heels got the best of us, so we kicked 'em off and carried them down to the beach. The salt air sobered us, at least to the point where we truly appreciated the silhouette of the giant palms against the burnt orange sunset. Her Royalness and I ended up shedding most of our clothes, giggling and running around in the ebb of the tide. Only when a tour bus arrived, spilling out a band of circus freaks onto the darkening shore, did we decide to head for home. Whether or not that was really what we saw, no matter, the fact that we thought we saw it, was enough. Drifting hazily back home to the Spanish style villa, we immediately plopped into the royal bed together. Smack dab in the midst of an inebriated attempt to invent some newfangled sexual position, we fell asleep in a tangle of white sheets and brown limbs. The following day, that glorious California sun seemed to scream "wake up!" as it burned my face through the French doors that faced the sea. We caught sight of ourselves, seeped in non-glamorous naughtiness, and broke the morning silence with groundbreaking laughter. Headache or not, it was an exhilarating way to start the day!

So, voila, the Yum Yum Boy has redeemed himself in my eyes with major life changes, and so once again we are back at it, trying to make our mark in the Guinness Book of world records for sexual intercourse. It seems we can't live without each other's skin and spunk. There it is in a nutsack, and on goes the sexcapades of our passionate cartoon character romance!

After picking me up at the airport, the YYB tossed me into the back of his SUV for a welcome home romp, presenting me afterwards with gifts of silver and scents. Damn my delirious desires, I should leave town more often!

The YYB bought tickets to see Dr. Andrew Weil at the Wordstock festival, which was an interesting afternoon, as I'm onboard with the holistic health approach to life...okay, so excluding the ciggies and vino that is. Dr. Weil spoke about integrated medicine and working towards incorporating Chinese, herbal and alternative medicine into all western medicine. Amen to that philosophy!

Good Advice from a Very Bad Girl

Another evening, we had a drastically different experience as we headed downtown to the Old Church. Church of the Perversely Wonderful was more like it. Chuck Palahniuk, the author of *Fight Club*, was to read from his new book, *Haunted*. He's a twisted and brilliantly funny man! Chuck started the night off hovering over several large cardboard boxes that sat stacked beside him on his little stage. When everyone was finally seated and quiet, he opened each box and pulled out armfuls of ersatz, bloody, body parts. Tossing them into an anxious and exuberant audience, he explained that the severed limbs all had relevance to the story he was about to read. Well, ol' Chuck was hilariously entertaining...and right about the body part/story relation. So, after getting my book signed, the Yum Yum Boy and I forfeited our appetite for dinner that night. Instead, we decided on heading home to devour one another's still-attached body parts. Delish, baby!

I happily received a letter from our U.S. Troops informing me that they have been my loyal fans for a long time, and that shamelessly, their entire unit wishes to be spanked by me. Wow, you hunky, military boys...and to all the troops fighting in Iraq, may the Goddess of Guttersluts bless you all. Now get those firm fighting fannies back home so you can get what's coming to you!

The summer is upon us like a whore on a sailor, and the heat of the season is likely to sizzle in more ways than imaginable. The Transient Trollop receives foot massages from manatees, sun block now causes cancer, Michael Jackson is an innocent pedophile, and the Catholic Church has a nazi pope. See, one just never knows what will happen next! But it's life, it's convoluted, and it's altogether priceless!

Mz. Conduct,

Oh, how very unprofessional and [sic] embarrassing. Your title on your web page is misspelt.....mz conduct's house of sin not MZ CONDUCTZ'S ....I'm laughing out loud!

Sheila in Australia

Dear SIA,

Mz. Conduct's House of Sin

Simmer down, honey. Not only do people in glass houses need to be attractive enough not to offend their neighbors, but also they should not throw stones.

For your information, I was fortunate enough to have a fan build my web site, entirely gratis. Being that he's a very busy boy, my fix-it list and I are entirely at his mercy.

Hmmm, I smell a tinge of envy wafting my way, but envy is one of the seven deadly sins, and being that this is the House Of Sin...sin on Sheila!

Dear Mz. Conduct,

I'm a guy who is just starting to explore sex, kind of a late bloomer I guess at nineteen. My dad (who is single by the way) and I both read your column! I figured you could tell me the trick to make a woman have an orgasm when receiving oral sex. Please, what's the reliable method, Mz. Conduct?

Orally Challenged

Dear OC,

Ah, a curious, little neophyte. It sure is a shark infested gene pool, I swear! Okay, sweetie, the first thing you should know is that the biggest sex organ is between the ears, and when you play that organ well, the sweetest music pours out!

There is no sure-fire method to making a woman orgasm, in any case. Keep in mind that all women are different in every sense: erogenous zones, degrees of pleasure/pain, and fantasy aspects. This is your mission, if you choose to accept, to communicate in all the various ways before you decide to do the dive.

Although some women don't enjoy oral sex, and many don't orgasm this way, generally speaking, the women who have the most difficulty coming during cunnilingus are ones who are uneasy about their lovers poking around down there, or are maybe uptight about their vaginas. But if oral sex just makes a woman yawn and figure out her grocery list (rather than tremble in disgust), chances are that her inhibitions are not the problem.

So, let's move on to technique. First: do you have one? Do you tongue sexy parts of her body, slowly working your way down from her mouth to neck (neck is a big turn-on for me, triggers a direct line of thrill-throbbing down to the clit, but that's me), nipples to her belly, to her thighs and groin? Or do you plunge right down there as if she had the last apple to bob for in the contest? You've got to spend time caressing her pink parts, which will most likely help to put her in the mood even before the lick-fest begins. When you do go down on her, how do you use your tongue? Are you just thrusting it in and out, or are you making sure to gently kiss, lick, and nibble the inner labia and clit as well?

Pay attention to her moans, even ask if she likes what you're doing and where. Some men think it's a great show of their manly abilities to stiffen their tongues and flap it around in there like a dying flounder. In fact, it's a great show of being clueless. Listen to her response. Slow it down until you're in touch with what's actually going on. Ask her to show you, if you fumble at finding the spot that feels the best to her. Watching each other masturbate can be very telling as well.

I take it when you ran this subject by ol' dad, that he didn't have any answers. Here's hoping you both can look, listen and learn about the woman you're with. Lick on, boys!

Good Advice from a Very Bad Girl

"I've come here to be drugged, electrocuted and probed, not insulted!"
–Homer J. Simpson

I had the most fabulous birthday ever, one that I had waited my whole life for. It was one of those 'it's only in the movies' birthdays. After being treated to lobster and an '89 Merlot, by my son and his dad, The Yum Yum Boy surprised the panties right off me when I walked into my house. He had me cover my eyes, but my ears heard Billie Holiday (my icon of icons) on the CD player, and out of the corner of my no-peeking sight, I saw about eighty tea-light candles flickering throughout the entire house! I immediately smelled the fragrance of what turned out to be the freshly plucked petals of three-dozen crimson roses. They'd been carefully scattered in the warm running bathtub that awaited me. A rose and a card sat on top of the leopard skin toilet seat cover. He undressed me, sank me into my tub o' flowers, and gave me the card. After my heavenly bath, he dried me off and wrapped me in my black silk robe, and guided me to a little tower of delightful gifts, all creatively wrapped on the dining room table. Next to that was a swank swank bottle of '87 Bordeaux and another rose. After we swilled the luscious vino by candlelight, and I opened my presents—sheer and naughty faux leopard thigh highs, cobalt blue wine glasses, a beaded necklace and a coolest of cool wine opener—YYB steered me through the flickering light to the bedroom, which was veiled in sheer red fabric. My bare feet relished the softness of the velvet petal pathway as I was led to the boudoir, which had been screaming our names all evening. There sat two long stemmed red roses on my pillow, alongside a love letter and an amazing poem. I blubbered like a schoolgirl who just had her pigtails pulled and liked it too much. Wow, this is what (almost) every girl dreams of! My brother says he'd never score any points with his wife with a feat such as this, as his wife is allergic to every flower known to man, detests candlelight and doesn't drink an ounce. Okay, well, we each have our own romantic fantasies, whatever they may be, and it's more than commendable when a man remembers what they are. I just know that one of my romantic fantasies was definitely fulfilled that night and I showed my appreciation to the YYB about six ways to Friday, honey!

Mz. Conduct's House of Sin

The Lion King took me to see one of my author heroes, David Sedaris, who I hadn't seen since he gave a free reading at a bookstore courtyard, about seven years ago. Now, he was at one of the biggest venues in the city and tickets went for thirty bucks a pop! He, like me, writes about everyone he knows and loves. He is absolutely hysterical and a true inspiration. If you haven't heard him read his stories on NPR, then I truly recommend any one of his many books. He used to be a housecleaner, like moi, but now lives in France with his boyfriend, going to auctions and having fabulous dinner parties. Sigh…one day daahlings, one day!

The Yum Yum Boy and I took home the Voluptuous Bar Vamp the other night. She's a bartender at our favorite club and has been hankering to bang us both ever since the day we met her. We've flirted, we've teased, but never took her up on her unsaintly offers…until now! We consumed oodles of Sheep Dip scotch and ended up playing with candle wax and ice cubes. As we held ice cubes in our mouths and ran the cold comfort all over one another's flesh, we then dripped cobalt blue candle wax over our exact same splendid body parts, watching the unique configurations take hold in the remaining candlelight. All the while, the Dells sang so soulfully "Oh What a Night." Indeed!

I was canoodling wickedly with my baby the other night, romping like thunder, and exploding my juices from here to eternity, when in a fit of maniacal bliss I reached above my head for support and promptly put my entire hand right through the window! Shards of glass flew everywhere and when my yummy boy stopped banging me long enough to exclaim, "Christ, honey, are you okay?" I wrapped my shredded hand in my skirt (conveniently at my head), and spit out, "I'm fine, don't you dare stop, mister!" We'll eventually fix the window, and my wounds will heal, but I'll have the sacred scars forever!

The Transient Trollop sent me a care package containing a disgusting, yet hilarious snack (what them folks eat in the southern parts of the states), a lovely can of, get this, hog brains and milk gravy! There's even a little picture of the concoction on the label. I put it in my Tiki-themed kitchen just to throw things off a bit. I should mention that she and her precious 'apple that didn't fall far from the tree' daughter also sent me a red vinyl and lace thong which looks great on, especially while holding the can of hog brains and milk gravy! Smooches to my girls!

Fret Boy and his fab gal pal came over and watched some really bad porn with us the other night. So bad that we had to turn it off! I'm sorry, but badly operated-on trannys just don't pull off the real deal. One tip: if you're going for the change and are going to be on film, save your pennies and get a decent job done! Of course, Fret Boy's microwaved cheese snacks may have contributed to the nausea, but who knows?

> Dear Mz. Conduct,
>
> Several months ago, I started chatting with a woman online. After a while we got onto the subject of cock size. I told her that I was 5 inches. She told me that I was too small. The other day, we chatted again, but she did not remember the cock size conversation. She did mention that her standard was about 7 inches and thick.
>
> So, now she wants to meet. I'm wondering if I should remind her of my size beforehand, or just let her find out for herself. The worst that will happen is that she won't let me have sex with her. I know I'm small so I can deal with that.
>
> What do you think?
>
> Small Fry
>
>> **Dear SF,**
>>
>> You seem to be obsessed with your premature penis and who knows, if I was a man, I might be too, but let people know you, and don't worry about reminding this woman about it. As you said, she'll find out herself and if and when she pulls your appendage out of your shorts and suddenly has a hankering for cocktail sausages, then so be it. Besides, small schlongs can be dreamy for booty sex! If she complains about your size, then bend her over and drive that wee weenie in her little pink pucker. Yes, some of us love anal sex too, honey, and there is more to a man besides the size of his cock…really! Be careful, your obsession will drive her away if nothing else.
>
> Dear Mz. Conduct,
>
> Your column makes my head spin, stomach flip, and blood boil! I crave your type of decadence, but I have no idea where to start looking for girls like you. How does a neophyte enter the world you live in? I must be discreet because of my job, and I'm very shy. Please advise me.
>
> Yours,
>
> Wanting More
>
>> **Dear WM,**
>>
>> Unfortunately, there aren't many girls like me in this world, and the shy boys rarely conquer us delectably decadent. You could try some of the Yahoo sites

or the polyamory sites like my friend's site, www.darklady.com. I've found quite a number of salaciously suitable folks included in these clubs and you can be as assured that you may be as discreet as necessary.

Dear Mz. Conduct,

Do you think that age matters when it comes to true love? I am significantly older than my girlfriend and people give us crap all the time. We're really happy, but it drives me crazy sometimes.

Geezer

> **Dear G,**
>
> Put your dentures in a drawer and gum that pink taco all the way to Mexico and back, baby! I have one short answer: hell no, age doesn't matter! I am in the same boat myself, always have been actually, just love those young-uns myself, as they're the only ones with enough stamina for me. See also: Chrissie Hynde and her husband who have a fourteen-year age difference between them. See also: Susan Sarandon and Tim Robbins who are twenty-years apart and have been together for what seems forever. It's not often you hear of such long lasting relationships, especially in the world of celebrities! Apart from the fame filled world, my dear friends, the Little Princess and her man, have a match made in heaven (at least in my little black book), and he's nineteen years her senior. So there! If ya have to pop a Viagra, then so be it! Goddess of Guttersluts, bless those little blue pills! People can be trite and focus on the trivial sometimes and maybe it's because they've never found what you have. You just keep rockin' on, grandpa, and put the meaningless critiquing where it should be…in a dumpster with all the mutated chicken parts behind a Kentucky Fried Chicken!

Good Advice from a Very Bad Girl

"They sharpen their knives on my mistakes."
–Tom Waits

Lately, I've been thinking of aging and the things that we (hopefully) learn along our life's journey. I am heading towards my fifth decade on this earth and noticing changes in my views, my body and even within my soul. The other day, I was rehashing the days of old, over the telephone and Bloody Marys, with the Transient Trollop. We remembered what a wild and wicked Gutterslut I truly was in my twenties. I was downright malicious deliciousness at it's best, or worst, depending on how you look at it.

When I first met the Transient Trollop, she and I were living in the same funky 1920's-built apartment in a shabby chic part of town. The T.T. shared a place on the fourth floor with a jealous lesbian lover, and I had just moved in to a place on the third floor. One evening I was attempting to entertain two boys who had stopped by with a housewarming gift and several bottles of wine. Suddenly realizing I had no wine opener, I remembered saying hello to the big, blonde that lived upstairs, so I ran up to see if she had an opener to borrow. When I knocked on her door, she hollered, "Entrez vous!" and was sitting in the middle of her living room floor with a two-foot bong in her hand. I looked at her and spouted saucily, "Somehow I know you must have a wine opener!" She let out her big booming laugh and confirmed my suspicions with a selection of three different kinds. I thanked her, explaining that I had two boys waiting and had to scoot. She blurted that if I ever had any extra boys, to let her know, although she would have to live vicariously through me because of her jealous girlfriend. We chuckled over that, and I grabbed a wine opener and headed back to my apartment…and the boys with the wine. Right then, I knew the Transient Trollop and I would be friends. That was sixteen years ago and we're still bosom buddies and thinking that forming an Old Lesbian's Club may be a good idea. We'll drink vodka and whisky from paper cups and wear our fuzzy house slippers and wee-small outfits that we really can't get away with anymore, and smoke ciggies and talk about what dolts and disappointments men really are. It's funny…the older I get, the mention of this fantasy club sure seems to gather more and more women who say, "Sign me up, honey!"

That apartment building held so many slutty, fun and deviant memories. I had forgotten about the TT living vicariously, so as she kept pointing out different boys in the building that I was certain to bed, I would shoo-shoo it off without a second thought. As time went on though I realized that she was right on the money with each suggestion.

I remember one afternoon, I was home cutting, ratting and dying my hair (it was the eighties after all), when the Transient Trollop called me on the phone to inform me of a hot young thang who was moving in right across the hall from me. She said I had better jump on that a.s.a.p. ! She said she had just ridden the elevator up with him and how she caught sight of his stomach when he stretched and "WEEEEEEEEE HA!" Too funny...and tempting.

Pondering the thought of his six-pack, I decided to go be neighborly, say hello and get a look for myself. She was right...he was deliciously distracting. I invited him over for a cocktail and he came knocking on my door just a few hours later. We had a fine get-to-know-you hour before our lips were locked and we were dry humping hot and heavy. He stopped suddenly to make a confession. He had a girlfriend in another city. Well, I had had about enough of jealous girlfriends, and honestly being 'the other woman' at that time in my life was no longer an option. So I told the beautiful boy that I appreciated his honesty, but we'd have to be just neighbors, and sent him home.

Three days later the boy knocked on my door again. Shyly, he mumbled that he just wanted to let me know that he broke up with his girlfriend. With eyebrows raised and a wicked smile brewing, I grabbed his hand and anxiously said, "Well, then, come on in, sweetie!"

We went at it like wild dogs on the fourth of July and afterwards he spoke (always a shame), to say, "Wow, sex can be weird" and I lifted my head from the

Good Advice from a Very Bad Girl

end of the bed, and remotely interested asked, "What does that mean, baby?" The boy replied, "Well, I've only had sex with one other girl in my whole life" in which I half heartedly and jokingly said "Well, me too." He gazed down at me with a sated smile and whispered, "Really?" and I so eloquently spewed "Oh, hell no, I was only kidding!" Well, the look on his sweet face just told me I should throw myself in the middle of the interstate and call it a day. That poor boy, I was such a bitchy little thing. Funny though, how he kept coming back for more...that is until he saw me entwined at a nightclub with another boy. I guess he decided he really couldn't deal with a wild woman like me. Besides, I think his parents sent him off to college.

So many concupiscent (hangovers and hood rings, I love that word) stories that conjure up from my past, but more of them next time, dear readers! In the meantime, stay true to your self and be sure to use and cherish each of your experiences as a lesson in this convoluted thing called life.

> Dear Mz. Conduct,
>
> Yet another call to duty for your honest and pragmatic mind.
>
> I am a straight guy, 34, professional, with conservative views on business and family while maintaining liberal social views. My girlfriend of six months and I have begun to get fairly serious. She is highly intelligent, very mature for her 24 years and voices conservative views in all aspects of life.
>
> We've waited 4 months before having sex. Recently we disclosed to each other the number of sexual partners we've had in our lifetime. Basically, she has slept with 51 guys, all after she was 19, and most of them were in her years at college.
>
> I'm no angel. Having sex for the first time at 16, I've slept with 36 girls in all. As a result of this knowledge I have been disturbed on some levels.
>
> One: I've always thought I wanted a virtuous girl to marry. The reality, though, is that I also need someone who is desirous, skilled and imaginative in the bedroom (or elsewhere.) Regardless, thinking of her with so many people triggers conflicting emotions. I find myself thinking about it quite often and even envisioning her exploits when we have sex. The weird thing is that these thoughts also turn me on.
>
> Two: I also dread meeting or running into any of her ex-partners at some college reunion or just out somewhere. I want to feel special with her, but my most important concern revolves around trust, commitment and discipline. I respect that she's been honest, when she could have easily lied, but I worry that if we have bad times, which is inevitable, she will want to seek comfort in another's arms.
>
> So Mz. Conduct, two questions...do I have anything to worry about with this girl, and if so, how would you address the issue without attacking her self-esteem or her?
>
> Hope you can help.

Mz. Conduct's House of Sin

Twisted about a Tart

Dear TaaT,

Okay, the first thing I'm tempted to say is, "just get over it, Boo Hoo Boy!", however, I happen to know first hand that it's a lot harder than that. I consulted the Yum Yum Boy on this matter, as he and I have had similar concerns. This is what he said, "You just gradually build trust with your partner and over time you find a way to put the disturbing thoughts in a place where they don't jeopardize your relationship. Don't sabotage the good thing you have now with dwelling on the past, it's just that, the past!" And I agree with him.

It sounds like you may be a bit anal-retentive with all things in your life, but this is one area you must be careful with. Decide if this is something that will always bother you, and if so, is it something you can work on and eventually let go of. If not, then call it quits right now, because she doesn't need to be reminded of a perfectly understandable, sexually abundant past just because you can't handle it.

Focus on the present and don't worry about the 'what if' in life, it's just wasted energy! You make each other happy now, build from there, and remember that virtue comes in many forms, honey!

Good Advice from a Very Bad Girl

Just as she was about to speak, there was a knock on the door. It was Sister Kimi, the dessert nun. "I thought you'd all like some sweets," said the adorable nun, pushing a tray filled with mouth-watering cookies and cakes. Cherry noticed she was wearing a habit that came to well above her shapely knees.
–Excerpt from *Mabel Maney's** The Case of the Not-So-Nice Nurse

When I was at the public library looking for a quick summer read and stumbled upon the aforementioned book title, I snapped it up with a devious smile. The back cover told of: two of America's greatest girl detectives as lovers, organza cocktail dresses with shoes to match, lesbians, and a conglomerate of nuns and evil priests. I felt overly obliged to check it out. (You see, I was a young, bossy girl, wannabe detective myself, with a group of neighbor kids who I easily molded into forming a club called, 'The Spy Guys'. Years later, I was sent away for an overactive imagination and raised by wicked nuns in an all-girl institution.) So, justifying my curiosity with the book in hand, I curled up on the lawn chair with a fruity cocktail, and read the whole thing. I giggled and snickered until I almost peed my non-existent under-panties! I'm going back to the library and get everything else Mabel Maney has written! This book is for all of you, fellow-recovering Catholics, who have a twisted and cheesy appreciation for a truly gay adventure! Mabel Maney is truly the Queen of queer hysterics!

Aside from the summer reads, Frisbee in the park (my ancient dog almost had a heart attack), and an occasional river trip, the Yum Yum Boy and I were fortunate to get a house sitting gig across town at a swanky hillside home. The global warming ordeal is working overtime here in the Northwest, so it's been sweltering. Needless to say, we were more than anxious to stay at this shaded home complete with wet bar and fabulous swimming pool. The first night there we realized that the pool seemed totally secluded, surrounded by thirty-foot pine trees. After evening cocktails and crab salad, inhaling the pine and herb of the night, we stripped each other naked and dove into the cobalt light of the pool. We always have a blast having sex under water, but this time it was better. The Yum Yum Boy grabbed my hips and held me up to his turgid tubesteak. For almost an hour he reminded us both that life is what you make it! The next night though, a thirty-something couple from next door stopped by to introduce themselves. With a subtle hint of sarcasm in her voice, the voluptuous woman said, "We heard you two by the pool last night and knowing the mundane people that live here, we realized the 'house sitters' had surely come." I started laughing, blurting out, "Oh, about a dozen times!" We instantly made new friends that night and shared the poolside. It was a great escape indeed.

When the Royal Diva escaped from the Northwest, she landed a weekly gig at Club Ripples in Long Beach, and is giving the drag queens a run for their money. She's getting monstrous tips from one certain gentleman each week, deservingly so, and gathered much enthusiastic appreciation by all of her fans. Since she's moved south, we have our cocktail hour by phone now, which is uniquely fabulous, as are we dahhlings! You can listen to her seductively sultry voice now, each weekday morning, from anywhere online, as she introduces an array of jazz tunes at the Long Beach radio station, KKJZ (http://www.jazzandblues.org/). When she plays Nina Simone, baby, I always know it's for me!

Another dear friend, who'd moved down south, graced me with a surprise call and visit this month. It was no other than the Distinguished Deviant! We met downtown at the club where the Yum Yum Boy works, then meandered over to our favorite strip club, the Peeled Onion. The night was hot and the girls were hotter! One dancer did her infamous fire dance, swinging long chains that held pots of fire like nobody's business! The smell of the kerosene and the way she moved made me light headed in ways that could only mean trouble. We invited her to our table after the show and I interviewed her for an article I was working on. At the end of the half hour, the YYB and the Distinguished Deviant each kissed her cheek, but I kissed a nipple…with her permission of course. All the way home I had to listen to the boys complain that life isn't fair. Hmmm, seems fair to me!

Good Advice from a Very Bad Girl

Donkey Boy, with his pooch in tow, came by for a 'little visit' recently, which turned into a night of debauchery, drinks, and draw poker. He wanted to make my computer sail like a cruise ship, and that he did, but my neighbor girlie came strutting over in her next-to-nothin' attire and quickly swept his attentions away from booting up to booty. I made a fresh batch of Strawberry lemonade with fresh mint from the garden. Okay, so I tossed in a bottle of vodka too. Donkey Boy and my neighbor girlie were hitting it off just dandy, when suddenly a stroke of exhibitionism hit the Yum Yum Boy. We wrestled around in the grass and soon showed them both what pornstars we truly are! After the batch of lemonade was gone, along with most of my memory cells, we all ended up in a heap on the lawn. With only the flicker of the citronella candlesticks—sporadically placed in the grass – there snoozed four snoring bodies, mingled and sated, in the hot August night. A marriage of bliss.

Speaking of marriage, boy, did the wedding bells ring this summer! Ding, dong, the single life is dead! I guess though it's all in the perspective…and the person you marry. Sometimes you marry the wrong people, however, I know in my heart that all my dear friends have chosen wisely, and will hopefully have an amazing and long life together. The Blue Sky Boy married his Southern Bella Donna, Mister Bo Dangles hitched his Ruby Girl, and Brain Boy and Cocoa Bean finally caved. Warm and fuzzy congratulations to all of my darling, daring friends! Now, with all that happy horseshit out of the way, I think I'll go marry my lips to that Yum Yum foreskin that lays in wait in my bed.

Dear Mz. Conduct,

I'm a long-time fan and think you rock! I have a question that I hope isn't silly, I'm a woman with knowledge where/how/of my G-spot. What I was wondering is, does the G actually stands for something?

Gigi

> **Dear G,**
>
> **Gee, Gigi, what I was wondering was, just how many times one can use the letter G in a G-spot question?**
>
> Okay, I'm just being flippant. The G in G-spot surely does stand for something. It stands for Grafenberg, a man (gee!), who basically discovered the spot. Here's the scoop: Masters and Johnson stomped on Freud's idea when they declared all female orgasms to be clitoral. Yeah, they were a bit off the mark

there. Somewhere around 1950, a German physician named Ernest Grafenberg—who decades before had developed the "Grafenberg ring", a primitive type of IUD—took notice of the urethra and what it had to do with an orgasm. No one paid any attention, the fools! Really, only in the last few years have a bunch of headstrong researchers totally invaded the medical and popular literature with their new discovery of this old and marvelous one. Whether the actual spot exists is still debated, and that just gets me…right in the G-Spot!

Dear Mz. Conduct,

How do I get my boyfriend to give me oral sex? I've been dating him only three months, but he says he's just not into it and I'm getting very frustrated now. I, by the way, make sure all his needs are filled! I feel like I'm becoming bitchier towards him now, and in someway resent him deep inside. What should I do?

Waiting in Washington

Dear WiW,

You should probably turn into Brazen Bitch, smother him with your cape and fly away! Let me tell you, he's not going to wake up one morning with some epiphany that'll compel him to launch his face between your legs and love it. Not going to happen. Ever! I imagine that some women can live without having their vaginas worshipped, but I am not one of them, and I doubt that you are either. Move on, he's not worth it. And however long it takes for you to change into your Brazen Bitch costume…in the meantime, don't you dare smooch that snake of his! I'm sick of all these women who whine about not getting what they want in bed yet they give the other person everything. Ugh! Now, I need an Ibuprofen and a cocktail!

*A special thank you to Mister R. who so kindly paid for my writings to remain on the Authors Den site www.authorsdenden.com for another year! Smooches to you, baby!

Good Advice from a Very Bad Girl

"The prettiest dresses are worn to be taken off."
–Jean Cocteau

A transformation of slutty feminist power has hit me like a brick in the butt. In my attempt to survive, I have considered (and been offered) a wide array of jobs in the sex industry. I've come to realize that I am not a prostitute in the general sense. Sure, with my phone sex job, I'm a voice whore, but I've found that it's damn near impossible for me to be blinded by money enough to perform sexual acts with someone I am not attracted to. Although I admire the women that can do this, and I definitely have a certain respect for them when their full self esteem is in place, I'm not one of them. The fact that they can control their duality as a sex worker is amazingly fantastic.

My latest endeavor as a topless housecleaner has proved to be part play and part work. It's interesting to me how many men feel powerful to have a bare breasted char girl come and clean what really isn't dirty. They watch me lustfully, as I bend over in my heels and skirt, and wipe invisible crumbs from their counter. It's not so bad to share the knowledge that they can never touch me, only themselves, and feather dust my way through their wifeless homes for an hour or two every now and then. I do feel the need to do a good job at whatever I do, and if the customer is happy when I leave, I'm satisfied too. So, I'm a voice whore and a dust whore...but I'm in control. I can live with that.

Last night unveiled another sick puppy on the phone sex line. Watching mommy in the shower is one thing, but when you want her to show you the inside of her vagina, that calls for a dip in a bucket of steamy feces, a straightjacket and a swarm of bees. Gumby in a gasmask, I so wanted to hang up, but it was such a long damn call and well, a girl needs her rent money. After that call came a voice note saying that the next caller wanted a virgin. All I said was, "Hey there, how are you tonight?" and they hung up. Apparently I can't even pull off a virginal 'hello, howd ya do!'

Mz. Conduct's House of Sin

My roommate, the Distinguished Deviant, remains fab! I get up in the morning, my coffee is made, the dishes are done and the lawn is mowed. Can't beat that with a single-tail whip. Of course, he adores me and we feel as if we've known each other forever. The Distinguished Deviant swilled his Pabst Blue Ribbon and lit a ciggie as he prepared to meet his starving artist comrades at the Loiter's Lounge. I fixed his rumpled tie and smoothed down his collar. It's like we're an old married couple already.

Greedgirl had a birthday bash the other night. The night was sweltering, balmy and mystifyingly dark, with the renaissance of a new moon in the sky. I dragged the Distinguished Deviant, the Yum Yum Boy, and myself (all scantily clad) to the big Victorian house. It was her royal princess-on-a-pillow party after all. Greedgirl sauntered down the winding staircase, making a princess-like entrance in her black, leather corset, sheer, purple, ballerina skirt, pink please-me heels, and her tiara...of course! Scads of cocktails and adoration were had by all and the haunting voice of Aimee Mann in the background made for a seductively sultry evening. We girls admired and kissed each other's nipples and worshipped the beauty of the boys we brought. Greedgirl gift-opening-time revealed her squeals of delight as she opened chocolates, books, make-up bag, pink leather flogger, and all sorts of princess purrrfect presents. One of my gifts to her was a snatch-shaped, strawberry and champagne scented bar of soap. So dirty, yet so clean!

The Yum Yum boy and I had big fun all over town, from drinking every alcoholic beverage known to man, guitar shopping, sand castle shows, watching *Harold and Maude* and *True Romance*, digging through old magazines at an ancient little bookstore, to making out in every public place imaginable. While walking in the sun, all over the city, we waved at the horse drawn carriage full of kids. They screamed that they liked the Yum Yum Boy's hat and my wild dress. We decided that we make a wild and beautiful couple. He's graced me with the most romantic of gifts: a cobalt blue hand blown water pipe, a two-page poem that made me cry a freakin' river, and two dozen mega fragrant roses. And nobody, and I mean nobody, has ridden Mz. Conduct—and Goddess of Guttersluts knows, there's been a zillion—like that cowboy. We are swirling in absolute naughty bliss and wankers on a Wheat Thin, I'm hankering for it!

Dear Mz. Conduct,

My husband and I have been married for over ten years. We have two children together and it seems our entire married life has revolved around them. Lately, my husband and I seem to be arguing all the time and snapping at each other in front of the kids. I don't have any clue why all of a sudden this is happening. I know you'll ask about our sex life, and I think it's okay, but we're both so tired at the end of the day that we just don't get around to it more than once a week. I want to make things better. Where should I start?

Southern Snapper

> Dear SS,
>
> A decade of raising kids can be taxing, I know, but you absolutely have to make sexual time for your marriage to survive. Be creative, and do what floats your libido boat, whether it's a romantic weekend alone at the beach or role-playing hooker and john night at a trashy motel or whatever. You both have to sit down and hash it out.
>
> There may be suppressed anxieties within both of your worlds, which neither of you want to bring up, even to yourselves. When you ask your husband why he thinks this sudden bickering is surfacing, really listen to what he's saying. Try to read between the lines as well, but be careful not to read too deeply, as you don't want to read things that aren't there. Be sure not to bring up the past and stay in the moment and be careful of what words you use. You don't want to lay blame, but you do want to solve this, so agree that you want to find a solution and work on it until you do.
>
> Sex is extremely important to connect with your loved one. It's not just the prolonged penetration...pumping, writhing, sweaty, hot bodies tangled into a pool of inordinate lust...lord love a lap-dance, I'm drifting off into reverie, sorry...but the intimacy of touch is also an important connection. After a long day, it's hard to instigate a wild romp in the sack if you're both exhausted. I've been in similar situations. To solve it, I would slip a note to my partner to meet me in the garage in 15 minutes. My man and I would scuttle our way through the power tools and cobwebs and climb each other like monkeys in a mosh pit. The sheer spontaneity and need for stress release made our sporadic sex all that much better. Mommy and daddy can take showers together once in awhile too. That soap on a rope never looks better than when wrapped around a pair of slippery, wet, ankles, honey. My point is, talk about how you will solve this situation and then follow through with it...all the way to heaven and back. Now, thank you very much, I'm as moist as a snack cake and worked up with esoteric escapades to spring on my own boy!

Dear Mz. Conduct,

Let me ask you this: If a guy comes over to my apartment for the first time and he adamantly doesn't want to pet my beloved cats, not because he's allergic, but because he simply doesn't like them, should I ever let him pet my real pussy?

Befuddled Barbara

Mz. Conduct's House of Sin

Dear BB,

Garfield in a garter belt, you're freakin' looney! On the other hand, I have to admit that if a boy I invite over and he doesn't like my dogs, it does clue me in to some negative things.

Sheesh, there is a human factor involved here and non-animal lovers are hard for me to understand personally. You can compromise though. A suitor can at least pat a critter on the head and eke out a bit of respect for your love for the beast and you can try to respect the suitor's indifference to the varmints and not make a big damn deal about it. If you can get by with him not smooching your feline friends and only slathering your koochie kitty with love then so be it. Purrrr where it counts.

Good Advice from a Very Bad Girl

"The piano has been drinking, not me, not me."
–Tom Waits

For my birthday, as a gift to myself, I've been weeding out the negative energies in my life and replacing them with all things new, untried, and positively positive. In that vein, I replaced my strap-on harness with the best leather one available, the double-headed dildo I gave away years ago for a wedding present, and all the patiently awaiting boys and girls out there waiting for me to be emotionally available once again. I'm back in true form, and damn if it doesn't feel fabulous.

Now, the weeding out process is just that. The dating scene is still and always what it was, unfortunately, but one must put on the garden gloves and trudge through the manure in order to find the blossoms that inevitably appear in spring. And it is spring after all!

My latest experiences with dating have tossed me a sad, soggy salad. I've gone out with men who felt guilty, men I intimidated, a guy who ran and threw up in a mid make-out session (too much liquor involved apparently), another who I lowered my standards for just to get laid—this one was compelled to take 'breaks' all night in order to keep up with me—I had a conniption fit and threw him out. One guy passionately talked about blowing up supermarkets all evening, and another bragged about his giant manhood, in which case I had no desire to view it after that. I felt as if I were in the frog jump Olympics, I swear. Then I found a prince! This beautiful punk prince rescued me from a horrible date I was on, found me the next day, wrote me erotica, and proceeded to bang me like a cheap screen door. Our second date was headed for the same slice of heaven until I completely screwed that, and every other date that may have followed, right out the door. Earlier, on the evening of our second date, I was on a business date with a lovely gentleman who fed me steamed clams, cioppino, and as much '96 Valpolicella that can be humanly consumed. I lost track of time and was hours late getting to the beautiful boy's house, as previously planned. Once dropped home by my business date, and blissfully inebriated, I called the boy to blather an apology, and explain my non-driving demented state. He graciously decided to take a taxi over anyway. Yay! Yeah, that was short lived, as only shortly after the beautiful boy's arrival, my ex-boyfriend started phoning repeatedly, trying to profess his undying lust in some drunken stupor. I finally turned off the phone, but the damage was done. If roles were reversed I would have been long gone, but he hung in there another night giving me unlimited orgasmic pleasure…for the last time. I can be such a nightmare, but my behavior shows me that I am only ready for me right now, and learn I shall from my actions, as we all should.

Two nights later, throbbing with lascivious thoughts, I decided to grab the bull by the horns, or the bull by his horny thorn. I called up the Tiki Trouble Lounge and asked for the waiter I met on New Year's Eve. When he answered the phone I hadn't time to explain who I was, as he remembered me clearly. Imagine that! It so happened that the next night was his only night off, so I invited him out with Cocoa Bean and Heady Hubby and I. We all met at the Fast Bar; a very cool bar seeped in blue neon and tall, red leather booths. I found out he was twenty-three years old, Christ on a cheese ball, and asked if he knew how old I was. His suave reply was, "It doesn't matter," and I was in even more lust. We had oodles of cocktails and headed back to my place, where my loins got the best of me. I straddled the hot boy and gyrated intensely on his lap. Cocoa Bean had her video rolling the whole time, and being the exhibitionist that I am, it got me hotter still. Soon, everyone left at my insistence and the boy unleashed his ample, pierced member into my clubhouse…all night long.

After a whirlwind of local affairs, I packed my purple striped suitcase, and decided on a trip to the east coast to drum up some shameless self-promotion. My famous artist uncle was turning ninety and I was turning forty-nine, and what a fabulous celebration it was! My aunt put on a huge party with over one hundred fifty artists, writers, and designers of all sorts. I headed for the open bar and soon made a big splash (and not just in my vodka), promising my first book to more folks than I can remember. I met the black side of my family (and loved them all), got a condensed education on history and art, saw the ghetto of Philadelphia, owls in flight, reunited with cousins I hadn't seen in forty years, and met some adorable men in many cities. A truly amazing trip!

Now I'm headed to southern California for a spell to celebrate Cinco de Mayo, which I'm sure will produce more stories to tell on my return. I have many more trips planned as well, as this year is about the celebration.

A shout out to the Transient Trollop on landing the love of her life, the madly sane Rooftop Rebel. I will include a train trip to visit them in the near future, and absolutely positively whenever she and I get together, if we don't land our ample asses in jail on a life sentence, we will definitely have wild stories to share. Stay tuned!

Dear Mz. Conduct,
Somebody was discussing tantric yoga and tantric sex the other day after an art class. Being that I was in a social circle of a mixed crowd, and a forty-year old woman, I was too embarrassed to ask what that was exactly. The same people mentioned your site, so I thought I could ask you and remain anonymously ignorant. Thank you, and just so you know, I am going to read all of your columns in hope to become more sexually aware, especially at my age.
Flustered in Florence

> **Dear FiF,**
>
> Don't beat yourself up over not knowing what tantric sex is, self-mutilation is not healthy, honey!
>
> Ironically, I just took a class in introductory tantric sex, and although I didn't personally learn much I didn't already know, I can certainly share my knowledge. My own definition is that it's an ancient philosophy connecting your sexuality and spirit and liberating social and physical boundaries within. A book that was suggested in class, and it's a good one, is *Tantric Sex for Women* by Christa Shulte. She explains tantra as "the complete acceptance and weaving together of all our feelings (even the so-called negative ones), and the forging of creative bonds with other people. The word tantra means network, connection, web and expansion. It is a word from the language of weavers, representing the string that is pulled through all the warp strings, binding them together."
>
> You have seven chakras, and by being in touch with them and the colors they bring, you can have an orgasm without ejaculating (and this means women too!), and you can easily have an orgasm without being touched in any genital areas. I've had many orgasms by just kissing or even by having my neck or knees touched. It's amazingly hot. This is how one author explains chakras: The word chakra is Sanskrit for wheel or disk and signifies one of seven basic energy centers in the body. Each of these centers correlates to major nerve

ganglia branching forth from the spinal column. In addition the chakras also correlate to levels of consciousness, archetypal elements, developmental stages of life, colors, sounds, body functions, and much, much more. Below is a brief description of each chakra.

Chakra Seven:

Thought, Universal identity, oriented to self-knowledge

This is the crown chakra that relates to consciousness as pure awareness. It is our connection to the greater world beyond, to a timeless, spaceless place of all-knowing. When developed, this chakra brings us knowledge, wisdom, understanding, spiritual connection, and bliss.

Chakra Six:

Light, Archetypal identity, oriented to self-reflection

This chakra is known as the brow chakra or third eye center. It is related to the act of seeing, both physically and intuitively. As such it opens our psychic faculties and our understanding of archetypal levels. When healthy it allows us to see clearly, in effect, letting us "see the big picture."

Chakra Five:

Sound, Creative identity, oriented to self-expression

This is the chakra located in the throat and is thus related to communication and creativity. Here we experience the world symbolically through vibration, such as the vibration of sound representing language.

Chakra Four:

Air, Social identity, oriented to self-acceptance

This chakra is called the heart chakra and is the middle chakra in a system of seven. It is related to love and is the integrator of opposites in the psyche: mind and body, male and female, persona and shadow, ego and unity. A healthy fourth chakra allows us to love deeply, feel compassion, and have a deep sense of peace and centeredness.

Chakra Three:

Fire, Ego identity, oriented to self-definition

This chakra is known as the power chakra, located in the solar plexus. It rules our personal power, will, and autonomy, as well as our metabolism. When healthy, this chakra brings us energy, effectiveness, spontaneity, and non-dominating power.

Chakra Two:

Water, Emotional identity, oriented to self-gratification

The second chakra, located in the abdomen, lower back, and sexual organs, is related to the element water, and to emotions and sexuality. It connects us to others through feeling, desire, sensation, and movement. Ideally this chakra brings us fluidity and grace, depth of feeling, sexual fulfillment, and the ability to accept change.

Chakra One:

Earth, Physical identity, oriented to self-preservation

Located at the base of the spine, this chakra forms our foundation. It represents the element earth, and is therefore related to our survival instincts, and to our sense of grounding and connection to our bodies and the physical plane. Ideally this chakra brings us health, prosperity, security, and dynamic presence.

So, you see this is a complex topic, but hopefully this will help you understand tantra a bit more. I suggest you read *Red Hot Tantra* by David Ramsdale for more history on this subject and there is a decent blog spot online at http://tantric-sex.blogspot.com/ which may help as well. The *Kama Sutra*, although stimulating, is a translation from one man's view, so as not to be confused with the actual historic origin. Good luck and chakra on, baby!

Mz. Conduct's House of Sin

"Speak in French when you can't put together English, keep your toes out when you walk, and always remember just who you are."
–The Red Queen from Through the Looking Glass

Thank you to the fans who've contributed to the column, and especially to the Dark Prince of the Islands, for his ever-so-generous gift. The Goddess of Guttersluts blesses your big ol' heart.

Sometimes being able to have a full-fledged orgasm just from a make-out session can be a curse. This was the case when my Rockabilly man and I took in a late night movie at a local art theatre. It was a depressing French movie which, once we stopped reading subtitles, was lost to us. Well, for the most part. The music droned on but nevertheless, wrapped in sopping kisses, seemed to heat my blood to the boiling point. I lost it loudly while a Parisian woman cried over a dead lover on the screen. For some reason the rest of the audience was bothered by this. Embarrassed, or as much as it's possible for me to be, I composed myself, nodding weak apologies toward the disgusted heads in the dark. Only a few minutes passed when the theatre manager discreetly knelt next to us and asked us to leave. Holding in shallow bursts of laughter, we willingly smooched our way down the aisle and right out the door. C'est La Vie, baby!

In the midst of my week, I had a fan fly out from the East coast on business. He asked to meet me and take me to dinner. Mastication is always an option for this gobble-minded girl, so as requested, I made reservations at my favorite swanky seafood place. Mr. Fan of the East walked into the bar—where I sat swilling and swiveling on a leather-bound barstool—his eyes darted to my lips, then down the long stretch to my black, lace covered legs. A gigantic smile broadened his handsome face, and the scent of expensive cologne tickled my nose. He bent down and kissed my hand, an excuse to gaze at my legs once again. Men are not slick that way, but I didn't mind, I was starving.

The bartender carded me, and visibly startled, he proceeded to broadcast my year of birth like a winning lottery number. I don't really mind that either, so I

Good Advice from a Very Bad Girl

gave him my card. Next, Mr. Fan of the East and I feasted on buttery steamed clams, fried calamari, melt-in-your-mouth oysters on the half shell...and then of course, I ordered lobster. I ate ravenously and was told I sounded like I was having an orgasm. Ha, if he only knew! We had a fabulous Napa Valley Cabernet, which made everything go down like heaven...except me that is. There was one hitch in the evening; he is a married man, and I don't date married men. I did make clear from the start, but men seem to have selective hearing at times, feeling compelled to insert one more extravagant offer—thinking perhaps it will change my mind. Not a chance! Even a Gutterslut can have some morals, loosely based as they might be.

After our incredible dinner, I took him to the biggest bookstore in the city where we spent close to an hour looking at retro style reading glasses for me, and travel logs for him. Next stop, the fetish shop across the street. Mr. Married Fan of the East was hankering to investigate the contents of the store, as the corset-clad mannequin in the window had a devilishly inviting glow. This seemed to be a virgin experience for him, so I had big fun leading him around like a wide-eyed, little monkey. I explained leather ball gags (and how some folks think I should wear one always), portable lipstick vibrators, strap-on harnesses, clit stimulators, and nipple clamps. He was cute, blushing brightly as we walked back out into the night. Six blocks in the crispy fall night and we arrived at my car. I thanked him for a wonderful evening. Saying goodnight, I blatantly avoided the kiss he tried planting on my cherry red lips, but blew him a big one, as I shot off in my car singing along with Sublime's "Bad Fish".

On a similar note, The Yum Yum Boy and I have discovered after all we've trudged though in nearly four years, that we still have flames between us. A heat seemingly stronger than anything or anyone can extinguish. This made me ponder some points as I wandered down the presto log aisle of the grocery store. Can two people, who've passionately fornicated for years, cease and desist such an entanglement and remain just friends? Can we start over again, entwined, but in a whole different realm? Minus sex, and without extreme intimacy, will it be possible to put aside the obvious, ever-present passion, and focus only on a fundamental friendship, a friendship that was previously tucked beneath the waves of the ever-flowing bed sheets?

Is it fathomable to build a real kind of security and respect? And if so, could we hammer it in with nails of honest intent, plaster it smooth without fears, and freshly brush it with paint from all colors of the rainbow, as rainbows make up the natural balance, the sum of the rain and sun? Hmmm, so home from the grocery store and still ruminating, I suppose this will unfold as an experiment in the lives of two human fireballs...sweltering infernos continuing to burn, but this time, trying not to burn each other.

In the meantime, The Lion King takes me strip clubbing, pays my gym dues, and keeps me in business cards, The Yum Yum Boy just designed and built me a splendid coffee table, Mr. R pays for a writer's site, The Webmaster Extraordinaire takes care of my own site, Dan the Man writes poems about me for another site, and tonight I have a date with the Good Doctor, who with his benevolent heart, has insisted on feeding me Curry and Cabernet and helping me put my book together. Thanksgiving is an all year round holiday if one counts their blessings daily, and well...life as I know it, is good!

> Dear Mz. Conduct,
>
> I have a question that has been bothering me for some time now. I guess I'll get straight to the point. I work at a hip clothing label, and all the employees (and some people in the public) know that the boss is having sex with the female employees.
>
> When I learned this I was outraged, and so I asked around to fellow co-workers to see what they thought. Well I was shocked to find out that almost all the males were appalled, while the women seemed to think it was 'okay'.
>
> So, are my male friends and I just cock-blocking? Suffering from penis (or 'getting it') envy? What gives?
>
> Concerned Co-worker
>
>> **Dear CC,**
>>
>> I've been in your situation before, but I banged the busboy and got over it! While it's really never a great idea to sleep with people you work with, let alone the boss, it happens all the time.
>>
>> In my experience, sleeping with the boss usually means someone wants to benefit in some way. Giving the boss a rise in his Armani slacks may get you a raise in your pay. That behavior, in my opinion, just shows a lack of character and self-worth, and you apparently have yours intact.

As far as what your little survey reveals, I can only guess the women who are boss-boppin' are participating either because the boss is hotter than Georgia asphalt, they're looking for a promotion, or both. Your male co-workers are probably just pissed because they want him themselves, or their diminutive status hasn't won their female co-workers over in the past.

Who knows? Don't fret about what's going on under the boss' desk or the designer sheets, honey. When someone files a sexual harassment suit (and it's inevitable) because they're replaced in the sack with the new dressing room attendant, you'll be able to keep your overly dignified nose in the air and out of the silly hipster canoodling. Now go sell something.

Dear Mz. Conduct,

I need some advice concerning a good friend/man I see sexually from time to time. He has a submission fantasy and wants me to find someone dominant to use him. I am extremely submissive myself and he and I both know I don't want to switch roles.

I found someone through the personal ads, but she is a pre-op transsexual, and I wonder if that would be over the top (no pun intended!). He is straight and I don't know if it would be too much for him. By the way, he is the one that first ordered me to have sex with another woman, and now I love it! He's had dildos in his ass before, but when I told him I'd love to see him suck a cock, he says "No, it'll never happen!" but it's almost like a challenge the way he says it. Should I trick him with the TS or look for someone else to join us?

Gender Quested

> Dear GQ,
>
> If he's such a good friend, I think there needs to be more communication going on between you two. You shouldn't have to wonder exactly what he means or be guessing about things. If he's leaving it all up to you, you'll have to take some slice of a dominant role, reminding him that you subbed for him, and now it's his turn. I think the TS should also be informed of everything as well. It's only fair, my dear. If your friend is indeed leaving everything in your hands (as a trusting sub should), then bring on whatever you think will tickle his Elmo, be sure to make him pay the tab, and have fun!

Mz. Conduct's House of Sin

"Elegance has a bad effect on my constitution."
–Louisa May Alcott

The Georgia Peaches have rolled their fruity asses downtown and I now have two new roomies, Punk Girl, covered in tattoos from Bettie Page head to combat boot toe—with a pet Chihuahua that she dresses up in vampire costumes, and a quiet little bald boy whom I rarely see. They are truly fab, and will take over my house when I move to a smaller, more affordable place.

Punk Girl is visibly high energy and immediately upon meeting her, told me—all in one breath—that her Chihuahua had a penis mishap the other day. He was humping his whistling, stuffed gorilla toy (apparently a normal occurrence), and his penis grew extraordinarily huge and wouldn't retract. She called the veterinarian for advice and discovered a hair had lodged itself inside the sheath, making it unable to go back in. She had to lube it up manually until it finally shrunk back inside the wee critter. I knew right then I liked this girl!

Trying to move from a house full of kitschy clutter into a one bedroom apartment truly sucks, but I desperately need some change, and it doesn't include stressing over shut-off notices, roommate drama and how I'm going to eat. I was so frazzled one afternoon that without noticing, I spooned a can of dog food onto my nachos. Only after sticking the plate in the microwave, did I realize that the disgusting smell was what it was. Thank the Goddess of Guttersluts I didn't put that mess in my mouth! It was that very same morning after all, that I woke up at the buttcrack of dawn, and while running across the dining room to pee, I slid my bare foot promptly into a humungous pile of dog diarrhea. Christ on a crescent roll! I tried to blame it on the Chihuahua of course, but the pile was larger than the little dog itself and I knew the culprit must be my fat, old bitch of a mutt. It was an anomaly, and after using every expletive imaginable and simultaneously plugging my nose, I investigated the situation. I found that my roommate had given my dog about forty pounds of lentil soup the night before. It's safe to say that this will not happen again.

Good Advice from a Very Bad Girl

I was on the job at the phone sex emporium when the Yum Yum Boy came sauntering in the room. He was grinning and wearing the leather undies I bought him, obviously trying to make me lose my composure—or what little composure one must have to maintain a jack-off sermon. We decided to incorporate a little reality sex with the spiel. It was pretty hot, I must say, and as I was screaming for him to pound my perfect mound, Whack-Away Willy, who I had on the line, was pounding his hand. I truly think we all came together. Unity is such a nice thing to strive for, don't you think?

The Royal Diva has been canoodling around the greater part of town, celebrating her freedom from a wickedly insane husband. Her spirit has not been depleted (although her ex would have liked that, as would mine), but instead it's soaring, honey! We often yak about the importance of keeping one's spirit alive and strong and not letting anyone pull you down to their pathetic level. She has lots of irons in her career fire, and I predict that she will be one of the greatest jazz divas of the northwest...maybe the world! She already is, to me!

The Yum Yum Boy surprised me a few times this month. One night, he pulled from behind his sexy back, a giant bouquet of flowers, and you know how I love my flowers! Another evening, when we'd been running around like headless chickens all day and realized we hadn't eaten, he tossed me in the truck and drove me to a swanky, sultry Cajun restaurant, where we relaxed over a long, romantic dinner of smoked fish, linguine and red wine. We've decided that we are incredible porn stars at heart, and make movies in our heads while the reverse cowgirl rides and the pony does its buckin'.

The YYB and I attended a house-warming party, and nuns with nipple clamps, did we warm that house! Our hostess, a tawdry little tart with red curls and a voluptuous form, had been an acquaintance we'd known for a just a few months. She and I would jokingly discuss how her husband and my boy would be fun to tie down and dick-tease into a fiery frenzy. They had both been naughty boys in the past and we, the vicious vixens that we are, felt they needed some discipline. As the night wore on and the crowd died down, little

Mz. Conduct's House of Sin

Miss Hostess and I wrote stern notes on cocktail napkins, "Get your tight little buns in the master bedroom—ten minutes!" We clandestinely slipped the napkin notes to our stallions while they mingled with the inebriated musicians still in a drum circle in the yard. It gave us just enough time to get there ourselves and dress ourselves in disciplinary garb. I left my knee-high leather boots on and stripped down to my thong and bra. Miss Hostess opened her closet, pulled out a black corset and heels. We lit seven large candles above the bed and propped ourselves on the big, red pillows that sat against the headboard. We waited. Fifteen minutes had passed when the boys walked in the room, confused and titillated. I told them to close the door and lock it and Miss Hostess reprimanded them for being late. They just stood there, smiling like Cheshire cats.

That sweet evening, we made them crawl on all fours, tied them up with stockings, and tortured their desire with girl sex and tongue baths and wooden spoon spankings. After an hour or so of this manhandling mayhem, and wet to our knees, the four of us ended up in an aerobic pile of reckless abandon. The full moon was in Aries and raging through our blood. Hours later, exhausted, I blew out the candles and we all fell asleep wrapped in our bad boys' arms. Now those are memorable party pals!

> Dear Mz. Conduct,
>
> I just have one simple question. I don't seem to know the right thing to do when my girlfriend cries. To me, there is no reason for her outbursts, and when she tries for an explanation, I don't understand. I think I'm a fairly sensitive guy and want to understand. How can I feel her emotions more, or at least so I don't end up sleeping on the couch so much?
>
> Confused on the Couch
>
>> **Dear CotC,**
>>
>> Quit your fairly sensitive whining and read on. I once consulted my wildly wise friend, a Ph.D. in genetic research, on this very subject. He informed me, that basically, there is one male hormone: it is either off or it is on. In females, there are two hormones and they have a complex dance of cycles and rhythms.
>>
>> In general, for all systems, females have a two to one ratio of hormones controlling many aspects of physiology. Remember, with one hormone there are two states, with two hormones there are four, etc. So, Christ on a crumpet, the four basic female hormones make us girlies 16 times more complex! We can't help it, just as you can't help the way you are made up either.

Anyway you want to look at it, being a man, you're not in the winner's circle, honey. Men tend to think with their heads (both of them), and women think more with their hearts. Of course, there are always exceptions, but the hormones have their own agenda, bottomline. Biologically, there is no possible way you can ever feel what she does, but that doesn't mean you can't empathize. We women have to realize this fact too, and not expect our boys to know what we're feeling all the time.

If your girl is having extreme and continual outbursts that you can never at all comprehend, even with this information, there may be a hormonal imbalance, or even a hypoglycemic problem. Many things can be controlled with diet such as the latter. Blood sugar can be an evil entity, believe me! The Yum Yum Boy knows when I haven't eaten or when I'm about to bleed like a stuck piggy when I start bitching about the lint on the carpet, or I see a lost dog in the dark, and start blubbering like a newborn. The hormone war may not be fair, but it is what it is. When she turns on the faucet, you can choose to backpack your butt off into them thar hills, or if your balls are big enough, stick around and be supportive the best way you can.

You may be outnumbered in the hormonal department, mister, but you'll score points by biting the bullet, making an effort to listen and comfort. Why do so many men head to the nearest bar and suck the suds down until they're numb? They're wimp-ass mo fo's in my little black book. I'll just bet my double-headed dildo that if you super-hero it out with her tears, she'll be more apt to understand your needs, such as gluing yourself to the nearest televised football game with one hand down your pants and the other in a bag of chips. It's your choice, and may the force be with you!

Dear Mz. Conduct,

I overstepped my boundaries on a date with a women and she furiously sent me on my way. She's really hot and I wonder, is there any thing I can do to get a second chance with this woman?

Wolfman

> Dear W,
>
> Great gobs of gonads! You obviously know that you crossed certain boundaries with this woman, and yet you don't seem ashamed or the least bit apologetic, just intent on getting 'another chance.' In my opinion, you blew any future dates with this woman and should take a serious look inside your pathetic self. Perhaps you'll realize (but I doubt it), that when you disrespect someone and piss them off enough that they blatantly tell you where to go, that's exactly what they mean. At this point, you will not redeem yourself, you can only learn by your mistakes. Send the woman a huge bouquet of exotic flowers with the promise of suicide, and then go knock your head against the nearest brick wall, you sociopathic pig!

Mz. Conduct's House of Sin

"He who asks a question is a fool for five minutes; he who does not ask a question remains a fool forever."
–Chinese Proverb

This is a slight diversion from my regular format, but I am celebrating writing my 100th column. So, I'll do what I damn well please! I decided to yak about a night out in Portland, as I get many emails from fans that are coming to visit or moving to this gorgeous city, and thought this could promote (or not) some of the places I graced with my presence on a single evening.

The balmy afternoon started out on a salaciously sly note, as I slid my thighs into my black lace body stocking, my crepe babydoll dress and seven-inch red, wet leather heels. I was being taken out to dinner by a local celebrity whom I'd never met before. My new roommate (resembling a young Peter O'Toole) had been his comrade and each time Mr. Big Wig called our house, he would hear my voice on the message machine. Mr. Big Wig—whom I promised I wouldn't mention by name—was captivated by my voice and was hankering to meet me. He and my roommate had planned to go out for drinks and they invited me along. I agreed, but mentioned that dinner at Jake's Famous Crawfish Restaurant (401 SW 12th) would be more to my liking. Jake's is the oldest restaurant/bar in Portland and the place to go for seafood. The atmosphere is a slosh of casual—sophistication with dark wooden booths and white tablecloths. Dress is everything from jeans and a tee shirt to Armani suit attire. I love it there. Mr. Big Wig accepted my plan and so it was set. My roommate and I met Mr. Big Wig in the crowd of a swanky, air-conditioned bar at Jake's. Mr. Big Wig was evidently quite taken with me—by the grin on his face and the glass of Merlot that suddenly appeared on the shapely, blonde waitress' tray. He'd heard I liked a good Cabernet and Scott the bartender had recommended one. There it was, a fat glass of an Argentine Cabernet called Terra Rosa and it was delightfully yummy.

Our waiter turned out to be an old friend of Mr. Big Wig, so the service was impeccable. I wondered how much of an actual tightwad Mr. Big Wig was when I ordered my lobster, my roommate ordered the top sirloin, and Mr. Big Wig ordered the fish 'n' chips. C'est la vie. I apologized for lack of conversation as I tore into the heavenly crustacean and enjoyed every minute of it, along with two more glasses of the Terra Rosa and the best sourdough bread around. At one point, as Mr. Big Wig plowed into his own meal, he hoisted a gargantuan glob of fish 'n' chips on his equally large belly, without notice. I called his attention to it and, embarrassed a bit, tried to wipe it off with water from his finger bowl. Perhaps trying to impress me, he announced that his shirt was made of silk, and flustered with the mess on the mound in front of him.

After dinner, we parted our ways and my roommate and I headed over to one of his favorite writer's wine bar, the Aalto Lounge on 34th and SE Belmont. A comfortably eclectic cove with a smoking room and back patio strung with Christmas lights. We sat at a round table with two friends we ran into. We ordered red wine, an ever-so-luscious semi-dry red wine from Spain called Amezola, and swilled under the stars. We discussed erotic films, as one of our friends is a reviewer of such. When it came to going 'round the table, telling bad jokes, I suddenly realized that the night was still young and I felt the need for a little more excitement. I excused myself and called my Yum Yum Boy to meet me. Ten minutes later, looking like sin-on-a-stick, my boy saunters in, holds out his tattooed, muscled arm for me to grab, and we high-tailed it to the nearby Dot's Cafe (2521 SE Clinton).

Dot's is fun and funky, kitschy and cool, walls full of velvet Elvises and posters from old television shows like *The Man from U.N.C.L.E.* and *Dragnet*. It caters to a younger crowd, but not entirely. Anyone with an imagination and zest for life should appreciate the conglomerated clash of knick-knacks. And the food, ranging from huge, black bean burritos to the Vegan Deluxe (hummus, tomatoes, spinach and sauerkraut, slapped between dark rye bread, spread with tofu sauce and served warm) is amazingly delicious.

Mz. Conduct's House of Sin

Dot's has the biggest cocktails around—with the smallest price tags—and that's what we had our eyes on. After all, my belly was still full of luscious lobster. My favorite is the Gin 'n Juice, which consists of Beefeater gin, lemonade, grape juice, crushed ice and a maraschino cherry and served in a pint glass... and it's four bucks. Yeah baby! The couple playing pool (free pool, by the way) was ogling the two of us and we smiled back with devilish intent. We figured that the tall, red haired girl—with an ass to die for—and the punkish shaggy-haired boy were either wanting to play other games with us or counting the body piercings we had between us. Whatever. We asked them to join us for a drink and they did. We all had a few more rounds then decided to head over to Common Ground Hot Tubs (2927 NE Everett). The place is in a beautiful, old Victorian house. The tubs in an outdoor, dimly lit, vine covered backyard. The ambience was inviting. Common Ground is a co-ed place that respects the individual's right to privacy—albeit in a public place. In other words, the business doesn't promote sexual play, and in the dressing area, has a hand-painted sign saying just that. So, we all stripped down, showered, walked outside and slipped into a bubbling tub of chlorinated comfort. During our soak, our feet touched one another's and I think we heated up that tub up and over the maximum limit. Bubbles were everywhere. My Yum Yum Boy and I nuzzled each other and the other couple just watched in wanton lust. Good enough for that evening. Exchanging numbers, we went out separate ways with the promise of "another time" to come.

Next stop, dropping off a keg and tap from a party I had the previous weekend. We got it from The Ship in the quaint little Multnomah Village. Real assholes there. When we informed then that their tap was leaky when we got it and needed a seal, just to let them know for the next person's sake, the woman at the bar refused us part of our refund. She insisted that we were the ones that broke it. It may be a cute little bar, but their attitude needs a serious adjustment. I wouldn't buy a French fry from them now. That ship has sunk.

Later that evening, the UNTYD band, our dear friends, were playing at a new club. We headed over to the ghost town called Vancouver and finally found the Back Alley. I was dressed for trouble with a capital T, and choked at first sight of this...sports bar in a mall? Yeesh! Too much light and not enough atmosphere, but the wait staff was turned out to be fabulous. Our waitress, Terri, was a cute little nymphet that catered to our every whim. Well, almost. I kept some whims to myself. The four-piece band was smokin' and heating the joint up with their tight and original rock and roll. It was just what we needed, of course that along with several Sapphire martinis.

During their break we went up and chatted and I gave them my card. I was pleasantly surprised when during their next set they dedicated a song to me! The song, appropriately called "So Bad" was a naughty little bluesy tune that would have rocked my panties off, if I had been wearing any.

With too many cocktails in our blood and never too much lust in our loins, my YYB and I went out to the parking lot where the lighting was better. We gave the back of my truck a whole new purpose. Two young girls screamed in disbelief, which only made it more deliciously tawdry. Then, off we drove, back to Portland just in time to see the sun come up.

Mz. Conduct's House of Sin

"Your dreams happen when you wake up."
–Anonymous

The bitch is back! My fiftieth birthday seemed to unravel a stream of airborne events that picked me up, carried me as high as the largest pines, and then sent me corkscrewing, head over heels, ass backwards into this wedded bliss. Yes, that's right, Mz. Conduct is married! Here is the story of how Mr. Conduct came to be.

Initially, as many friends have pointed out, I didn't even want a boyfriend, simply a decent man/boy to bang me like a cheap screen door several times a week and get the hell out. After hanging with Romeo in Black Jeans, whom stimulated my mind but didn't share my overactive libido (and like most all of my exes, has remained a dear and true friend), I felt I needed more. The next candidate came along and although cutting the mustard in the sack, left me still with a void in the intellectual department. He broke up with me after I revealed that I had a romp with the Yum Yum boy (oh well!), but then forgivingly asked me back a few days later. I relented, as this was all there was for the moment and he was very sexually talented (always a difficult thing to dismiss for me.) But then a man I met years ago, and wasn't ready to take on at the time, for some of the reasons men may try to entangle you, i.e. being the philanderers that they can be. However, in the meantime, this man was honest with me, respected me for seeing through so much crap and not taking it. He shared his relationship battles and bulges, as people do so easily with me, knowing full well that I would not be party...except as the Mz. Conduct advisor guru. We kept a distant contact always. A year flew by, with polite, inquisitive emails from him, and once again an offer to swill cocktails together, I finally agreed. I stood him up. Not intentionally, but for the simple reason that I was all over the map at that point, (as with many points in my life), and in the back of my mind there was always an unready, strange intensity I felt with/in him. Couldn't quite figure it out, but I didn't try too hard either.

Another year of his same remote inquiries came and went. Then soon after my "Ohmagawd, I'm half a century young!" birthday, he once again offered a night out, a celebration no less. Christ in a corset, I decided I would finally get it over with, maybe figure out what the baffling connection was, or maybe not. It was a warm, dizzy, half moon night and my boytoy at the time was working out of town, so why not?

When I flounced in to meet him, at the apropos Starry Sky Club, I was dressed in a black, short, babydoll dress, my prick-me-pink ruffled bloomers and red cowgirl boots. I was, as always, doused in my orange cinnamon oil, and fashionably late no less. I saw him sitting in a booth, bespectacled...writing, and my heart did a little black flip. Covering nicely—as I rarely ever get swept away by such boyish charm—I sat down and ordered a vodka and lime. Brat that I am, immediately informed the wait person that I wouldn't be paying for anything, it was all on him. That's the moment when he knew he wanted to spend the rest of his life with me, he says. Well, of course!

Later, after five hours of sordid storytelling, and gazing into each other's same sea green eyes, I told him it was time for me to go. He walked me to my car, looked at me under the fluorescent moon and told me I was trouble. Okay, so you don't have to be a Rhodes Scholar to see that, but it was the universal whisper that let me know that he was trouble too. That, and the way he grabbed me by my pigtails, yanked them hard (oh baby!), and slammed me into the side of my car, kissing me like a nomad finding an oasis. He drank me in. I let him, as I allowed myself to swallow his energy too. Twenty minutes later, I forced myself to drive home. Alone. All the while feeling like a hurricane just hit my heart. I knew then that I had been his all along.

The next morning, waking up in our own beds, we realized the mutual mesh of emotion which had taken us both over. There it was, refusing to be ignored, insisting on forever.

So, after making our lives more available for one another, we met again. We drank Veuve Clicquot, shared our souls and a zillion parallels, we dove head on into unknown yet somehow familiar waters. We haven't surfaced yet.

Mz. Conduct's House of Sin

Don't get me wrong, the ups and downs have reared their ugly heads, but we are two peas in a precious pod, and we both know we can't change what we can't change, that all of our vicious past shenanigans have made us exactly who we are. Neither of us would change that. We have what is necessary: Respect, honesty, total acceptance, trust, security, communication, laughter, creativity and support, uninhibited play, experimentally open...and finally a man who can keep up with my insatiable self! Or in any case, he may die trying, we'll see. As he puts it, "Sweetheart, you fuck like a banshee on PCP." Uh...ya think?

A month later he proposed to me, under the next half moon. We are halves of each other and the half moon seemed to hold that meaning too. I moved in to his house, which by the way was a brothel in the 1800's. You can imagine how tickled I was at that fact! I then ripped out thirty feet of overzealous blackberry bushes and planted a now flourishing garden, sprouting flowers in all the colors of the rainbow, orange mint, green beans, herbs and passion vines. Next project, he and I planted a thick, green backyard lawn, where not only did we continuously canoodle on, but several months later were married legally in the same consecrated spot. Mr. Conduct in his tailored black suit, skinny vintage tie and I, in a made-for-me short, blood red, cabaret dress, both of us barefoot, we said our "I do's" in the sandalwood air, cool champagne baths mixed with the heat of the evening, and under yet another half moon. I am told daily, by the groom, that I am not a handful, but two handfuls, and thus, the love of my life, the crazy, creator monkey, the sexiest beast and beast master, Mr. Conduct was born!

We had a houseful of loved ones, family, and several exes on both sides attending, as they all told us they knew, that from the moment they saw us together, we were already married in our hearts. The Transient Trollop arrived with the Rooftop Rebel (and a large dead salmon), Raphael came bearing a case of vineyard heaven, Mr. Bo Dangles and his lovely wife showed up, as did The Lion King and his angelic other. My son even flew out from law school! Homer K.

Good Advice from a Very Bad Girl

was there, Punk Girl and her Pretty Boy Toyd were joined at the groin as always, Romeo in Black Jeans came bravely stag, and oodles of other unwritten characters celebrated with us. Much appreciation to my adoring fans that sent well wishes and gifts...you are part of the reason I write!

The bash was fabulous, with only the minimal drunken escapades: Mr. Conduct's brother tossing his stomach contents all over the back of my truck, a friend of Mr. Conduct's nudging another guy, sleazily saying "wouldn't you have loved to bang her (pointing to me) at least once before she got hitched?" and the other guy turning to him and saying, "dude, that's my freakin' mom!" Embarrassing laughter ensued. And then there was yours truly introducing my new mother-in-law to someone as Mr. Conduct's wife. An uninvited guest unloaded her cocktail on my son's friend, I made out with two girls, and while insisting on changing a light bulb, fell off the porch and bruised up my ample keester. Other than that, and a small gardening accident which caused me to have a shredded forearm on my day of wedded bliss, things were absolutely perfect.

Mr. Conduct has formed a new band, with Punk Girl rockin' out the vocals, and her Pretty Boy Toyd on drums. I have an article, bio and picture in the September issue of Playgirl, so things are progressively creative around this old brothel. Mr. and Mz. Conduct are making the neighbors run to purchase ear plugs...in so many ways!

> Dear Mz. Conduct,
> I seem to have an ongoing problem or pattern, and I can't figure it out! I am an intelligent, pretty, 32 year old woman with a career (although I change gears sometimes), my own place and a loyal dog and cat. I have no problem meeting men and even having boyfriends—for a little while anyway. All these guys seem great and seem to like me, they tell me how cute I am, etc. until all of a sudden they either admit that they are still hung up on their exes or they aren't ready for a monogamous relationship. There is always something! This is driving me crazy and I don't know how to break this pattern! Please help me? I know you'll have an explanation.
> Loose 'Em Lucy
>> Dear L.E.L.,
>> All I can say is that you seem to need the approval of these boys you're meeting, which most likely bleeds through and is uber unattractive. Men like

Mz. Conduct's House of Sin

bitches. Now when I say that, it doesn't mean that you have to be a pissed-off, snappy, unkind woman, I simply suggest that you pull out your good bitch. Be full of confidence, don't give a hoot about approval (only your own), and be sure of what you want and how to get it—or at least know what you don't want. That's a start. Once you feel secure with that, and you venture out into the world of dating, you will put forth a different energy for others to pick up. I'll bet my double-headed dildo that you will attract different, more suitable men. You seem to let the men be in charge of where your life is going (relationship-wise), and my advice is to never, ever let that happen. Now, go summon up your inner bitch while I perfect mine.

Dear Mz. Conduct,

I am a guy who's interested in being with a couple (man and woman), and finally met some people online that I feel I click with. We were planning a meet when they sent an invite to 'felch.' I'm not sure what to tell them because I don't know what that is. I don't want to ask them and sound like a vanilla dork. Help?

Donny Dumbo

Dear D.D.

Okay, without passing judgment, that's disgusting! Yeah, okay, I've been a fluffer in a Bukkake* show, so whatever, but felching is licking cum out of another person's asshole, dude! Sometimes people cum swap while kissing after ass banging, and sometimes sick folks even use straws. Hey, to each his own, but it's sure not safe sex, so remember that, if nothing else.

*In feudal Japan, many moons ago, if a Japanese wife was unfaithful to her husband and this was discovered, she'd be tied to a post in the centre of the village and all the local men would masturbate over the woman. This was not the law, but sort of the unofficial, accepted punishment for infidelity. Sex play parties sometimes perform this under safe conditions.

Made in the USA
Charleston, SC
02 March 2013